THE QUALITY OF MERCY:
THE LIVES OF SIR JAMES
AND LADY CANTLIE

The Quality of Mercy:
The Lives of Sir James and Lady Cantlie

Jean Cantlie Stewart

London
GEORGE ALLEN & UNWIN
Boston   Sydney

**George Allen & Unwin (Publishers) Ltd,
40 Museum Street, London WC1A 1LU, UK**

George Allen & Unwin (Publishers) Ltd,
Park Lane, Hemel Hempstead, Herts HP2 4TE, UK

Allen & Unwin Inc.,
9 Winchester Terrace, Winchester, Mass. 01890, USA

George Allen & Unwin Australia Pty Ltd,
8 Napier Street, North Sydney, NSW 2060, Australia

First published in 1983

British Library Cataloguing in Publication Data

Stewart, Jean Cantlie
  The quality of mercy: the lives of Sir James and
Lady Cantlie.
1. Cantlie, *Sir* James   2. Cantlie, *Lady*
I. Title
616.9′88′30922   RC961
ISBN 0-04-920066-6

Typeset in 10 on 11 point Baskerville by
Inforum Ltd, Portsmouth
and printed in Great Britain by
Mackays of Chatham

Contents

List of Illustrations

Foreword

This is the story of an idea – the story of man's duty to his neighbour.

Now and again men and women are born who do not act for material gain, either for themselves or for their families, but are moved instead by some feeling of perspective or sense of destiny in their hearts which makes them act only for the well-being of their fellow men.

To these people mercy is not a dated word but a reality which brings them to the side of a man wounded in battle, or a victim knocked over by a passing vehicle, or a patient far from home in a hospital bed.

This idea, which is as old as the story of man himself, was expressed in the parable of the Good Samaritan. Finding a man set upon by thieves, he gave first-aid by pouring oil into the wound, provided transport by setting the man upon his beast, and ensured his welfare by putting his hand into his purse and paying for the sick man's keep.

This rendering of medical and first aid, nursing and welfare, fill the unfolding chapters of this book. These pages record the achievements and the endeavours of unselfish men and women who held fast to an idea until success was secured and then straightway pioneered fresh paths for the benefit of humanity, demanding further work and sacrifice. The lives of Sir James and Lady Cantlie are two among many in a period of great service to the nation and the world.

I would like to thank those kind subscribers, individuals and organisations, who have helped me with practical support, encouragement and information.

I would like also to thank all the librarians in the libraries in which I did the research for this book for their unfailing kindness and expertise – particularly I would make mention of those overseas, in Paris, Brussels and Hong Kong. I am most grateful to all the friends who helped in checking the manuscript. I would like to make grateful mention of my uncle, the late Lt General Sir Neil Cantlie, Director General Army Medical Services, who wrote *A History of the Army Medical Department* and gave me every encouragement and support in the idea of rewriting this biography which he originally wrote in 1939, since when much new material has become available. I wish that he had lived and been able to help me with it for his advice would have been invaluable.

Jean Cantlie Stewart
Cupar, Fife
23 May 1982

To my son and daughter-in-law

It was my son's skiing accident in the Cairngorms and the subsequent almost miraculous rescue arrangements which led indirectly to the writing of this book.

CHAPTER ONE

Early Days

It is a distinctive feature of the culture of the north east of Scotland that a man never forgets his clan or the place of his birth. In the last century so many young men travelled the world from these villages that it is fitting that any biography should have its origins firmly rooted in these beginnings. The days of Empire are now associated in the minds of many people with the amassing of fortunes and the 'thin red line'. It is no longer remembered that men and women of good will brought education, medicine and the benefits of Western science and civil-isation to the farthest corners of the earth, working ceaselessly and unselfishly to better the conditions of their fellow men.

James Cantlie, author, surgeon, one of the originators of first aid and of tropical medicine, and friend of Sun Yat Sen, first President of China, to whom the latter owed his life, was born at the farm of Keithmore, Dufftown, in the parish of Mortlach and county of Banffshire.

The parish of Mortlach lies in a hollow amid the hills – *morlag* in Gaelic means the great hollow. To the west the Spey flows through the pastures of Aberlour, to the east Deveron rises in the windswept heather of the Cabrach, to the south the massive, often snow-capped Cairngorm mountains form a barrier crossed only by an eighteenth-century military road linking rivers Dee and Don with the north. From Tomintoul the road twists northwards through Glenlivet, Ben Rinnes towering above, and leads into the village square of Dufftown, built by James Duff, Fourth Earl of Fife,[1] below which, down by the Dullan Water, stands the Church of Mortlach, founded in AD 556 by Mortlag of Bangor, friend of St Columba. Each entrance to the hollow is guarded by a feudal castle. High above a moat with the Fiddich burn tumbling beneath, the battlements of Auchindoun stand stark against a stormy sky, commanding the westward approach from the Cabrach and the southern pass from Glenlivet, trodden by the feet of pilgrims on their way to Mortlach. Across the bowl the cannon holes of ruined Balvenie, home of the Stewarts of Atholl, guard the road to Keith, and from its windows can be seen the castle of Kininvie which signalled the approach of enemies from the Spey. Keithmore, one of the two feudal manor houses of the parish, stands on a plateau looking up to the castle of Auchindoun and down to the village of Dufftown. Once protected on three sides by farm steadings and a wall, it bears the Duff coat of arms commemorating Adam Duff of Keithmore[2] who built it in 1688 with thick walls and small low windows to withstand cannon shot.

Hither in the nineteenth century came William Marshall, composer of Scottish violin music, factor to the Duke of Gordon and great uncle by marriage of James Cantlie. He added on a Georgian front and a walled garden behind.

James Cantlie was born in 1851 in the bedroom where Marshall composed many of his lovely airs. Perhaps he may have heard those melodies lingering in the house, for whenever he heard a Scottish tune James would hum or whistle or add his musical voice to it, while the same rhythm of the burns echoed through his own prose and poetry. 'Marshall,' wrote Cantlie,

> dwelt in Strathspey itself. The great part of his best known springs were composed at Keithmore in Banffshire. The neighbourhood he lived in was alive with the ripple of the burns, the murmur of the Fiddich and the sough of the Spey. It was their whisperings, their forte and piano sounds, that gave Marshall the key-note to his inspiration; for this music was but an echo of nature and sprang from the very essence of the environment in which he lived. I was born and brought up in the very house of Keithmore, home of the ancestors of the Earls of Fife, where Marshall wrote 'The Marquis of Huntly', 'Miss Forbes' Farewell', and 'A' the airts the Winds can Blaw', a host of reels and strathspeys which mak' us crack our thumbs, tak' the floor, be we auld or young, and hooch till we gar the rafters dirl and maist raise the roof.[3]

James was the eldest son of William Cantlie, who was born in 1810 at the farm of Clunymore. William, sixth child of James Cantlie and his wife, Helen MacInnes, for whom Marshall composed an air, married Janet Hay and moved in 1850 to Keithmore. He was a young man of energy, determination and ability. His laird, the Duke of Gordon, introduced him to the Prime Minister, Lord Derby, as the biggest Tory in Banffshire, referring to his massive size and independent principles. Like many north east Scots his regard for learning was undaunted by the poverty caused by his father's early death. There were insufficient funds, despite help from an uncle who was a Writer to the Signet in Edinburgh, to send him to the university when he became a prize winner at Mortlach School. These were the days when clever boys passed straight from the parish schools to university and the ratio of graduates to the population was one in six. Fifty years before General Wolfe had learnt mathematics from one of these parish schoolmasters when stationed near Inverness, and in 1827 Greek was available in all but two of the Aberdeenshire parish schools. This gave a command of style and grammar which Dr Johnson acknowledged in an otherwise critical account of Scottish life. William, determined to carry on with his education, started evening classes for the village lads at which he could instruct himself by instructing others and, with this start, he became assistant to a land valuer and auctioneer in Dufftown. There his experience in buying crops and cattle helped him to pioneer new farming methods and to found his own 'Eliza' strain of shorthorn cattle from a heifer picked out by his 10-year-old daughter. His training gave him also an understanding of money, and when a branch of the Aberdeen Town and County Bank opened in Dufftown, he became its manager. In those days London prices arrived only once a week for half a crown, but William lived to see the penny post and two mails a day, one of which brought *The Times* from London. With his powerful voice and ready wit he was sought after as a speaker at meetings and dinners and was invited to stand for parliament, an invitation which he declined to the disappointment of his friends, for he had a gift of humour and genial kindness which made him an excellent mediator between opposing groups.

It is this sense of humour and capacity for warmth and fun which gives the north east Scot the courage and bouyancy to face his struggle for existence amid upland rocky soil and severe winters. 'Only by permitting a sense of humour,' wrote Sir Arthur Keith, 'to play on the grim face of necessity, can life be made tolerable to a people oppressed, as we northern Scots are, by the seriousness of our earthly pilgrimage.'[4] One of James's first memories was of a storm with drifting so deep that the house could only be reached by a tunnel through the snow, snow that lay on the fields that year from Christmas till May. Keithmore means in Gaelic 'a big wind', and James's character was moulded by these early influences. During his childhood he listened many times to that eerie silence betokening wind muffled by the heaviest falls of snow which cut off farms and houses for weeks on end. He had battled against its icy blast on his way home from school to Keithmore when, breathless from the cold air and wet blanket of snow forming over his nose and mouth, he had learnt to fight off the hypnotic effect of the white emptiness of 'blind drift' which entices its victims, exhausted by plunging in snow to their thighs, to surrender themselves to its tempting embrace, to give up and lie down. Unconquerable will then alone ensures survival and thus steadiness, determination and drive are characteristic of this sturdy race. Remoteness as well as the dangers of these rigorous winters imposes upon people the necessity of learning another lesson, the need to keep together and share the little that there is. Further south there is warmth in the soil and the sun; in the north it is only in the hearts of men. This interdependence demands that other people must be helped and that they must not be placed in a position of inferiority. The courtesy of the clan insists that a man with a crust must share half with the man who comes knocking at the door. 'You're very welcome' removes the obligation in 'Thank you' and the maintenance of good relations is regarded as more important than money. 'What do I owe you?' is still met today with 'Ye're nae owin' me naething', or 'I'll see you again', or by underquoting and relying on the payer's generosity. All his life James followed this simple philosophy with a kindness springing from the heart. His patients of every nationality were all members of his clan and he liked to doctor them for nothing. Once, after a serious operation, the rich and foreign husband of a patient inquired about the fee; Cantlie suggested twenty-five guineas. The husband was furious. 'Do you think my wife's life is only worth twenty-five guineas? Here is a cheque for a hundred.' These severe winter conditions and the clear mountain air of summer taught Cantlie another lesson which he stressed all his life, that people, particularly young children, should wear warm protective clothing in winter and shade their heads against a strong sun. Frozen blood carried back to the heart brings collapse and death, and although the topee is now out of fashion, anyone who has suffered sunstroke knows the strength of the sun's rays, particularly in the East. Lastly, the distance from medical help in a remote mountain farm meant that a knowledge of first aid was essential to help both men and animals. The man who acts in an emergency must be trained to improvise and use the objects at hand. Afterwards, in demonstrations of first aid, Cantlie used the props he knew in his youth, a pitch fork stuck in the ground to make a tent out of a groundsheet, a piece of wood for a splint, ropes of straw for a field hospital bed.

The life of a parish revolves round its church and every Sunday, crossing the churchyard where Malcolm II defeated the Danes and, in thanksgiving, temporarily created Mortlach a Bishopric, the Cantlies entered the dark interior pregnant with history. Around them was woven the story of the parish, here the tomb of Alexander Duff and Helen Grant of Keithmore 'he being nearly and lawfully descended from the most noble Thanes of Fife', there a wall plaque with the name of Leslie of Kininvie, and on the roll of ministers that of Tough, now Touche, famous in financial circles throughout the world. In a dark corner of the church another plaque told the story of the lepers who in early times watched the service from outside through a lepers' squint, so great was the fear of their contamination. James carried the pain of this exclusion with him always, and during his later work in China it was the lepers of Hong Kong and the Canton colonies who were always closest to his heart. What the family could not then know was that the window facing them was later to commemorate Lord Mountstephen, brilliant son of the parish, whose generosity to medicine and first aid was renowned. When James was 12 his cousin, also James Cantlie, emigrated to Montreal where he married Eleanora, sister of Lord Mountstephen who, together with his Morayshire cousin Donald Smith (later Lord Strathcona), built the Canadian Pacific Railway and united an awakening continent from coast to coast. James Cantlie of Montreal won a reputation for himself for integrity in business, his word was his bond, and 'lovable, courteous and upright' his epitaph. Thus two James Cantlies founded families on either side of the Atlantic who have remained firm friends ever since in spite of the ocean which divided them.

Every weekday morning, his school bag on his back, James walked three miles to Botriphnie School in the village of Drummuir where the Minister, the Reverend Donald Stewart, was the schoolmaster. This was not uncommon in landward areas, for the connection between church and school went back before the first Education Act of 1496;[5] but the lairds' contribution to the parish schooling was imposed by John Knox, who made them provide the schoolmaster's house and half his salary, the remainder being paid by tenants in oatmeal. Standards varied between schools and parents keen on education chose those where they were highest. James was fortunate to be educated during the flowering of Scottish rural education, when the standard in north east Scotland was second to none owing to the munificence of the Dick Bequest which paid higher salaries to graduate schoolmasters who had taken a further qualifying examination. Since increases were paid on a sliding scale according to the lairds' contribution generous lairds, like the Gordon Duffs at Drummuir, attracted schoolmasters of the highest quality, who were held to be *ad vitam aut culpam*, and soon only a graduate could secure a position in the three north east counties. There were no frills in the school day, the older scholars helped the younger ones with their work; no fees were paid by poorer pupils, others paid according to the difficulty of the subject; the pupils brought peats for the school stove and the boys chopped the wood. In the winter, hours were from sunrise to sundown and in the summer from 7.00 a.m to 6.00 p.m; those, like James, who studied classics arrived an hour earlier. This habit of early rising and the love of teaching stayed with James all his life. It was a system of state education never again matched and before James left Botriphnie its excellence was marred by the Revised Code of 1861 which required that grants were only paid at pass standard regardless of the difficulty of the subject.

At 13 James went as a boarder to Milne's Institution at Fochabers, a small eighteenth-century town beside the Spey laid out around a green, tree-lined square and built by the Duke of Gordon to replace the old village of small thatched houses clustered round the castle walls. The church, with Grecian portico and pillars, and the Town House, with arched Georgian windows, gave the town an air of elegance, while on the other side of the road a door opened as if by magic to reveal the lake and castle beyond. This Duke was the husband of the romantic Lady Jane Maxwell, friend of Robert Burns, who raised the Gordon Highlanders with her kisses, introduced Scottish dancing to London and presented her son at court in full Highland dress. She must have blown one of her famous kisses down the corridors of time for the boy from Dufftown, who arrived raw and country bred, quickly absorbed the sophisticated spirit of this unusual town. James must have been one of the Duchess's most devoted recruits, for he later endured the banter of his fellows in Aberdeen University by attending classes in a kilt, bonnet and cloak. Starting as a Volunteer Surgeon in the London Scottish, the territorial regiment of the Gordon Highlanders, he raised the Volunteer Medical Staff Corps; he danced and held classes for reels and strathspeys wherever he went in the world; and no toast to the 'Immortal Memory of Robert Burns' was complete without his address in Doric.

Milne's Institution had been started by a young man with a mind of his own who was dismissed from the castle for refusing to cut his hair. Emigrating to America he made a fortune which he willed on his death to found a free school for the children of his home town of Fochabers and two orphanages in Louisiana. Nine years after James's arrival in

the school a Royal Commission commented upon its excellence, by
which time many boys paid fees and boarded during the week as James
had done with the headmaster, who in his day was Dr Robert Ogilvie, a
classical scholar and LLD of St Andrews and Aberdeen. Although
James became a prize-winner, as a younger boy he was more interested
in wild life and games. Indeed a zest for adventure nearly cost him his
life when, seeking birds' eggs for a competition, he was chased by
gamekeepers. Terrified of being caught he plunged, to his pursuers'
horror, into the Spey where it was wide and deep and after a struggle
against the current, and kept up by his kilt floating round him, he
reached the bank and afterwards sat all day in dripping clothes rather
than risk discovery. His broad shoulders, deep chest and strong arms
made him a forceful batsman and boxer, although his enthusiasm was
temporarily cooled when he stunned a fielder with a hard drive and
knocked an opponent unconscious with his only punch of the fight.
Cricket he returned to later with pleasure, but the fear that he had
killed his opponent and his dislike of inflicting injury on others caused
him never to box again. Free afternoons were spent following the Spey
to its mouth at Garmouth, where he lay watching the ships in the
harbour and, although his father restrained his enthusiasm to go to
sea, his love of boats and the lure of distant horizons remained with him
all his life.

At 15 James passed the Bursary examination and entered the University of Aberdeen in 1866, attending classes in the Faculty of Arts at
King's College. In appearance he was of medium height, with a fair
freckled complexion and lively blue eyes; in character he was open-
hearted and generous with a streak of impetuousness which led him
sometimes to decided but unorthodox opinions. He quickly made
friends among his fellow students, one of whom was Mitchell Bruce
from Donside, Aberdeenshire, with whom he set up lodgings in the
Spital Brae. Here in Old Aberdeen, where St Machar's Cathedral is
built on land round which the River Don curls like a shepherd's crook,
the students were surrounded by the architectural economy of line of
the seventeenth century, 'a granite city, symbolic as well as unique'.
Bruce and Cantlie were moderately well provided for, but there were
students who could not even afford candles and studied by the light of
street lamps. This tradition of poverty at Scottish universities goes back
to 1325, when the Bishop of Moray gave the first bursary to poor
students to attend the Scots College at the University of Paris. It
continued unchanged when universities were founded at St Andrews
and Aberdeen in 1451 and 1494, and 400 years later privations at the
four Scottish universities were still general and tragedies not uncommon. There were students who died of starvation because too
proud to ask their parents for more, when their sack of meal ran dry,
while others, having achieved early academic distinction, died young.
'Many of us', wrote the writer Robertson Nicol, born in Aberdeenshire
in the same year as Cantlie and a fellow student at Aberdeen, 'had our
constitutions permanently impaired by lack of good and adequate
food. Far too large a proportion of my fellow students died early.'[6]

Cantlie described how he knocked up his tutor in the small hours in order to study the classics and how his tutor's bed was then taken by a poor student without lodgings who thus snatched a few hours' sleep.

Vacations for Cantlie were spent at Keithmore, and journeys thither were undertaken by train, passing through Huntly and Keith. Cantlie wrote a description of one of these journeys, illustrating the reticence, good breeding and perhaps superstition which prevents north east Scots from asking direct questions:

Entering a carriage, I sat down, took off my bonnet and put on my smoking cap. I wore a Highland cloak and carried a parcel of books and a Blackwood magazine in my hand. In Huntly all left the carriage except the passenger opposite me, and as Huntly Station is roofed and it was too dark to read, I put down my magazine and said, 'It is a fine day' (the traditional north east greeting). He replied, 'Aye', and after a pause, 'You're not getting off here?', 'No,' I said. 'Ye'll be gaun as far as Rothiemay?' 'Yes.' 'Are ye stopping at Rothiemay?' 'No.' 'Maybe ye'll be stopping at Fife Keith?' 'No.' 'When ye leave Keith which line do ye tak? Do ye leave by Mulben hand or do ye haud on by the Craigellachie hand?' 'By Craigellachie, but I'm not going as far as Craigellachie. I'm stopping at Dufftown.' 'Do you belong to Dufftown?' 'No.' 'When ye come to the Square, which hand do ye tak?' 'I am going to the left.' 'Guid sake, I'm going down that road ma'sel,' 'I'm going to Keithmore.' 'Guid be here! Ye'll be Jeemes?' 'Aye, I'm Jeemes.' 'Well laddie, I never saw ye, but I gaed for the doctor to your mither the nicht ye were born. I was cattleman with your father for twa years.'[7]

Like all dutiful sons of the north east, time in vacation was spent working on the farm, but Cantlie's mind was now turning to medicine, and when not on the farm or fishing in the Fiddich burn or the Spey he roamed over the hills in search of rare plants, an interest in botany which returned to him in China when he learnt all he could of herbalist medicine. Back at University he now began combining arts and science and graduated MA with Honours in Natural Science in 1871. His medical studies in Aberdeen lasted, however, only one year, for in 1872 Mitchell Bruce, who had obtained a post on the staff of Charing Cross Hospital, asked Cantlie to join him in London for the summer session, sharing his lodgings in Gray's Inn Place and attending lectures at Charing Cross Medical School. It was not unusual for a young man to divide his studies in this manner; it had been done by Dr Benjamin Golding, founder of Charing Cross Hospital, who had started his studies in Edinburgh and ended them at St Thomas's Hospital. Bruce felt that Cantlie's ability required wider outlets than a medical practice in Banffshire offered and he feared that Cantlie's family would persuade him to stay near home. Cantlie took his friend's advice but, loyal to his *alma mater*, he decided upon the unusual plan of taking classes at Charing Cross Medical School and sitting the examinations in Aberdeen, undertaking the journeys by sea, when the salt wind blew away the stale smells of Holborn and Charing Cross. His London life changed him very little in manner, appearance or character. He did not alter his speech or mannerisms, or become aggressively nationalistic in outlook. He remained his high-spirited, natural self, working and playing hard, benefiting from new experiences, out-going, extrovert and unself-conscious.

In 1873 Cantlie graduated MBCM at Aberdeen University with Honourable Distinction and went to Keithmore to celebrate and discuss his future. He had by now taken a junior post as instructor in the Anatomy Department at Charing Cross, believing as always that the best way to learn is to teach, and having thus firmly set his foot on the ladder of success his parents were ready to give their blessing for his return to London. Again his own record of that journey gives a second-to-none description of life in the Highlands at that time:

> On boarding the train at Boat of Garten, I and another passenger were hustled in, bag and baggage, by the guard who seemed in a great hurry. Then away we went at such a fine pace that I couldn't sleep. In half an hour we stopped at a station and the guard called out, 'Onything to tak' on here the nicht, Geordie?' 'Na, na, I shifted them off wi' the last.' The whistle sounded sharply and away we went with much bustle and hurry. At the next station the process was repeated. I tried to lie down and sleep, but in vain. Presently something appeared to be wrong with the train, as after much bumping and clanging it stopped on the line. The carriage door was opened and the guard appeared standing on the line with his lamp held up to my face. 'Anything wrong, Guard?' I asked. 'Nae, there's naething wrong.' 'Is this a station?' 'Nae, it's nae exactly a station, but the engine-driver's sister is getting married doon by here and we're a' gaun doon. Would you like to come?' Of course I would like to come. I was not twenty-two years of age for nothing. My fellow passenger thereupon was awakened, and the engine-driver, the stoker, the guard, the brakesman, a Post Office official, and we two passengers, after banking the fires on the engine, made for a distant light showing from the windows of a house. At two o'clock in the morning we entered to the sound of the Reel o' Tulloch on the pipes. I danced thirteen reels on the mud floor until four o'clock, when the guard came round saying, 'We'll need to be going now, sir.'[8]

Arriving back at Gray's Inn Place, Cantlie was greeted by Bruce with the news that he had been appointed Demonstrator of Anatomy at Charing Cross and, as the two friends went off to celebrate at Romano's and the Alhambra, Cantlie must have felt that the world was at his feet. He turned to his companion:

> 'Bruce, what is that motto you have on your signet ring?' 'Why, Jimmie, that's our family crest, a setting sun with the word fuimus – we have been. The Bruces, you know, were once a great family.' 'Well, Bruce, that motto wouldn't suit me. I haven't got a crest but

I'm going to invent one now and it will be a rising sun with the word erimus, we shall be.'⁹

But the motto on which his life was really moulded was that of the Duff family on the wall of his home at Keithmore, *Virtute et opera*, 'By virtue and hard work'.

CHAPTER TWO

Charing Cross Hospital and the Start of First Aid

It is not only Londoners who fall in love with her charms. As Bruce and Cantlie walked home from the Hospital to their lodgings in the flagged passageway leading to the peaceful charm of Gray's Inn, they met the full tide of human existence which, said Dr Johnson, was at Charing Cross. After the silence of the hills and the provincial kindness of Aberdeen, the anonymity of London could have been overwhelming, but to Cantlie there were simply more people to become his 'ain folk'. One of their homeward routes lay along the Strand, where wealth jostled with squalid poverty. The street was crowded with dray horses, hansom cabs and costers' barrows. On the pavements were fashionable young men and women, street minstrels and sellers, and girls with fruit baskets on their heads. The mansion houses, whose gardens had once led down to the river, had now been replaced by the elegance of the Adelphi, product of the Adam brothers' genius. In 1873 the Strand was at the height of its fashionable life; during the day travellers poured into the new Charing Cross Station which had replaced Hungerford Market opposite the Hospital, and in the evenings in the restaurants, theatres and music halls the whole world feasted and laughed. These were the days of Henry Irving, of drama at the Lyceum, Shakespeare at Drury Lane, ballet at the Alhambra, Nellie Farren at the Gaiety, dinners at Romano's, Gatti's and Simpson's.

Charing Cross Hospital, with its Grecian pillars and portico, stood on the corner of an island site, a watershed between two worlds. If the friends followed the shorter route home to the north east, they passed through narrow streets where in the night vice and riotous living abounded until sleepers awoke to the cries of the fruit market in Covent Garden. Here and eastwards to Ludgate were the slums of London, prototype of Dickens's novels, where disease-carrying rats, made homeless by demolition, entered the restaurants in search of food. These were the results of too rapid a change from rural to town life bringing with it infant mortality, bad air, over-crowding and insanitary conditions. In the area of Covent Garden, once the home of the élite, and of Charing Cross, Disraeli's 'two nations' met as one. Cantlie identified himself with both; the one challenged his sense of vocation, the other his capacity for enjoyment. At the end of his working day he researched into the effects of lack of fresh air and exercise and the presence of vermin on a city population, warning that most Londoners would not survive in present conditions into the third generation, while at the same time he became an ardent concert- and theatre-goer, starting a students' dining club in the Strand.

The site of Charing Cross Hospital had been chosen in the midst of this flood of humanity by Dr Golding who in 1815 put up his plate on his house in Leicester Square and treated free all sick persons who could not afford fees. They came in thousands, and by the time the Hospital came to rest on its island site 36,000 patients had been treated. Meanwhile, with a committee of twelve, Dr Golding drew up a plan for the Hospital of vision, compassion, sound organisation and financial good sense. It was to promote 'not only the welfare of the poor but the improvement of the Healing Art and the Good of the Community at large'; young doctors were to give medical attention without fees to the sick and needy and in return would learn from seeing 'diseases in their multifarious forms and complications'. There was to be a School of Theoretical and Practical Instruction in Medicine and Surgery within the Hospital so that, as well as walking the wards with their masters, following the custom of learning then in practice, pupils would attend lectures given by 'every Professional Officer of the Establishment . . . upon the subjects . . . for which he [was] most qualified'. The School would be free for students of 'respectable but unfortunate families' who could not pay fees. Medical aid was to be available for everyone, including the families of soldiers and sailors and 'poor distressed foreigners'. Attention was to be given to the well-being of the patients; a careful diet would stimulate their appetite and clean bed linen restore their self respect.[1]

The plan was Christian and the Hospital a Christian community. On Sundays Bruce and Cantlie attended the Church of St Martin's, once literally 'in the fields' and now looking out on the swirling traffic of Trafalgar Square. The association between Church and Hospital was close. At Christmas, choir boys in red cassocks filed into the wards to sing carols and Cantlie, benign and bearded, played Father Christmas, a role he loved to fill all his life in many parts of the world. The Hospital chaplain conducted morning prayers in the wards and held a Sunday Service in the chapel. This was the inspiration for the courtesy which diffused the atmosphere of the Hospital. Serenity of mind was seen as a key to recovery and the spiritual needs of the patients were met and their anxieties comforted. Those who were cured were encouraged to give 'humble and hearty thanks to Almighty God', those very sick were helped to be 'patient under affliction', and those hopelessly ill were given spiritual strength and courage. This vision was in no way new. Dr Golding was inspired by the monastic foundation of St Thomas and had seen the example of one of its benefactors, Mr Guy, who thought so little of himself that he dined off newspaper as a table cloth and so much of his fellow men that he founded a hospital for them, Guy's Hospital. The inspiration for these hospitals – the candle in the window or the good neighbour going out to seek and succour suffering – is as old as the story of the Good Samaritan, which Cantlie always quoted as the finest example of first aid. But the idea of a school within a hospital which awarded degrees in medicine was in England quite new. Here the prototype was the Scottish university and infirmary at which Golding had been trained. Certainly in other London hospitals there were schools in which masters took pupils and trained them in the day-to-day tasks of medicine, but the only examinations they could take were those of the Society of Apothecaries and the Royal College of Surgeons. Oxford and Cambridge universities awarded medical degrees but gave no practical training, so that their graduates attended hospitals on the Continent or in London. The idea of the Medical School of Charing Cross was to integrate for the first time teaching, research and practical medical care under a dean and in 1839 its certificates were recognised as degrees by the new University of London. Its birth was timely, for London was now the centre of an Empire and great demands were made upon her and upon the medical profession as responsibilities grew for the health and welfare of Her Majesty's subjects overseas.

By the 1870s and 1880s it would be difficult to have found a hospital with a greater spirit among its doctors and students than Charing Cross. Its position alone gave it a feeling of vitality, for it rubbed shoulders with the busy world which roared at its doors and drew life from the stimulus of its surroundings. Its popularity showed in the rapid increase of student numbers during Cantlie's period as instructor. The brilliance and originality of former pupils such as David Livingstone and Thomas Huxley set a standard for young men to achieve. Dr William Hunter in his historical account of the Hospital wrote that 'the period 1872–1877 was one of the most formative in the history of the school, and with the important developments of the time must be connected the names of Dr Greer, Dr Silver, Dr Mitchell Bruce and Mr James Cantlie'. An anonymous poem in the *Charing Cross Gazette* which runs:

> Though young we are we still can show
> A list of men whom nations know.[2]

carries all names but Cantlie's – for why? He wrote it.

Appointed Demonstrator of Anatomy and later House Physician, House Surgeon and Surgical Registrar successively, Cantlie by this time had built up a reputation not only as a teacher and doctor, but as one who threw himself into all the activities of the Hospital. Both patients and students loved him, the students for his energy, versatility and sense of fun; the patients for his great kindliness, ability and the gift of communicating, as if by electric current, his vitality and the will to live. Whenever he came into the ward, the sun came out from behind the clouds. He combined an unusual degree of responsibility towards others with a capacity to enjoy life to the full. He had a power of amusing persons of all ages; he was a friend to turn to when anyone wanted cheering with story or song, mostly rendered in native Doric with fitting gestures, for he was a born actor; but when people saw that below his good nature there lay a deeper sense of purpose, a dedication of self to the service of his fellows, then to their liking was added a greater regard. It was his sympathy and compassion for human suffering, combined with his buoyant cheerfulness and humour which made him a favourite after-dinner speaker; and it was the dedication of all his abilities to the love of his vocation that made him a great doctor.

Aspiring surgeons usually spent some time learning dissection by teaching anatomy, but it soon became clear that Cantlie had an unusual gift of imparting knowledge, so that to his crowded classroom came candidates for the Army and Navy examinations, students for Primary Fellowships, chronic failures from other hospitals, and women pioneers of medicine. Turning down an offer to become Demonstrator of Anatomy at the newly formed School of Medicine for Women, Cantlie agreed instead to coach them at weekends for the University of London examination. Immediately a girl pupil won a scholarship and first prize in anatomy. The examiners were amazed until told that Cantlie was her teacher, whereupon they shrugged it off as commonplace with the comment, 'Oh that accounts for it'. The secret of his success lay in his love of passing on knowledge and his enthusiasm for his subject which swept his pupils along like a river in spate. Added to this he had a gift of using imagery, colour and visual aids, perhaps partly inspired by the matchless seventeenth-century engravings and the museum at Charing Cross. But what made him famous as a teacher was his flair for drawing comparisons from everyday life, so that his pupils said of him that he 'humanised anatomy and made the dry bones live';[3] the amusing stories he told which made the facts stick fast in the pupil's memory and, above all, the way he instilled in his students his own sense of purpose and dedication, so that the great pains he took with their instruction became their conscience and their spur. One dark night, remembering a topic not covered in his lectures which might come up in examination, he took a hansom cab to Camden Town to see one of his students, a young man whose knowledge of anatomy was not the best and who was sitting the Navy Medical entrance next day. The landlady told him his pupil was out. Cantlie, however, was forearmed. Producing an upper jaw bone from his pocket – in after life he once took his ward Marjorie Usher in a taxi to a first aid lecture with a skeleton to be used in demonstration sitting between them – he opened *Gray's Anatomy* at the correct page, laid the bone on it and scribbled the words, 'You will read these pages on your arrival home tonight, as soon as you get up in the morning and a third time after breakfast'. James Porter followed his advice, passed into the navy and became Director-General of the Naval Medical Service. It is not difficult to understand the popularity of a teacher who takes such pains with the instruction of his pupils.

As well as learning dissection candidates for the Surgeon's examination also spent time in the Casualty Department, gaining experience of fractures and bleeding and benefiting from the shift system of staffing which left time for study. Dr Golding had sited his hospital at Charing Cross because he wanted it to become 'one of the great casualty hospitals of London'. He replied to those who argued that the area was too congested, that it was this congestion that produced the large number of accidents which his hospital would treat, and that the movement of these patients to remoter London hospitals caused unnecessary suffering. Here in the large, square, white-tiled Casualty Department Cantlie developed his interest in first aid, for to the Hospital came victims of every sort of emergency and accident, those collapsed by drunkenness and starvation, women in childbirth, road victims, theatre casualties and accidents in factories, on the railways or in the homes. At this time Cantlie nearly lost his own life by contracting septicaemia in the dissecting room immediately after an attack of typhoid. He was left with a permanently weakened right shoulder, site of two abscesses, but, as always, optimistic, he continued with his studies and afterwards said of it that he handled a gun better than before. Two years later in 1875 he became a Fellow of the Royal College of Surgeons. He had an ideal temperament for the task, confidence, calmness, optimism, imperturbability and infinite patience. His shoulder did not trouble him and the impulsive side of his nature, unwanted in the operating theatre, simply dropped from him like a discarded garment.

After five years at Charing Cross Cantlie sought and gained the post of Assistant Surgeon, not without opposition, however, since he was the first Charing Cross man to apply for an honorary post. Mitchell Bruce pointed out to the Dean that 'the very existence of our place depends on our bravely supporting the first Charing Cross man who has come forward for an Honorary post'. 'Charing Cross,' Bruce continued in his diary, 'would otherwise have been rent in twain.' The appointment turned out as anticipated; the following year, spurred on by Cantlie's teaching and example, every Charing Cross man passed the examination of the College of Surgeons. Because consultants and housemen in hospitals are constantly on call, hospitals tend to be 'in' societies where it is important to negative internal disagreements and generate a loyal spirit of good will. The constitution of Charing Cross thus provided for annual dinners to foster the spirit which the doctors were working to develop in the Medical School, and at Cantlie's suggestion the students gave dinners in return, inviting him to take the chair and on special occasions asking the Household Cavalry Band to provide the music. Societies abounded in the Hospital, literary, musical, dramatic and sporting. If a society was in existence Cantlie joined it, if it was not he started it, becoming its chairman or secretary. Usually in the chair for concerts, in 1883 he initiated 'Smokers', amateur music halls, where he acted as compère and performer, either acting or singing. The Hospital had acquired the Polygraphic Hall in 1869 and let it as a theatre which it looked upon as its own. With this dramatic background Bruce and Cantlie started Punch and Judy shows for the children who, some on crutches and many bandaged, forgot their suffering in their delight. The student Christmas amateur theatricals and pantomimes were given good press reports: 'The Cobbler Crepin was most amusingly and cleverly portrayed by Cantlie who entered thoroughly into his task and played in a hearty genial fashion with an amount of humour that would have told well on any stage and an entire absence of self-consciousness.' The Students' Club Matinee was soon presenting performances at Toole's Theatre with Cantlie as the bluff old Admiral who 'looked the part well and fully realised the spirit of the character' and the press, as well as commenting on the production, always alluded to the enthusiastic applause with which Cantlie's appearances were greeted. It was a popularity which lasted all his life and enabled him to raise much enthusiasm for public service.

With prodigious energy he still found time to contribute articles to the *Charing Cross Gazette* and medical journals, to write chapters for medical books and to translate foreign research. Charing Cross encouraged international research by teaching its young doctors foreign languages, so that Cantlie, who had studied German in Aberdeen, attended lectures and clinics in Germany with Bruce during the vacation, and later contributed an addendum on yellow fever to Scheube's *Disease's of Warm Countries*. Trained nurses had arrived in the Hospital in 1866 and Queen Victoria, carrying on the close interest which the Royal Family had taken in the Hospital, had bestowed on them the honour of wearing the Guards' Ribbon. Cantlie described in a *Gazette* article how much responsibility a nurse lifted from the doctor, and how much help she gave in observation and diagnosis, as well as bringing comfort to the patient. 'She relies more upon symptoms as her guide [which, as he pointed out, are often the first to show], whilst the modern Physician trusts more and more, as investigative methods are extended, to signs.' He described how this same Nurse M. taught him to appreciate the use of alcohol in illness. Realising a patient was dying she went out and bought a small bottle of brandy which she gave to the patient who recovered.

In his writings Cantlie combined this gift for minute observation with dramatic clarity and simplified without losing detail. Never taking anything for granted he always asked the question 'why?'. 'Why is the mechanical less wonderful than any other explanation?' Thus he explained how the movement of the diaphragm aided the stomach's action, how a full stomach and duodenum pressed upon and emptied the gall bladder, how the stronger current of the arteries aided the weaker flow of the veins which run beside them, how nerves which require to be stretched lie coiled in a spring, how the left-hand side of the body is heavier than the right because of the weight of food in the intestine. This latter, he claimed, was the reason why the left foot was chosen to beat time to music. He made his points by over-statement and poured them out with profusion that defied criticism, saying, 'I have determined to set mine forth, criticise them as you may'. He wrote as he spoke, like most north-east Scots, in short, simple, classical sentences, with images and examples from everyday life, employing the question and answer technique used in his teaching:

The nerves are like telegraph wires, laid on between station and

station; the originating battery, the brain, sends an impulse along the
wires, the nerves, to work a machine at the other end, the muscle. We
have absolute command of the one set (voluntary muscles), but not of
the other (involuntary muscles); we can lay down our pens when we
like, but we cannot stop our heart's beat; we can push away the
tempting fluid, but cannot prevent its absorption or stay its digestion
when once swallowed.[4]

He splashed all his words with colour; to show the way the muscles run
through the body he turned to a cut of butcher's meat, illustrating
the different fibres in yellow, white and red. The individuality of
his style was its urgent pace, which never sacrificed balance or
meaning.

It is difficult to believe that chance alone should have caused this
man to be asked to write and edit from an unfinished manuscript the
first book on civilian first aid in the world, a book which was to run into
hundreds of thousands of copies; or that an apparently chance en-
counter should have led him later to be described as the 'finest teacher
in Europe' of first aid. In August 1878 Surgeon Major Peter Shepherd, a graduate of Aberdeen, called at Bruce's lodgings on his way to
the Zulu War and gave him an unfinished manuscript called 'First Aid
to the Injured', commissioned by the St John Ambulance Association.
He asked Bruce to see that it was finished if he never returned, for he
was leaving for South Africa within the hour. After he had gone
Cantlie asked Bruce, 'What's first aid?' 'I don't know,' replied Bruce,
'but let me read the papers and I'll tell you.' After doing so he threw
them into Cantlie's lap saying 'Here, Jimmie, you take them; this is
more in your line than mine'. Shepherd was killed at the massacre of
Isandlwana, before the victory of Rorke's Drift as he gallantly dis-
mounted to give aid to a wounded man. All he had finished of his work
was a two-page cardboard leaflet which he distributed on board his
ship to South Africa.

The St John Ambulance Association had been created the previous
year by the Order of St John of Jerusalem, whose work for the faith and
service of mankind went back to the Crusades, 'promoting and encouraging all that makes for moral and spiritual strengthening of
mankind and all works of humanity and charity for the relief of
persons in sickness, distress, suffering and danger without distinction
of race, class or creed'. The Roman Catholic Order had brought its
mission to England in the twelfth century when St John's Gate was
granted to it in Clerkenwell. Dissolved by Henry VIII, the English
Order was revived under the Protestant faith in 1831, reacquiring St
John's Gate in 1874. Like the Catholic Order, which had moved from
Malta to Rome during the Napoleonic War, it devoted itself to Christian faith and charity, caring for the sick and wounded in war and
nursing and providing diets for the sick poor in time of peace. It had
approached the London hospitals in 1872 asking for doctors to train its
nurses, but with the exception of Dr Pollock of Charing Cross and Dr
Sieveking of St Mary's, the medical profession 'was not friendly to-

wards its objects', fearful lest this type of voluntary work should dilute professional standards.

These two men were sympathetic because, for one thing, two years earlier, they had become founder members of the National Aid Society for the Sick and Wounded in War (later the British Red Cross Society). This had been formed in 1870 during the Franco-Prussian War by a group of men in London, prominent among whom was Colonel Lloyd Lindsay (later Lord Wantage) and Mr John Furley (later Sir John Furley) in response to a call from Henri Dunant. Dunant, a Swiss businessman travelling in Italy in 1859, found himself by chance on the battlefield of Solferino where he did everything he could to bring relief to the wounded, earning the title of 'the man in the white suit'. Deeply moved by the suffering of the wounded he returned to Switzerland and formed the Red Cross with its emblem of the Swiss flag reversed, drawing up the first Geneva Convention of 1864 to bring aid to the sick and suffering in war. Although the National Aid Society sent teams of doctors, nurses and medical supplies to both sides in the Franco-Prussian War and was ready to do the same in any further emergency, it did not see for itself a training role, so that ambulance men such as Furley and Dr (later Surgeon General Sir Thomas) Longmore, who had been identified with both movements, turned to St John now to fill the need. Hence their approach to Sieveking and Pollock. The question, however, remained unanswered. Whence would come the instructors?

An outbreak of typhoid in 1873 in the colliery town of Coalville in Leicestershire brought matters to a head. The Order sent nurses and was brought into contact with the dangers faced by men and women in the pits. Accidents occurred in confined spaces on steep gradients, poisonous dust was endemic, explosions a constant threat; medical aid could not be fetched quickly nor be asked to travel long distances underground. Thus was the need for civilian first aid both recognised and born. The order first provided two-wheeled litters similar to those of the Prussian Knights of St John and then set up an Ambulance Department to train volunteers in first aid. But still the question remained unanswered, who would provide the instructors? This time the Order turned to the Army Medical Department which, concerned at its own lack of trained medical personnel among the Volunteers, saw the opportunity to teach first aid as a way of getting more trained medical recruits. In 1877, therefore, it sent Surgeon Major Francis Duncan as Supervisor of the St John Ambulance Department (now called the Association) and Peter Shepherd and Francis Falwasser as instructors. They 'greatly contributed to the success of the movement', and twelve centres were formed in six months, others following in Derbyshire and the Midlands. Shepherd, who instructed in the docks at Woolwich and on 13 August 1978 the police at Scotland Yard, was commissioned to write a manual, while Falwasser, who instructed at Chelsea, prepared a syllabus.

What St John Ambulance Association really wanted was to see civilian doctors instructing civilians, while at the same time the Army

Medical Department realised that unless the resistance of the medical profession to voluntary ambulance work could be broken the Volunteers would never get the trained medical personnel they needed. Whether the act of the Army Medical Department in sending these army doctors overseas was one of folly or wisdom must remain a matter for conjecture. But the obvious choice in looking for a successor to Shepherd was to approach Pollock of Charing Cross or Sieveking of St Mary's. Shepherd chose to approach Charing Cross, and thus if it was chance that brought him that day to Bruce's flat it was an extraordinary act of fate, for Cantlie's gifts equipped him to meet the challenge of the manual and the lectures. He stepped into Shepherd's shoes, delivered the lectures and finished the manuscript which he presented under the subtitle, 'For Use of the Metropolitan Police and other ambulance classes now being organised by the Order of St. John in all parts of England'. In four years over 50,000 copies were sold and it had been translated into all the leading languages. With characteristic unselfishness Cantlie referred to Bruce and himself as 'the kind and able coadjutors' in the Introduction and left the matter there, until years later Bruce revealed the extent of Cantlie's authorship (as Corbet Fletcher recounts in the second edition of his book, *The Annals of the Ambulance Department*).

The greatest need was for the instruction of the police, since they were responsible for tending and transporting to hospital victims of street accidents. 'Scarcely a day passes,' said a Middlesex coroner Dr Hardwicke, in February 1878, 'in which I am not called upon to witness the clumsy and atrocious way in which the sick and wounded are attended in the streets of London. The ignorance displayed by the police ought to be removed forthwith!' Cantlie found the Metropolitan Police at Scotland Yard his most enthusiastic and energetic recruits. By the end of 1878 300 had been trained and their relationship with St John was so close that the Assistant Commisioner instructed them that 'when aid is offered in rendering assistance to persons injured from a certificated pupil of St John's the offer is to be accepted'. A year later they transported to hospital a total of 4,000 casualties and a Supplementary Report of St John on 4 February 1879 spoke of the 'gentleness and knowledge of the trained constables'. Meanwhile the movement was becoming nationwide. Meetings at the Guildhall were attended by Militia Volunteers and police chief constables who linked up with centres formed in the colliery towns. Cantlie travelled the south of England lecturing at Woolwich and the Soldiers' Institute at Portsmouth, to the navy who had started classes at the Admiralty, to the Birkbeck Institute, part of London University, and to other centres in London and Sussex. He also joined Dr Manders of St Mary's who was teaching railway employees at Paddington: 'At some stations,' commented the press, 'it has been no unusual circumstance for classes to be instructed or even examined in the intervals between the arrival and departure of trains.' Meanwhile requests came from women for training in accidents in the home, and Cantlie gave them instruction at Lavender Hill, Milton Mount College and the Working Women's

College. At last the trickle of instructors was becoming a flow. In 1879 Sieveking of St Mary's was promised support by seven London hospitals and the Army Medical Department appointed as an instructor Dr Hunter (later General Sir Guyer Hunter), who was to play a considerable part in the raising of the Volunteer Medical Staff Corps.

A training centre for the Metropolitan Police, with Cantlie as instructor, was set up in Hyde Park and, under his supervision and demonstrating his methods and improvisation, the police provided one of the teams for the first public open-air demonstration of first aid and ambulance held in Hyde Park under the auspices of St John. This display was part of a Medical Congress and Sanitary Exhibition held in London in 1881. Cantlie was a member of the Committee and suggested giving an ambulance demonstration at South Kensington. The idea was turned down, but when attendance flagged he was called at the last minute to provide such a demonstration by Sir John Elkington. He plastered Piccadilly and Regent Street with boards and on the day 5,000 people attended. A patient simulating a broken leg was treated by the police, who applied truncheons to each side of the broken limb using their badges to secure the truncheons to the knee and ankle and their belts to tie the two limbs together. Other teams were provided by St John and the Militia Volunteers. A doctor who had been watching came up afterwards and asked Cantlie in a German accent, 'What are those pieces of wood?' Cantlie explained that the splints were policemen's truncheons. 'Ach,' said the German, 'I see. I am Dr Esmarch. I have taught the world military ambulance, now I know how to teach civil ambulance.' Dr Esmarch, one of the best known continental medical men and Professor of Surgery at Kiel, assembled classes on his return to the university to teach this new branch of medicine. A Russian and a Spaniard, also spectators, went home and started the teaching of first aid in their countries. Thus this first display had wide and international results.

Cantlie summed up the purpose of instruction in first aid in a chapter in The Health Exhibition Literature of 1884. It is

To tell the bystander in simple language what to do to stop the flow of blood, to prevent a broken bone doing more damage, to restore a person from a faint, and to render such assistance as will allay suffering and prevent more serious complications until such time as the doctor arrives . . . If it is objected that a little knowledge is a dangerous thing, if to tell a mother how to save her child's life be teaching her doctoring, then the sooner she is taught the better. Again it is not a little knowledge that is to be told you; it is complete of its kind, and there is nothing beyond it that is necessary for you to know upon the subjects dealt with.[5]

Instruction had to be built upon the maxim that it was just as important to know what not to do as to know what to do. Cantlie pointed out that people who knew how to act in an accident would be more likely to avoid them – the start, in fact, of preventive medicine:

To prevent accidents occurring in our streets, factories and mines would be to teach people to take care and caution while crossing a street; to warn the worker that the sharp saw which revolves as he pleases may one day be his death; and to teach the miner to keep his safety lamp shut. In the house and home also the most simple things may become the instruments of death.[6]

Royalty gave the movement their support. Princess Christian became President of a Ladies' Group in Windsor and Prince Albert attended classes at the Polytechnic. Members of Parliament also took a personal interest. Dr R. Farquharson, MP for West Aberdeenshire, speaking of the two-wheeled Furley litters said, 'If you were to take one of these carriages to Charing Cross the eloquence of those interested in the Association and the support of the medical profession should enable us to popularise it'[7], while Colonel Duncan, MP, watching Cantlie instructing at the Working Women's College, referred to him as the 'originator of the system of rendering first aid to the injured'. St John's Annual Report of 1887 spoke of Cantlie's 'invaluable services to the Metropolitan Centre', commenting upon the untiring energy and devotion exhibited by the members of the medical profession: 'the large-hearted enthusiasm with which they are ever ready, at any personal sacrifice, to benefit a cause, the guiding principle of which is identical with that which inspires their own humane and noble calling ... The work is political in its highest sense, the function of helpful, loving and unselfish citizenship.'

CHAPTER THREE

The Volunteer Medical Staff Corps

Cantlie's work for St John had brought him into contact with the Army Medical Department and he now for the first time turned his attention to first aid on the field of battle. In 1882 he joined the London Scottish Volunteers as Assistant Surgeon. With the uncertainties created by the Turkish–Serbian war of 1876, the War Office was becoming increasingly concerned about the lack of trained volunteer medical personnel. There was no separate ambulance corps in the Volunteer Army as there was an Army Medical Department for the Regulars. Instead, each regiment had its own surgeons and stretcher bearers so that at reviews and march-outs, when a separate ambulance corps had to be formed, these men left their regiments and formed a temporary corps of Volunteer Medical Officers and stretcher bearers. Some surgeons, like Cantlie, were dressed in the kilt, others in the gay trappings of the Lancer or the ponderous uniform of the Life Guardsman. The stretcher bearers also were in a motley collection of uniforms, here a red coat or grey uniform, there a spiked helmet or Scots cap, the kilt, or the broad red stripe of an artillery man. This arrangement meant that every man with a stretcher was a bayonet less in his battalion, and when sixteen men were attached to a bearer company from one battalion, the colonel had reason to grumble. Moreover, men from one regiment objected to being commanded by a medical officer from another, and regiments with only one surgeon, who saw him drafted away, were left without a medical man at all. 'All these anomalies had to come to an end, but it could only be by the formation of a properly organised bearer company, and that meant agitation, legislation, the creation of a new department and a special vote by Parliament of the necessary supplies.'[1]

That they came to an end when they did and were replaced by one Volunteer Medical Staff Corps was due to the conception of the idea in Cantlie's mind, born of a turn of fate which took him to the Guildhall one snowy night in 1883. Mr Andrew Maclure, a London Scottish Lieutenant, whose stretcher bearers had formed the ambulance at the Windsor Review of 1881, had not only undertaken to train the volunteer stretcher bearers, but also saw the importance of placing the responsibility for their training and organisation upon the Volunteer Surgeons. In March 1883 he asked Cantlie to deliver first aid lectures to a Volunteer ambulance class and to witness the subsequent stretcher drill. 'The origins of many a great enterprise are all too apt to become snowed under in the flakes of official memoranda, and were it not for Cantlie's record it is probable that Maclure's contribution would have suffered a similar fate.'[2]

'Maclure held a meeting of Volunteer Surgeons in the City,' wrote Cantlie in an account in the *Charing Cross Gazette*,

> with Surgeon General Sir William Longmore, Army Medical Department, in the chair and seventeen Volunteer Medical Officers present. Mr. Maclure stated the objects he had in view and how they were to be accomplished; and throwing the onus of organisation and development on the Volunteer Surgeons waited for their reply. He had not long to wait, for first one and then another got up and asked what business Mr. Maclure had to teach them their profession. Who was he? Was he a surgeon? What right had he to call them here today to lecture them as to their duty? It would have been pardonable had they been conversant with drill and ambulance organisation, but when interrogated by Mr. Maclure on how to render first aid to the injured, the display of ignorance was such that it called Sir William Longmore to his feet to say that he was, for the first time in his life, ashamed of his professional brethren. Longmore was a man from whom a rebuff of this kind ought to have had effect. He had devised all the exisiting organisation in the Army Medical Department at that day. Out of the chaos of the Crimea, he developed the perfection of the medical services in the later Egyptian Expeditions. There were two or three Surgeons present who left the meeting determined to mend matters.

One was Surgeon Platt, later a surgeon in the VMSC, who had taken a lead in all Volunteer ambulance matters and whose bearers at the Brighton Review of 1881 had first attracted Cantlie's attention. Platt now threw in his lot with Maclure, and Maclure's Volunteer Ambulance Department began to take a place in the hearts of the Volunteers. Maclure was given an office at Whitehall and issued his orders from the War Office. According to Cantlie this resulted in a fair number of London battalions possessing trained stretcher bearers, but the stumbling block remained the attitude of the Volunteer Surgeons, most of whom did not know how to organise stretcher bearers or ambulance drill. Without their co-operation no ambulance corps could be brought into being. If historically the VMSC represents a movement of national and military importance, on the human side it shows how much can be accomplished through the vision of a man imbued with the will to do, and the soul to dare in the face of long odds.

'While I was instructing,' wrote Cantlie of that night in 1883,

> and watching stretcher drill I was struck with the usefulness such instruction would be to medical men. The Medical Curriculum gave us no such knowledge, the lifting of patients, the carriage of the injured by road and rail formed no part of our instruction. One

night, whilst trudging westwards through sleet and slush after the class was over, the idea of teaching medical students stretcher drill came into my mind. Gradually the vista opened, I saw those medical students applying their knowledge to the movement of patients in hospital. I saw these young men scattered throughout the country when their hospital career was finished, carrying with them a practical knowledge of ambulance and becoming Volunteer Surgeons and instructors of stretcher bearers in the battalions to which they belonged. I believed also I saw a connecting link whereby the surgeons might be gathered together into a coherent body instead of existing as separate units; the genesis in fact of the Volunteer Medical Association. Moreover, it seemed possible thus to supply trained lecturers for the St John Ambulance Association. The mind travels fast, and in a few seconds the work of years was mapped out; and that these ideas proved no castles in the air the future proved.

Cantlie invited the Regular Army Sergeant Instructor to come to Charing Cross Hospital and teach the students stretcher drill. He told the students of his plan and asked them to join the drill. Seventy-two joined that afternoon and for the first time the words 'Attention', 'Lift stretcher', 'Lower stretcher', echoed round the Medical School, words which were soon to be heard in most of the country's medical schools. The drills were held three times a week and as their efficiency increased so did their popularity. One day, at the end of his anatomical demonstration, Cantlie was handed a card bearing the name Surgeon Major Evatt, AMS, Royal Military Academy, Woolwich. Evatt, a distinguished soldier with experience of field ambulances in the Afghan Wars, explained that he had been sent by Maclure because he too was interested in the development of the volunteer ambulance movement. Over luncheon at Romano's the two men laid the foundations of the Volunteer Medical Association and arranged to call a meeting of the Volunteer Surgeons in the Board Room of Charing Cross Hospital. As a result the Volunteer Medical Association was formed, with Surgeon General W. G. Hunter (later Sir Guyer Hunter, MP) as Chairman, Surgeon Major Evatt (later Surgeon General Sir George Evatt) as Vice Chairman and Cantlie as Secretary. Meetings were held at Charing Cross until June, when the National Aid Society offered their rooms at York Buildings, by which time fifty-one Surgeons were on the General Committee and all the medical schools had representatives on either the Executive or the General Committee, although Charing Cross at this stage was still the only hospital with trained medical students as Volunteers. Meanwhile Cantlie obtained permission for his students to drill within St George's Barracks under the eye of the Guards and procured, through Maclure's influence, an ambulance wagon, stretchers and tents for a parade on Wimbledon Common.

'As time went on,' Cantlie continued,

and the month of July came round, I was anxious that the trained body of bearers should be seen by the public and by someone in authority. After reflection I fixed upon no less a person than Lord Wolseley. It is the custom of Charing Cross Hospital to hold the annual distribution of prizes about the month of July, and at the committee meeting beforehand I got one of the teachers to propose that Lord Wolseley should be asked to preside. This was unanimously agreed to and I then unfolded my plan, which was that the distinguished soldier should inspect the hospital stretcher bearers at St. George's Barracks before distributing the prizes. The day for inspection arrived. During the intervals of waiting the drills had been frequent and exact, but I was anxious as to the result of the day's work; not only as to how we should execute our movements, but also as to the effect on the men I wanted to get at, namely the staff of the London Hospitals. At the last minute all the carefully laid plans were nearly destroyed. It happened that in 1883 the Charing Cross cricket team was of excellent calibre; so good, in fact, that they were to play the final for the cup against King's College. To my chagrin, it turned out that the match was to be played at the Oval on the day fixed for the inspection by Lord Wolseley. To the Oval every one of the students was going as player or spectator, and the ranks of my company seemed about to be bled to the last man. I was in despair and bethought myself of what could be done. I fell back on a simple plan. I appealed to their appetites, and asked the whole company, seventy-two in number, to luncheon at a restaurant in close proximity to the parade ground. The importance of the work outbalanced in my mind the value of a horde of luncheons, and the result of the day's work I deemed to be full of vital consequence to the future of the V.M.S.C. At the adjournment for luncheon at the Oval I reminded the members of the company that their luncheon was ready and the omnibuses outside the ground were in readiness to convey them thither. Thus I secured their attendance. And now we had to run the gauntlet of the afternoon's inspection and criticism in St. George's barrack square. The students' uniform consisted of jackets, low hats and Red Cross brassards worn on the left arm, not much for a lad to be proud of, but the drill and discipline had told, the ranks were well dressed and the smart appearance of the company called forth unanimous praise. From such recruits one would expect excellent results; young, hopeful, intelligent, well clad and well shod, they looked capable of anything.

Lord Wolseley arrived and inspected the ranks, which were drawn up in open order. There was little to inspect, as the men had neither uniform, arms nor equipment. Such an anomalous squad I am sure never before passed the distinguished soldier's criticism. No wonder his first question was 'Who are these men? Are they St. John Ambulance? Are they Volunteers? Do they belong to the Red Cross Society?' No, was the answer to each question. I could merely say, as we passed down the ranks, that they were medical students of Charing Cross Hospital trying to improve themselves in ambulance drill. A few minutes afterwards I was able to tell him the scheme for the formation of a Medical Staff Corps for the Volunteers, and that it was thought wise to commence with medical students, as likely to form the future officers of the Corps; and that should they become battalion surgeons they would be able to take up their appointments with a full knowledge of their duties. In shorter time than I take to write the account Lord Wolseley's keen ear and sharp intellect took in the statements, and grasped their meaning. He foresaw the importance of the work. He mentioned the difficulties of creating a new department, the necessity of a special grant. In a word, the future of the Volunteer Medical Staff Corps, its possibilities and difficulties, lay like an open book before his clear perception. The ranks were closed, the squad told off as a bearer company and presently thirteen stretchers were at work. The members of this first company parade executed their movements with a precision and care which won applause from all present. Whilst the members of the Company bound up imaginary wounds on the drummer boys lent by the Guards, Evatt, ever on the alert, was among the spectators, instilling the principles of the idea into the men we wanted to get at, the staffs of the London Hospitals with medical schools attached. So well did his words tell that more than one Hospital Surgeon left the ground asking, 'Why should not every Medical School have an Ambulance Company?' We knew then that the day was won, that the work so far was a gain and the future of the Corps a question of push and time. It was all so novel and fresh; the large crowd; the successful soldier; the success of the parade; the glorious weather; the hopefulness of the future of the movement.

At the prize-giving afterwards at Charing Cross Hospital Medical School Lord Wolseley spoke in glowing terms of the parade and unfolded the idea of the VMSC to the large assembly present so that next morning people read the words Volunteer Medical Staff Corps in the national press. Mitchell Bruce recorded in his diary, 'This movement, which promises to be of national extent and importance originated entirely with Cantlie. He has fought the battle single-handed and we can now say he has won it.' But as with all new movements success was not certain until finance was assured. Offers were not long in coming. On 25 July Sir William McCormac sent for Cantlie and told him that the National Aid Society had granted £250 towards the training of ambulance companies. Cantlie now realised with gratitude that, should the government not receive the corps into the Volunteers, the NAS would allow them to enlist under its auspices and train an ambulance of medical men and hospital assistants ready to help in national emergencies. The *Globe* newspaper welcomed such a plan, pointing out that the 'funds of the N.A.S., instead of lying idle, would be usefully employed in supplying the ambulance material for the bearer companies, which the new organisation seems able to enlist'. Cantlie knew however that, while appreciating the moral and financial support, the Volunteer Surgeons would wish to stand, if it were possible, side by side with their regular brethren in the Army Medical Department.

Expressing his thanks, Cantlie was obliged to ask permission to cut the meeting short, as he was leaving for Egypt within half an hour. He was one of a party of twelve civilian doctors and six regular officers from the Army Medical Department who had volunteered to go to Egypt to fight the cholera epidemic. Sent by Lord Granville, Secretary of State for Foreign Affairs, the party was under the command of Surgeon General W. G. Hunter, who posted Cantlie to Kafirzayat in the Delta area where the unchecked ravages of the disease had already accounted for a third of the population. This was due to a shortage of hospital attendants and medical assistance, to the appalling sanitary conditions, ignorance and squalor in which the local people lived, to their custom of burying corpses by the simple method of ejecting them into the Nile, which was also used for drinking purposes, and to the fact that they concealed their cases. Cantlie recounted the story of how in the first village he could find no cholera cases at all. Puzzled, he at last found an Egyptian soldier who trusted him and took him to a house with a case, although even then he had to find the boy under a pile of hay. When the patient recovered he had 200 cases in twenty-four hours. Experimenting with remedies, Cantlie found that lead and opium brought the greatest relief to sufferers. The epidemic was brought under control in two months and he returned to London in October with an expression of thanks from the Egyptian Government: 'The Ministry of Foreign Affairs has pleasure in acknowledging the zeal and devotion which Dr. Cantlie has continually shown during the trying time of this unfortunate epidemic, and in the name of the Egyptian Government expresses its unqualified satisfaction.' He also received a warm letter of personal appreciation from the Duke of Gordon. The Egyptian expedition showed the adventurous streak of Cantlie's nature, and it gave him his first experience of tropical diseases and awoke in him again the lure of ships and travel and the fascination of the East.

Before leaving London Cantlie had become unofficially engaged to Mabel Barclay Brown, whom he met during a camp with the London Scottish on Wimbledon Common. His decision to join the Volunteers thereby led him to the most important decision of his life. Mabel Barclay Brown was then 22 years of age, tall and slim, with the fairest of flaxen hair and smiling blue eyes. Her grace and frankness captivated Cantlie, who lost no time in paying a call at her father's house in Putney. As he walked home with a friend he remarked, 'I'm going to marry that girl.' His friend murmured congratulations, when Cantlie said 'I'm not engaged; it's only the second time I've seen her.' Her father, Robert Barclay Brown, was also in the London Scottish. Her mother, Ada Bayliss, was from Worcestershire and there were two other children of the marriage, a son and a daughter. Robert Barclay Brown, a large-framed, large-hearted man with a curling beard, magnificent in the kilt, had come south from Montrose, bringing with him a family business in ship building and repairing which went back for centuries – an ancestor, James Brown, had been forced, while prisoner during the Napoleonic Wars, to design a yacht for the Empress Josephine. On

Cantlie's return their engagement was announced. It was characteristic of her unselfishness that she had encouraged him to go to Egypt and carry out what they both conceived to be his duty. Mabel Cantlie always said that as a child she had three wishes: to see the Pyramids, to sit on the Great Wall of China following the example of her grandfather, James Bayliss, and to sail round the world. She lived to see them all fulfilled. During the winter she joined her fiancé in all his activities; her name was added to the cast for Christmas theatricals at Charing Cross and she became a member of St John Ambulance Association. As far as the Volunteers were concerned, much depended on her attitude to her future husband's voluntary work. 'I shall never forget,' wrote Cantlie,

> telling Evatt of my engagement. In October 1883 we were in the throes of doubt and trial. Each medical school had yet to be attacked and the work was only in its infancy when I announced my engagement. He regarded it as the greatest calamity and actually wrung his hands in despair. After a little thought he said, 'The future of this movement depends on this woman. Can I see her?' She was quickly introduced and within fifteen minutes Evatt's despair was turned to joy and he bade us farewell that afternoon with a light heart. When Volunteer matters were to be discussed and the Director-General or the P.M.O. Home District or Surgeon Major Evatt called and found me not at home, they heeded it not, for they found a better half capable of discussing propositions with keenness and intelligence.

Two natures so dissimilar yet linked together in such lasting and deepening affection it would be hard to find. The one supplied what the other lacked and each was to the other a constant inspiration. This living comradeship supplied to certain defects in Cantlie's character, as none other could, their necessary corrective. To his Celtic restlessness and impetuosity his wife brought stability and poise; to his occasional extravagances of speech or behaviour, the dignity of rectitude and restraint; to his lavish and even reckless generosity, a heart as kind but a sense of proportion; to his large tolerance of his fellows, discrimination, good judgement and sound sense. Cantlie had that acute sensitiveness to the feelings of others characteristic of members of a clan; he avoided arguments by appearing to agree with an opponent against his better judgement, though he had the knack of gaining his point when words gave place to deeds. Mabel Cantlie was more resolute, often brusque in speech and action; she never allowed personal considerations to weigh against matters of principle, was never pleasant at the expense of truth. James had the genius, the vision, the drive, the impetus and the flair for organisation and leadership, but a loving trust of human beings that was not always deserved, so that it was a weakness as well as a strength. Mabel's sense of duty was also based on religious feeling which brought her joyousness and serenity of spirit. It was in keeping with Cantlie's good nature that he should be self-effacing to a degree which many of his friends considered a fault. Many times in his life of public service his initiative was responsible for the formulation of a brilliant idea and its culmination in success: he would then step aside and let others take the credit. But Mabel Cantlie was jealous for his prestige and she strongly resented these injustices even when, as was generally the case, she could do nothing to prevent them. As a hostess she excelled and, as her social gifts widened the circle of their acquaint- ances, she strove loyally to bring him indirectly the recognition that he would never seek for himself.

On Cantlie's return from Egypt in October 1883, Evatt explained his plan to raise recruits from medical students of other London hospitals by means of a lecture tour. This brought into the movement University College, the London Hospital, St Bartholomew's, St Thomas's, the Middlesex and Guy's – St Mary's joining the movement when it became a Corps. During the winter, meetings of the Association were held and on 13 February Sir Trevor Lawrence, MP, introduced a deputation of Volunteer Surgeons, civilian doctors, teachers in London medical schools and members of the ambulance association to Lord Harting- ton, Secretary of State for War. The deputation said that, while the Volunteers possessed regimental surgeons, they had no medical department or hospital corps to organise divisional bearer companies or field hospitals. The deputation stated that there would be no diffi- culty in starting such a medical corps which would stand in the same relation to the volunteer forces as the Army Medical Department did to the Regular Army, but that it would need a capitation allowance and ambulance training material. Lord Hartington expressed his favour, but promised nothing until Parliament debated the army estimates. He allowed the deputation to hope, however, that the idea would be favourably entertained in the next session, and he spoke so encourag- ingly that Cantlie and the other members left with firm hope of recog- nition and confidence in the future.

While awaiting a decision from those in authority, the obvious next step was to bring together the seven hospital companies in which there was an understratum of feud and rivalry. The trouble was, as Cantlie recounts, that

> Every Hospital wanted their own separate company, and, with but a few exceptions, the prejudice seemed insurmountable, not only with the men themselves, but with the members of the Hospital staff at many Schools, who had set their faces against amalgamation. Under these circumstances, I believed that a uniform was the only means of breaking down the barrier and bringing about cohesion in one battalion. But how was the money for such a uniform to be raised? I happened in these straits to come across Mr. McGill of the firm of Pipe and McGill in Maiden Lane. I informed him we wanted a uniform and asked him to supply patterns of cloth similar to that worn by the Medical Staff Corps of the Army. Gradually it came about that I made a proposal to this effect; [like all north-east Scots Cantlie thought it bad manners to ask directly for something, instead

he cast a fly and waited for the fish to rise] I said that my object was to get Government recognition for the Corps, and in the meantime I wanted them clad in uniform for two reasons; first to induce the various hospital companies to come together, and secondly to make so good an appearance that the Government dare not refuse us recognition. I pointed out to Mr. McGill that the sum I meant to spend for the good of the nation was more than I dared risk, and that, did we not get recognition, it was a question of my going bankrupt on principle. I believed that, did the public come to know how such a catastrophe came about, it was certain a question would be asked in the House and the matter brought up. Mr. McGill saw my arguments, believed their cogency, and pushed on the clothing of the men with all speed. Nor has he lived to repent it. He got, thereby, an introduction to every Medical School in London and extended his private business accordingly.

The uniform was modelled on the army pattern, but there were some points on which there was discussion: the Regular Army Medical Staff Corps undress uniform cap was the ordinary forage cap worn by the line regiments, while the Scientific Corps, Engineers and so forth wore the round cap.

The War Office, I was told, would not allow the round cap. It was not allowed for the Regulars, and therefore would be vetoed for the Volunteers. However, as we were not yet under military authority we got the round caps and wore them. When the time came for laying them aside the same story was repeated, and then came the tussle. I pointed out to the authorities that . . . its not being allowed in the regular army was no reason why the volunteers should not have their just due. That rather than give way, we would enrol ourselves under the National Aid Society . . . Whatever the reason may have been the round cap was allowed us.

'As the summer wore on,' Cantlie continues,

the drills were attended by more men in uniform, until only recruits appeared in civilian dress at Battalion Drill. There was, however, still friction; the old separate Hospital notion had not died out. Companies had to be equalised in Battalion Drill and men had to fall out of their own Hospital ranks and join those of another with fewer men. Hospitals with large numbers asked what was the good of getting sufficient men together to form a Company when at parades their numbers were bled to supply the efficiency of less energetic Officers and students of other Hospitals.

Cantlie decided that what was needed was to

inculcate into the students a higher loyalty, an esprit de corps more binding them even their respective hospitals could provide. . . . In such circumstances, my mind turned again to an inspection by some prominent person as the only means of diverting the thoughts of the students from themselves and infusing the battalion with a feeling of common interest. Who was the great one to be procured? . . . After Lord Wolseley's inspection, when we were elated with the success of the parade, I had determined to infringe further on his Lordship's good nature, and accordingly wrote asking him if he could bring it about that the bearer company he had inspected could go to Windsor and appear before Her Majesty the Queen. Lord Wolseley had replied with his wonted courtesy that he did not think the time had arrived for such a step, but that on a future occasion, when we were better equipped he would consider it. In my present dilemma my mind reverted to another inspection. I therefore wrote now to Lord Wolseley concerning the matter, and reminded him of my request and of his reply the previous year. Day after day went past and no reply came. The middle of July was approaching and still I heard nothing. A few days more and the fulfilment of my scheme would be impossible owing to the breaking up of the schools. The horizon was dark, when it was suddenly lit up by a letter from Lord Wolseley announcing that he had forwarded my letter to Windsor, but that Her Majesty the Queen found it impossible to grant my request for the present year. However, at Her Majesty's request, he had sent on my letter to Her Royal Highness, the Princess Louise, Marchioness of Lorne, to whom he had spoken on the subject previously. Accordingly, I had a letter on July 16th from the A.D.C. announcing that Her Royal Highness had consented to see the Hospital companies, but that the only day possible before the 24th when the schools broke up was the following day, the 17th, at 2.30 p.m. Here was a dilemma! The intimation that Her Royal Highness was coming was most gratifying, but the time! The men were not in barracks, to be called together by a bugle. They were attending at different hospitals and living in houses and lodgings, scattered all over London. It was 9 p.m. on the 16th when we got the news, but as moments were valuable we did not discuss the matter, but set to work and dispatched letters and telegrams in all directions. I enlisted a number of Charing Cross Hospital students for the evening and their willing hands did giants' work. At 1 a.m. I went round the various daily papers and had it announced in the notices for the day that Her Royal Highness, Princess Louise, would be present in St. George's Barracks to see the Ambulance Companies paraded for inspection. The inspection came off, not entirely satisfactorily, but the men looked well in their new uniforms and went through their work creditably. There was a fair gathering of onlookers and after the parade the Marquis addressed the Companies and in a capital speech gave an account of the possibilities of ambulance work. With a hearty cheer in honour of Her Royal Highness the inspection ended and once again the members dispersed for their holidays.

Cantlie was now told by the War Office that it would be necessary to find lay recruits, for a Corps formed only of medical students would not meet with approval since they would only be in the ranks for about two-and-a-half years. 'But where to find such recruits?' Cantlie asked himself,

I had lectured for a good many years in ambulance work at the Birkbeck Institute [now London University] and got well acquainted with a few of the more prominent students to whom I unfolded my plan. With enthusiasm they set to work to spread the idea, so that within three weeks fifty men were enrolled. After careful thought I decided to take advantage of the cordial atmosphere of a smoking concert to unfold the news [Cantlie was uncertain how popular the idea would be with the medical students]. I therefore asked the Birkbeck Company to come to the students' room of Charing Cross Hospital Medical School half an hour before the time of the concert and to stay to the concert afterwards. As the medical students assembled with their friends from the other Schools they found stretcher drill proceeding, but did not recognise the Birkbeck men. I enlightened them and tried to get the onlookers to admire the drill, but my announcement was received coldly. The students began to whisper among themselves and retired out of view to converse. . . . At last one or two spoke out and said that were any but medical men to belong to the contemplated Corps they would resign. I knew this was coming, it was no good pointing out to the lads of seventeen that the Corps was an impossibility unless laymen belonged to it. . . . When the drill was over and the concert began it was difficult to get harmony. The Birkbeck men sat in one corner, the medical students in another. At last one of the former gave a capital song and proved an excellent musician; affairs went on more smoothly and at the end of the concert the two sets of men were favourably impressed with one another.

Thus the most critical moment in the life of the Corps was successfully passed and a further company of lay recruits was later enrolled at Woolwich. Meanwhile the War Office had also advised that the movement must include hospital medical schools and universities all over the country and Evatt had set out on a lecture tour to bring these students in as recruits. Cantlie accompanied Evatt on almost all of these tours. Owen's College, Manchester, and the Yorkshire College, Leeds, were accomplished in an afternoon and evening, with the two men returning on the midnight express. Edinburgh, Aberdeen, Dublin and Belfast involved more time. In Edinburgh, the Principal Medical Officer of the forces in Scotland was Lord Wolseley's brother, and the medical students already made up two of the finest companies of the Queen's Edinburgh, of which the Lord Advocate was the Colonel. This did not prevent him from encouraging the students to join the new Medical Corps which he promised to present with an ambulance wagon. The result was 'a magnificent body of men in the blue uniform of the V.M.S.C.' Leaving for Aberdeen, Cantlie's *alma mater*, at 5.00 a.m.,

they met a committee already formed to raise a branch of medical
students for the Volunteer Medical Association. At Trinity College,
Dublin, where Evatt had trained, the doctors were well received and
Evatt's words drew much applause on account of their remarkable
powers of address and persuasion. Cantlie records that as a result of
this visit the medical students of Trinity enrolled as a company of the
VMSC – a great achievement, as Ireland had no volunteers – and at
Queen's College, Belfast, there was the same satisfactory result. A
further company was also raised at Maidstone. Press reports in these
towns commented on Evatt's talks on military ambulance and Cantlie's
lectures on peace-time first aid, in which he pointed out how much
civilian doctors could learn from the military about the movement of
patients and organisation of hospitals, and the *Lancet* made particular
mention of the evils of separating military and civil medicine.[3]

The last qualifying step having been taken, Cantlie was told in
February that a grant for the VMSC was in the army estimates for the
year and throughout March he was in the War Office daily. On 3
March a request was made to Hunter from the Medical Department of
the War Office to nominate an officer for the command of the new
Corps and Hunter returned Cantlie's name. On 1 April 1885 the
Volunteer Medical Staff Corps was gazetted with a constitution of four
companies, an adjutant, a quartermaster and a surgeon commandant.
'The title of Surgeon Commandment,' Cantlie continues,

> was a well-chosen one, as it got over many difficulties of rank . . . The
> definite relative rank of the Surgeon Commandant was never
> determined. The uniform arrived the night before we started for the
> Easter manoeuvres, and the rank the tailor had conferred upon me
> quite scared me. After deliberation, I thought it better to remove the
> star; there was no time to change the facings; and I issued forth next
> morning not knowing exactly what I was, and waiting for remarks.
> Everything was hurry and bustle for the Easter manoeuvres com-
> menced on the 3rd, two days later. The evening of Wednesday, April
> 1st, found the outpatient department and the boardroom of
> Charing Cross Hospital converted into an equipment store. In one
> room were greatcoats, in a second side arms, in a third belts, in a
> fourth water bottles, in a fifth haversacks and in the boardroom the
> men were sworn in. After assembling in front of the Hospital the
> Corps was marched to the Chapel Royal, Savoy, where the service
> consecrating the Corps was held. At 6.30 a.m. on April 3rd 115
> Officers and men of the V.M.S.C. started for Brighton. Entraining
> from Victoria to Three Bridges they marched fifteen miles south
> and camped for the night. Next morning the advancing columns
> fought a defending force, which action provided its complement of
> wounded, and they completed the march, reaching Brighton late on
> Saturday evening. By this time the distance began to tell upon the
> weaker members and the wagons had their complement of sick and
> wounded. Those who were not entrained for London were trans-
> ferred to a Station Hospital upon arrival in Brighton. Easter Monday

arrived and the troops assembled on the Downs for the march past. All the V.M.S.C. men turned up, giving the contradiction to the forecasts of many friends who said that surely I did not know what I was doing when I undertook to proceed to Brighton with a hundred medical students. Did I think that I would manage to hold them together from Saturday till Monday? Never did a body of men behave better and never was officer more proud of his command than I was of the V.M.S.C. on that Easter morning. Three mounted Officers led the unit and, as the rear of the combatant battalions passed the flag staff, the new Corps of the Volunteer Forces was displayed to the Duke of Cambridge who took the salute. No sooner had we slackened our marching-past rigidity than we were stopped by the Duke and his Staff. After a short, sharp, scrutinising glance at the halted companies, he said, 'I believe you are a new Corps?' 'Yes, Sir.' 'When were you enrolled?' 'On the first of April.' 'Good God, extraordinary!' As the Duke rode away the Earl of Fife (later the Duke of Fife) extended a friendly hand of congratulations.

One last obstacle had to be overcome, the procuring of a band. Perhaps the sight of the Duke of Fife reminded Cantlie of his north-east Scottish connections, for whoever heard of a 'Moray loon' engaged in any activity from fair to funeral without the stir of the pipes or rhythm of a band. Cantlie decided that, although the Regulars still had no band, the VMSC who, according to the press after a military camp at Aldershot in August, showed considerable musical prowess, would endeavour to secure one. At their first annual inspection, he wrote, they had marched past to the 'tuck o' the drum' and the effect was not exhilarating and the marching not steady.

I made up my mind to have a band by next year. I found out, however, that permission for its formation was not likely to be forthcoming; in fact there was not the slightest hope. The Medical Staff of the Army had eight years before subscribed between £8000 and £9000 for a band, but when they asked permission from the War Office the petition was refused. Nothing daunted, I not only found a bandmaster but also a band ready to hand, and it was merely a question of clothing them in our clothing and the thing was settled. Again, however, the War Office gave me no hope. Director General Crawford was afraid the request was futile. General Elkington could find no precedent and the door seemed shut in my face. All the time I was getting the band into uniform. As a last resort I deter-mined to go to the War Office, and, with a map of the distribution of the Volunteer Forces in Great Britain, which I had drawn up, to boldly face Lord Wolseley, bent on attaining my end. The map I exposed to his scrutiny and in a few seconds he gave me valuable suggestions which I duly noted. [The map would have showed for one thing how scattered the Volunteer Medical Forces were.] I asked if the Volunteer Corps were allowed bands officially, and, when this turned out to be the case, I ventured to add that the V.M.S.C. was a

Volunteer Corps, therefore we could have a band. 'Certainly,' said Lord Wolseley; but, on further thought, he added, 'I cannot see what a doctors' corps wants a band for – and, besides, the Duke of Cambridge won't allow it. He would not give it to the Regulars.'

Cantlie described to Lord Wolseley how useful the band would be at inspections, concerts, theatricals and social gatherings, pointing out that the Volunteers were only held together by the unity of good fellowship and that the band would act as a focus, whilst, in addition, a band in a hospital encampment would 'enliven the monotony of hospital life and cheer the weary patient'. To Cantlie's delight Lord Wolseley suddenly said, 'Well, put in your application and I will back it up'. 'That very afternoon,' says Cantlie,

> I sent in the application to the Director General, who promised to forward it. It was certainly urgent, as the day was Tuesday, and on Monday I had arranged that the band should appear and play at St. James Hall, when our prize-giving took place. On this occasion the War Office put through the work speedily, for by Friday I had permission to raise a band. It was already at hand, and when the Director General and General Elkington came to the prize-giving on Monday, they were confronted by the band in the uniform of the Corps playing them welcome. Not only had we got our band, but, more important still we had established the principle of a Medical Corps having a band, and in 1887, although I was away in China, it would have been a great satisfaction to me to have been present at Aldershot when the V.M.S.C. band played the Regulars to Church.

In due course the Regulars acquired a band which was maintained voluntarily by the officers until 1938 when it was officially recognised. It could now be truly said that the VMSC had taken firm root amongst the recognised units of the Volunteers, and on the creation of the Territorial Army in 1907 it became the Royal Army Medical Corps (TF).

Undoubtedly it seemed the time had come to slacken the tempo of Cantlie's life. At least, surely, that is what Charing Cross Hospital must have thought. Alone among the London hospitals they had been in the vanguard of both the St John Ambulance and Volunteer Corps movements. They had seen their boardroom turned into a committee room for the Corps; their hospital into a quarter-master's store, a drill hall and temporary barracks; they had seen one of their most promising young surgeons lecturing all over the country to St John Ambulance centres, to the police, to men and women in factories and the home and writing the Association's first aid books; and finally securing recognition for the VMSC and becoming its first surgeon commandant. Now surely it was time for him to rest on his oars as regards public work and direct his attention to hospital and private medicine and his own career. His marriage had taken place to Mabel Barclay Brown on 30 July 1884 at St Martin's-in-the-Fields, and they had returned from their honeymoon to a house in Suffolk Street, Pall Mall. He seemed, to the dismay of his friends, who recognised his genius but not its direction, to be dashing off at tangents, sacrificing his income for non-remunerative work in the public sphere when he should have been settling down to an assured future in a Harley Street practice. Such philanthropy was all very well as a side line, they argued, for although they foresaw he would go far, they little guessed how far he would go or how great a sense of purpose there was in his life. What they saw was that there was nothing in him of the canny Scot with regard to money or the generous giving of his time to others and, indeed, but for the wise counsel of his wife, his generosity might have dissipated his energies and ruined his finances. Sooner or later circumstances exert a powerful influence on most men. Cantlie took and moulded circumstances to his own use, and as soon as one challenge had been met he rose to another. Now, having walked through the blizzard of difficulties surrounding the raising of the VMSC, he paused for a moment and walked out again to climb a further summit and meet another demand of human need. Like the poetess he seemed to be continually asking himself, 'Does the road wind uphill all the way?' and giving the same answer, 'Yes, to the very end.' He was already fighting another crusade, and this time he was fighting alone.

CHAPTER FOUR

Hong Kong and the College of Medicine for the Chinese

In his work for first aid and with the Volunteers as well as with the poorer patients in the hospital Cantlie had noticed that the physique of Londoners was poor and had asked the question why. To find an answer he now turned his attention to the subjects of hygiene and physical fitness, and made as a result a number of startling observations on London life. He saw the crowded slum dwellings surrounding Charing Cross. He observed that among poorer patients none came from London families who had survived beyond the third generation, and those of second generation families were often small and sometimes misshapen. This he attributed, one hundred years ahead of his time, to lack of ozone in the atmosphere. He pointed out that during a thunderstorm or snowstorm ozone is released into the atmosphere, but that the further men are from the sea or from the country the less ozone is available, that smoking chimneys consume it, but that even without these the sheer conglomeration of men together means that air is many times breathed and ozone is at the minimum. These ideas he put forward in a public address delivered in 1885 in the Parkes Museum, entitled 'Degeneracy among Londoners'. In drawing the attention of the public to the foul air of London he was too far ahead of his time for anyone to understand. The newspapers loved it and it raised sufficient protest for him to have to publish the text to avoid misinterpretation. During his early first aid work he had clung to the traditional anonymity of doctors, but once his open air demonstrations had begun it became more difficult, and when he raised the VMSC this anonymity was torn from him. The journalists wanted news and Cantlie was news, headline news. 'From whatever quarter the air is blowing,' he said, 'the outer circlet of, say, half a mile of human beings, absorbs the fresh air, and not only so, but adds various pollutions to it, so that the air breathed within a given area centred around, for instance Charing Cross, has not had fresh air supplied to it for, say, 50 or 100 years.'[1] Lack of ozone, he went on, was the reason why Londoners did not get sunburnt, and why exercise taken in the heart of the city did not do as much good as in the country. 'The city shop-keeper,' he pointed out, 'has not the advantage of fresh air entering his abode, and, tied up all the hours of sunlight, can only take exercise after dark and in a polluted atmosphere.' The result, he asserted, was catastrophic. 'When my attention was first drawn to this subject, I started with the premises that a Londoner was one whose grandparents come under the category; but I had to stop as I could find no such specimen. The boy who becomes Lord Mayor is pictured as invariably coming from the country; and leaving pantomime aside take note of the Lord Mayors who were born in London. Few. Very few.'[2] He then went on to categorise and analyse the defects of second generation Londoners, and to give examples from patients he had treated.

He was a voice crying in the wilderness, but this did not deter him from following the lecture with another at the YMCA Exeter Hall in the Strand in October 1885 entitled 'Life in London Hygienically Considered'. Again the national newspapers were delighted; 'the address stands out as the most unique form of platform literature that we have come across'. Henceforward the provincial newspapers were also to print his utterances. He repeated his previous theme but went further: 'Why should we not have fresh air brought to London in pipes?' And this time he added another novel notion, 'The sloping pavements of London streets, which slope so much as five inches in ten feet, make it impossible for a man to walk straight, and so as we cannot walk level in London we have to twist our spines in order to balance and thus become liable to curvature.'[3] Had Cantlie his tongue in his cheek? No. He overstated his case in order to draw attention to a social evil, but the result was that now, in addition to being reported, he was also lampooned by *Punch* and by *Fun*, who wrote an entertaining lyric on his controversial theory:

A tale which causes mental pain has reached our ears from Mincing Lane,
A man who has his office there but sleeps in Brixton's purer air,
Has made a rule, the rumour saith, on no account to draw a breath,
For fear that he should not survive, between the hours of ten and five,
On Tuesday last, while thinking hard and consequently off his guard,
He took in air, the merest pinch, three quarters of a cubic inch.
And now has taken to his bed and looks upon himself as dead.[4]

His friends worried about Cantlie's provocative statements and so did his mother who heard his lecture on a visit to London. When walking home afterwards, mindful of the great appreciation shown by the audience, she said, 'Well, Jimmie, I'm thinking these London folk are fine easily pleased'. He often told the story to show how a Scottish mother cuts her family down to life size, without realising that her mother's Highland heart was probably also saying, 'Keep with the clan, Jimmie, don't get out there on the hills where the snipers will get you'. In his voluntary work with St John and the Volunteers he had the clan with him, in just the same way as he had in his professional work as a doctor at Charing Cross, but now he was on the hills alone and he did not understand how vulnerable he was.

Again there was protest and this time he bowed before it and 'held his wheest'. He had his career to make. The following year he was made Senior Surgeon at Charing Cross and Keith his eldest son was born.

During this time he made a number of contributions to medical knowledge which foreshadow the detail and clarity of his later Red Cross *First Aid Manual*. One was on veins and circulatory troubles in Quain's *Dictionary of Medicine* and two articles, one on the ligature of the caratoid, iliac and femoral arteries and another on injuries of the cranial nerves, with particular attention to the eye, in Heath's *Dictionary of Practical Surgery*. His mind, however, was also on his work with St John and the Volunteers, for in the same book there is an article on 'Ambulance in peace and war' and another on 'Management of the sick room' which shows his knowledge and love of nursing, an interest which, like first aid, stayed with him all his life.

The routine life of the London practitioner and surgeon did not provide sufficient challenge or satisfy his love of adventure. He had not forgotten his boyhood dreams inspired by the ships at Garmouth or the lure of the East and his interest in tropical diseases, encountered in Egypt. During the Christmas recess of 1886 the Cantlies were staying with Mitchell Bruce, who had received a letter from Dr Manson saying that he wished to come home from Hong Kong and find a replacement for himself in Dr Hartigan's practice there. Not mentioning a name Bruce asked Cantlie if he knew of a substitute and after discussion in which no candidate came to mind, Cantlie said, 'Well, if it is Mackie's practice in Alexandria or Manson's in Hong Kong I'll go myself. I know Mackie, for I was with him in Egypt. Manson I have never seen, but I know his reputation.' The next day a cable was dispatched and upon receiving the answer the die was cast. Mabel Cantlie would now fulfil her ambition to sit upon the Great Wall of China like her ancestor James Bayliss. Cantlie, whose respect and affection for Charing Cross Hospital and for the ambulance movement was both life-long and mutual, did not resign from either until he knew that his family would settle in Hong Kong; he took sabbatical leave of absence for six months and set off into the unknown. 'Having taught young medical men,' he said, 'for some seventeen years and having seen them depart abroad for the Army, the Navy or the Colonial Service, I was imbued with the spirit of seeing for myself and learning something of the diseases they talked about at home.'

The Cantlie's view of Hong Kong as they sailed into its harbour on 27 July 1887 was one of breathtaking beauty. Myriads of small islands ringed by yellow sandstone rose out of a sapphire ocean, here and there shading to the green of glacier water. To the north, like the backdrop on a stage, wispy mists blew among the mountains of China, less enveloping and more mysterious than the mists of Scotland. They must have felt that, like Keats, they had unlatched 'magic casements, opening onto perilous seas, in faery lands', not forlorn as the poet saw them, but bustling with activity. Forests of masts – junks, steam vessels and sailing ships – filled the sheltered, magnificent harbour into which the mainland town of Kowloon jutted like an arc, dividing the barren peaks and fertile valleys of the New Territories and China from the verdurous wooded hills of Hong Kong island. Twin-sailed junks and sampans plied their way to and fro between the town of Victoria and

'Kowloon side', together with the new steam ferries which also linked Hong Kong with the Portuguese colony of Macao on the tip of the isthmus leading to Canton, entrance port to the province of Kwang-tung in South China. For 300 years Macao had provided a base for the East India Company and for the British merchants and missionaries who in 1841 had moved to Hong Kong, ceded that year to Britain after a naval victory in the First Opium War. (Kowloon and the first part of the New Territories had followed twenty years later.) Voices were raised in the British Parliament and press and among the doctors and missionaries, against the selling of Indian opium to the Chinese but it was the only commodity, apart from gold and silver, which the Chinese traders of Canton would take in return for silk and tea, and the Colonial Surgeons' reports show that, until the 1890s, the dangers of taking the drug were seriously underestimated. Hong Kong had always maintained a thriving Chinese community of about 2,000, well and honestly administered, in which scholars from China had taken refuge so that the seeds of Western culture found fertile soil in which to flourish. The London Missionary and Morrison Education Societies, both from Macao, were now joined in Hong Kong by James Legge of Huntly, Aberdeenshire, who founded a Chinese Theological College and took three Chinese boys back with him to the Duchess of Gordon's School, thus strengthening the links between China and north-east Scotland.

Standing at the ship's rail, the Cantlies would have seen naval craft riding at anchor in the approaches to the dockyard, for since cession the Royal Navy had based its far Eastern Fleet in Hong Kong and between it and the Chinese people had grown a lasting regard and affection. Stepping ashore they would have been engulfed in a crowd of purposeful activity, typically Chinese. Men and women packed the pavements and streets, never jostling, never hurrying so fast as to break the rhythm of life, always laughing, the serene, patient faces of the older women betraying an acceptance of life, a philosophy timeless and enduring. The Peak, with its three summits, dominated the island. The flag of Government House flew from above and behind the Central Square, where the Supreme Court and Hong Kong Shanghai Bank looked out on flower beds and neatly mown grass. The houses, mostly constructed by Jardine Mathieson of Canton brick with tile rooves, were built on top of one another, first floors opening on to back streets which mounted steeply to the ring of trees surrounding the tram station at the top. The Peak tramway was newly installed, two carriages on a pulley system soon to be familiar at ski resorts but then, according to Mabel Cantlie's diary started in that year, 'quaint and unusual with everything at an angle'. The following year the Cantlies moved to the healthier air of the Peak, but now they stayed 'below' not far from the consulting rooms, and thus became more quickly acquainted with the Chinese who, in spite of their urban surroundings, remained a rural and seafaring people.

The sights, sounds and smells of the East hold Europeans in thrall. Chinese banners hanging on poles from houses, festooned streets along which straw-hatted Chinese towed rickshaws and pushed bar-rows, while shoppers bought wares from open markets or small crowded shops and passers-by ate meals at street restaurants using chop sticks and exquisite china bowls. Cantlie always walked to his consulting rooms for he never rode in a rickshaw, and friendliness fast replaced the first feelings of unfamiliarity. These people had charac-teristics of his countrymen at home in Banffshire. Both were rooted to soil or sea; both reared in poverty, but secure within rules of courtesy and hospitality, which here were bound to the family instead of the clan. As in the Highland glen, traditional individuality and independ-ence were linked to interdependence and good neighbourliness; politeness was paramount; a visitor must be offered a chair and food and drink, which he must accept in order not to give offence; friends and strangers alike must not be allowed to lose face and must be put at their ease. In the doorways of the shops and single-roomed one-man businesses, Cantlie would have passed the familiar groups of men that he would have seen in Dufftown, lending a hand to speed the work, while at the same time swapping news, so that the 'bush telegraph' operated at lightning speed, keeping informed ordinary people and secret societies all over the island. Early in the morning and late at night the industrious activity continued for, to the Chinese, as to the north-east Scot, their work was the most important part of life, and they plied their trade or studied their profession with single-minded concen-tration. Even the infants handled tools beside their fathers and brothers and here, under the Eastern sun, the women also were out in the streets, ironing or watching the children as they worked or played. Children were everywhere, tranquil, happy children, for Chinese children hardly ever cry. They accompanied their parents by riding on their mothers' backs and when they wanted to sleep they lay down in a box at the back of the shop or living room. As in the Highland but and ben, the box bed stood by the kitchen stove, a hole in the roof let out the smoke, a palliasse lay on the floor instead of a bed; only here in Hong Kong there was filth as well as poverty, a pot in the kitchen instead of outside sanitation, the only household drain being that from the kitchen sink to the public sewer; and a dangerous indifference to overcrowding and disease.

Five years before Cantlie's arrival the British Parliament had insti-gated their most recent survey on the overcrowding and sanitation of Hong Kong, which had resulted in the setting up of a Sanitary Board under Dr Ayres, the Colonial Surgeon. Cantlie, who had taken the Diploma of Public Health in London before leaving, was invited to be one of its members. The Board had no legal powers and was in an awkward position, for the ordinances authorising housing improvements were not popular with the *laissez-faire* Chinese who took to the streets in mobs if they were put into effect. Trained not be aggressive in the home they adjusted to overcrowding, and the hot sun enabled the worst conditions in houses or among the boat people to be transformed into personal cleanliness by quick drying laundry. If the Board pressed its advice too hard upon the Governor, then the Government ran into trouble with the Chinese which displeased the merchants; yet Dr Ayres prophesied the outbreak of an epidemic if conditions remained un-altered, warning that drains under the houses leading to public sewers were often blocked with sand during rainstorms; that some houses were not connected with any drainage at all, that some had polluted wells; that there was no ventilation between houses and that in the slums sixteen people were sharing 437 cubic feet (while Britain was aiming at 300 per person). There was also dry earth sanitation and house-to-house scavenging for manure used in vegetable growing, and householders stored food under the wooden floors within reach of rats. In all these circumstances it was hardly surprising that the death rate was high. Just how high was hidden by the fact that older Euro-peans and Chinese returned to their country of origin.

Right from the start there had been a reputation for ill health on the island. A 'most severe and fatal sickness' (probably malaria) together with dysentery and diarrhoea decimated the troops in the first year of cession. The settlers came near to discovering the cause of malaria for, seeing that outbreaks of fever occurred after digging or heavy rain, when there were pools of water in the sandstone or granite rock, they shut out the damp by hanging blankets round their beds, thus protect-ing themselves from mosquitoes breeding in the pools. Manson, whom Cantlie had arrived to replace, was a graduate of Aberdeen and had made a great breakthrough in insectology and tropical medicine in Amoy and Formosa where he had traced the insect bite as the cause of elephantiasis and filariasis; from this discovery followed the later proof that malaria was transmitted in the same way. Manson had already made two contributions to the life of Hong Kong island; he had started a dairy herd which, coming soon after the fresh water supplied by the building of the Pokfulam dam, helped to cut down disease, and he had been mainly responsible for starting the Hong Kong Medical Society one year before Cantlie's arrival, where doctors were able to demon-strate and record the diseases of patients, isolating new ones and suggesting cures and alleviates to each other. This helped to cut down the work load carried by the Colonial Surgeon, who doctored the Civil Service, police and convicts, administered the Government Hospital and Lock Hospital for infectious diseases, prepared the Annual Report and had to undertake private practice to supplement his income. This Annual Report was, until the start of the Hong Kong Medical Society, the only record of diseases which, by the time Cantlie arrived, included beri beri, Asiatic cholera, hydrophobia, small pox, venereal disease, yellow fever, dengue, sprue and the whole range of 'Hong Kong' fevers – simple, continuing, remittent, intermittent and enteric. Malaria was given its name in the Report for the first time in 1888. The diseases directly connected with overcrowding were enteric, diarrhoea and dysentery; and tuberculosis, both pthisis and pulmonary affections. Leprosy was not mentioned, not because it was not present in Hong Kong but because lepers were returned to the mainland if they re-ported sick and so suffered the disease in silence.

The greatest problem in administering and improving the health of the island lay in how to persuade the Chinese to attend Western hospitals and to learn about Western medicine and science. Whereas in education and Christian ethics missionaries had made strides, in medicine they met an insuperable barrier. The Chinese would not give up the potions of their herbalist doctors, they would not report themselves ill to the Western doctors and preferred to go to their death houses to die. The first missionary hospital was closed within five years for lack of patients as was also the Seamen's Hospital, in spite of generous financing from Jardine Mathieson. In 1872 the Government had accepted the Chinese preference for their own medicine, and built for its practice the Tung Wa Hospital in Tai Ping Shan, one of the worst slums in Hong Kong, where sometimes there were pigs in the upstairs of the houses. It was clear to all thinking people that no progress could be made to improve the island's health until the co-operation of the Chinese was won and they could be educated in Western medicine and hygiene. The question was, how could this be done. It was Dr Young of the London Missionary Society who first broke down the barriers. He set up a Dispensary for the Chinese in Tai Ping Shan which was so successful that in 1884 it was decided to turn it into a hospital with funds given by Dr Ho Kai, a distinguished Chinese and medical graduate of Aberdeen, barrister-at-law and member of the Inner Temple, in memory of his rich English wife. Just five months before Cantlie's arrival the Alice Memorial Hospital opened on the intersection of Aberdeen Street and Hollywood Road.

Thus the first part of the problem had been solved, provided that the Chinese continued to support the Hospital in the same way that they had attended the Dispensary. The important question remained, however, of how best to persuade them to be educated in Western medicine. As with the story of first aid, it was fortunate for the teaching of Western medicine to the Chinese that already on board ship Cantlie was laying plans for the formation of a hospital school for Chinese students. His teaching in Charing Cross and for St John's had been his life, and he could not face the future without it; 'I regretted giving up teaching, as that was and is my chief enjoyment in life, so on the way out I contemplated how I could minimise the loss and the College of Medicine was the result.' Within thirty-four days of arrival he called a meeting of medical men on 30 August at the Alice Memorial Hospital to discuss how to promote the study of medicine for the Chinese. The site of the meeting and the men he approached beforehand were the key to its success, Doctors Ho Kai, Manson, Jordan, Gerlach, Young and Chalmers (the last two from the London Missionary Society) and Mr W. E. Crow.

According to the minutes of the Senate of the College of Medicine for the Chinese, 'The Chairman called upon Dr. Cantlie to state the object of the meeting called by him. Dr. Cantlie stated that in conjunction with Drs. Ho Kai, Manson and Jordan he had issued this notice of a meeting to obtain the collective opinion of those engaged in the practice of medicine and in scientific work in Hong Kong. After some discussion it was unanimously resolved that "a College of Medicine for Chinese be established in Hong Kong". The Chairman then asked to see the scheme drawn up provisionally by Dr. Cantlie as a basis for deliberation.' The opening preamble of the final text of this first draft stated that 'A College of Medicine for the Chinese, Hong Kong, is founded for the purpose of teaching the Science of Medicine in all its branches and to grant licences to practice in its name to Chinese and to such others as may wish to avail themselves of the privilege of the College. The licence granted by the College certifies the ability of the Holder thereof to practise Medicine, Surgery and Midwifery.' It was then proposed by Cantlie and seconded by Jordan and passed unanimously that the present meeting, with power to add to their number, resolve itself into the Senate. The Senate was to consist of professors and lecturers who would, as in Charing Cross, give their tuition free. Dr Chalmers, representing the Hospital, offered its accommodation free to the College for lectures and demonstrations. Students were to be charged fees, but scholarships were soon forthcoming from generous citizens such as Mr Belilios. The government of the College was to be vested in a court, the first members of which were to be Drs Young, Manson, Cantlie and Chalmers and Mr J. J. Francis, QC, Standing Counsel to the College. As in Scotland, the Court was to include a rector chosen by the students, although in the first instance the rectorship was offered to Mr Frederick Stewart Lockhart, the Colonial Secretary, with Dr Ho Kai his assessor.

The press report which reached London in November ran as follows:

A College of Medicine for the Chinese has been opened in Hong Kong. Probably this news will be not altogether surprising to those who remember that Mr. Cantlie, the organiser of our V.M.S.C. quitted his surgical and professional duties in Charing Cross Hospital early in the year and attached himself to the staff of the Alice Memorial Hospital in Hong Kong. Enthusiastic and energetic, once arrived in Hong Kong he conceived the idea of utilising the material at hand in the medical school and called a meeting of scientific and professional men on the 31st of August. There has now come home news of the College of Medicine with Dr. Manson as Dean and an able staff upon which are utilised the services of a Government chemist and botanist, of a section of the Army Medical Staff Corps and of the Alice Memorial Hospital Staff. Ambulance Training will be fully appreciated by the Chinese.

This report in the *Daily News* of 16 November 1887 is interesting for three reasons. There seems to have previously been some doubt as to whether Cantlie or Manson started the College of Medicine for the Chinese, although it is absolutely clear from the minutes and other sources, including the press, that Cantlie called the first meeting and proposed a Medical College on the same lines as Aberdeen and Charing Cross. But the press in this instance refers to 'the medical school' as if there was one already in existence; so the confusion may have arisen because the Hong Kong doctors may have had for a month or two an embryo school running in the Alice Memorial Hospital on the same lines as those previously in existence in the early London hospitals with no formal lectures, constitution or examinations. The second reason it is interesting is because it shows that right from the start the chemistry of Western medicine was to be fused with the herbalism and botany of Chinese medicine; and the third reason is because the report states that the army medical staff were to play a part in the school. Cantlie taught the Chinese students first aid and ambulance work both in St John and the Volunteers and later introduced first aid into the teaching of tropical diseases, while service doctors played a significant part in the conquest of disease in the colony.

On 1 October 1887 the inaugural opening of the College was held in the City Hall and Major-General Cameron, the officer administering the government, explained that the aims of the College were 'to promote medical science among our fellow citizens and to involve the grand object of spreading the gospel of medical science through the whole of China'. Chinese lack of enlightenment in medicine and sanitation in no way reflected upon their high intelligence, he said, but was because they had never turned their attention to these subjects. The plan was 'to form agencies all over China and to see what we can do to alleviate all that immense amount of bodily suffering there is in the country'. Manson, in his address as dean, restated these aims but added a warning that licentiates who went into private practice in the Chinese Empire would have 'to overcome native prejudice and fight the vested interests in the native profession . . . The task in front of the medical reformer is herculean . . . At his back the whole of European science, before him three hundred million to whom to give it.' Manson, having confessed to an earlier hope that the Taiping Rebellion of 1850 (which had been put down by General Gordon at the request of the Peking Government) might have brought a new dawn for China, said that now in his mature judgement he accepted the rule of the Manchus, thought 'the action of the governing class after the Taiping Rebellion was correct', and admired the skill of the Peking Government. 'There has not been nor apparently will there be any sudden reform . . . and therefore no sudden revolution or other cataclysm.' His prophecy proved false. Listening to him in the audience was one of the newly enrolled students, Sun Yat Sen, first President of China.

Sun Yat Sen holds a unique position in the history of China for he drank from the watershed where Christian traditions blended with the ancient wisdom of the Chinese classics. He had a gentle, idealistic disposition which made him both vulnerable and invincible; he was an honest, courageous boy, who endeared himself to others by unselfishness and sincerity of purpose. His rural childhood gave him tranquillity and patience, from his parents he learnt morality and goodness, at school he memorised ancient Chinese texts, whose complexity demanded such single-minded concentration that since poverty allowed only one wick at home in the evening he read his books by moonlight or sat in the living room humming to shut out the noise. At 13 he joined his elder brother in Honolulu and entered an Anglican School, learning about Magna Carta, Parliament and liberty under the law. He went from there to an American College, where he was taught about the American and French revolutions and where under the influence of the missionaries he was baptised. He said that he saw no break between his early Confucian training and the principles of Chinese humanism, Lao Tzu and Buddha and his Christian baptism of 1884; it was simply the difference between rigid law and the grace of forgiveness. His immediate reaction to his baptism, however, was a boyish one, for he was a high-spirited lad who hated sham and injustice. He went home and in company with other boys smashed the arm of an idol in a temple to prove its impotence. The villagers were furious and his parents sent him back to an Anglican College in Hong Kong, from which he went to Queen's College and then to a missionary medical school attached to Canton Hospital. Hearing of the new College of Medicine in Hong Kong and believing that through medicine he could best aid his suffering countrymen, he enrolled and became its most conscientious and brilliant student.

The Alice Memorial Hospital, in which the students had the back wing, must have looked to Cantlie very different from Charing Cross. The Georgian elegance and classical pillars were replaced by the square lines and shuttered windows of a typical Victorian settler's house; but the area chosen for the hospital was familiar in the sense that it had been picked because it was in the most over-crowded part of the town, where the covered booths of Aberdeen Street fell steeply from Bonham Road down to the sea. Here the bright colours of the Chinese banners hanging from the window poles were obscured by the drab washing hanging round them; old men and women, with expressions born of fulfilment and suffering, sat beside stalls waiting for customers with whom to barter wares. Here was a group playing cards in the sunlight, their wide straw hats shading the upturned packing case used for a table, and there the chop sticks and china bowls of the street restaurants gave an improbable refinement to the disturbing poverty of Tai Ping Shan. But, as always, the hope of the Chinese – 'today is not good, tomorrow will be better' – bubbled over into beauty and everywhere there were flowers adorning the window boxes and dark interiors of the houses, their scent mingling with the smell of fat frying in the kitchens and open air cooking stoves. Cantlie never looked back to what lay behind except to apply the same high standards to what lay ahead. The challenge was formidable and only the most robust of constitutions could have survived the mistreatment he allotted to himself in order to alleviate the human suffering that lay everywhere around him.

There were in those days in Hong Kong no trained nurses and Cantlie appointed two Chinese students, one of whom was Sun Yat Sen, to nurse one of his gravely ill patients, a Mr John Humphreys. The students received no remuneration for their work, and so grateful was the patient for their excellent care that he awarded the Watson Scholarship out of which the College authorities gave both students free tuition and a monthly allowance. Alone among the doctors of Hong Kong Cantlie had had seventeen years of experience of running a hospital school. The leisure time activities of the College bore a marked resemblance to those of Charing Cross. There were the same 'Smokers', entertainments, societies and games, tennis, cricket and rowing. Cantlie taught his Chinese students cricket – an example of two-party government – and gave Sun Yat Sen his first instruction in croquet, a game springing from the Middle Ages which demonstrates the importance of blending competition and mutual aid and which Sun was still playing in his last home in Peking. There was also instruction for the Chinese students in first aid both for the St John Ambulance Association, which Cantlie started in the island, and for the Volunteers, which he joined as Surgeon Captain. Sun was one of the best ambulance recruits just as he was a brilliant student in his examinations and clinical work. Cantlie said he found the Chinese students 'willing, earnest in their endeavour, quick to understand, retentive of memory'. Repetition is the essence of school life in China, and the effect of this is to develop a retentive memory to a degree unbelievable to those who have not come into contact with oriental students. 'In one professional examination for the Diploma of the College', wrote Cantlie,

> the questions were answered perfectly, but on comparing the papers it was found that the answers were identical. The examiners, new to Chinese methods of instruction, insisted upon another paper being set as they believed that the students had copied from each other. A fresh paper was set and a careful watch kept; again the answers were correct and identical in every point, and it was only when the text book recommended to the class was referred to that the explanation was forthcoming. They knew the large text book of some five hundred pages by heart and could answer any question put to them, word for word, from the book.[5]

The standards of the College were, according to Professor Lo, a Chinese historian, as high as those in Britain, 'all due to Cantlie's teaching. Cantlie was a great scientist and teacher, sincere and good for his students, all his students were very happy to study under him. He did not teach them science only, but science in general, giving them a wide knowledge of Western science, particularly the work of Harvey, Jenner, Hunter, Darwin and Lister.'[6] Cantlie's most profound influence on Sun, Professor Lo points out, was the teaching of Darwin's theories of natural selection, as a result of which Sun became the first Chinese doctor or scientist to accept Darwin, believing that the best could survive only where there was competition both in the animal and human world. Professor Lo also claims that Sun modified Darwin by what he called the theory of mutual aid, believing that there is a natural bond which draws men together, and that teaching can draw out this desire.

In October 1888 the College held its first annual prizegiving.

Manson was ill and Cantlie summed up its ideals in his own address, reported in the *China Mail*:

> What is wanted is to bring the people of the British Empire to see the importance of having a medical and scientific educational establishment in Hong Kong; to consider this attempt to introduce science amongst the Chinese as a civilising agency of primary importance and to look upon it as their moral duty to extend the advantages science has brought themselves ... Will not the people of the Western Empire send an emblem of peace to this ancient people instead of implements of war, will they not send the blessings of modern research for the alleviation of human suffering ... Let science be the association, and a bond of respect will be formed between the peoples such as no superiority of war could command.

The Governor in reply spoke words of tribute to Cantlie's work and of prophecy for the future:

> I need hardly say that I have listened with great pleasure to the favourable report of the College which has been read by Dr. Cantlie to whom not only the foundation of the institution but the success of so much is so largely due. I regret exceedingly the absence of Dr. Manson, whose name I observe is at the head of what may be called the works of the institution, but I am glad to observe that Dr. Cantlie, whose enthusiasm and energy have already done so much has proved a worthy substitute for the occasion. Nothing will keep Hong Kong abreast of the advance in the age of medical knowledge better than teaching the young. This will be the centre of learning for the Chinese Empire. It will further good relations between the English and the Chinese.

Then to the Chinese students he spoke words which were visionary in their foresight:

> Remember that you are only on the threshold of knowledge. Rough country lies ahead. You must overcome obstacles, troubles too great to be borne, but you may buoy yourself up with the hope that honour sooner or later will come to you. Honour that will not end with your life but will grow afterwards.

It was almost as if he had seen to the end of a road and knew what lay ahead.

Cantlie's first act as Dean of the College, in which position he succeeded Manson, was to draw up a draft Bill of Incorporation and in order to facilitate its acceptance as an Act, to ask Mr Francis if he would act as its emissary in England. The plan failed and incorporation had to wait until 1907 when Dr Ho Kai successfully steered it through the Legislative Council in Hong Kong. Meanwhile, however, Cantlie invited Li Hung Chang, Viceroy of Canton and later Grand Secretary of the Chinese Empire, whom Manson had treated for suspected cancer, to become patron of the College. Li wrote the following words of encouragement, which were included in a letter published in the *China Mail* of 18 October 1889:

I remark that your countrymen devote themselves to practical research and base their scientific principles on the results of investigations, thus differing from those who rest content with theories. The happy results which ever attend the treatment of disease on scientific principle are evidence of the advantage to be derived from the constant study of Anatomy and Chemistry, and the consequent illumination of the dark path of knowledge. There is no doubt that when your admirable project is achieved it will be appreciated and imitated and that it will through your students be a blessing to China.

CHAPTER FIVE

Hong Kong Surgeon

To read the record of Cantlie's work in Hong Kong, whether in the official papers, the newspapers, the minutes of the College of Medicine, or those of the Hong Kong Medical Society, in his own publications on medical research or in the diaries, leaves one amazed that one man could have been in so many places and switched his attention so rapidly from one subject to another. First, the founding of the College of Medicine for the Chinese; secondly, his work to alleviate the human suffering everywhere around him, whether as surgeon, doctor or nurse, for the lack of trained nurses imposed an extra burden; thirdly, his public work on the Sanitary Board, his vaccination for smallpox and his successful proposals for the founding of an Institute for making fresh lymph; fourthly, his research into tropical medicine and tropical surgery, then in their infancy, the papers and books he wrote and his wife translated, the demonstrations he gave in the Hong Kong Medical Society and the laboratory work he did in his own house with germs cultivated by his wife in home-made soup in the kitchen; fifthly, the Peak Hospital which he opened and in which over 1,000 patients were treated during his time in Hong Kong; sixthly, the St John Ambulance work which he began and the Volunteer ambulance instruction which he carried on in the colony; seventhly, his contribution to the social and educational life of the island, the debating, literary and scientific societies he started, to say nothing of a club for Highland dancing; eighthly, his work during the bubonic plague and afterwards as a member of the committee set up to examine the workings of the Medical Department; and ninthly, his final achievement, just before he left Hong Kong, the founding of a Hong Kong Public Library, free for all citizens. 'Cantlie,' said the *China Mail*,[1] 'is in several places at once unwearied in well-doing.'

He wished to make the advantages he had received as a boy available not only to the people of the colony, but to as many people of the Chinese Empire as he could find the time to reach. While advising others to find time for recreation he worked incessantly; while they rode in rickshaws he ran beside them. His was a programme that would have killed most people and sometimes it came close to killing him. He knew that in that heat his health would suffer without exercise, so in order to keep fit he jogged alongside the rickshaw at the coolie's pace. The older residents said he would get heat stroke and die, but he survived, perhaps miraculously, while writing papers warning Europeans that they should exercise in the evening cool, after which they should bath and rest. His inspiration was his love of his fellow men; he could not refuse anyone anything. Mabel Cantlie's inspiration was the love of her husband and her belief in him which transcended everything. Many wives would not have tolerated his hours of work. During a cholera and typhoid epidemic, or at a confinement or difficult operation he would be out all night or to the 'wee sma' hours'. Her diaries show how wearisome she found the time without him and how worried she was about his health (she always called him Hamish, Gaelic for James): 'Hamish looks worn out with all his work . . . Hamish out all night with cholera . . . Hamish had only one hour's sleep . . . Has still a dreadful amount of work . . . Hamish stayed all night but the baby did not come . . . I feel very anxious about him.' She never complained but found much at home to occupy her attention; Keith, their eldest son, was a year old when they arrived in Hong Kong, Colin was born in 1888, and Neil in 1892. In 1889 the Cantlies built a house on the Peak at Mount Kellett, where their hospitality to visitors to Hong Kong was, according to Sir Arthur Keith, bottomless.

These were the days of free trade and the Pax Britannica, when Western science was pushing back the frontiers of knowledge, and the peoples of the world wished to share in the dawn of this new civilisation. Hong Kong was the hub of this new trade and culture; protected by the encircling arm of the China coast and by the Royal Navy, it provided hospitality in one year to 4,000 visiting ships and 23,000 junks. This tiny island, this jewel set in the mistiness of the China seas, was thronged with people from all over the world, who came in brief or prolonged stays, or as settlers, making their own contribution to its economic and social life. Believing that, in spite of her husband's long hours of work, they should not isolate themselves from its social life, Mabel Cantlie attended balls and dinners at Government House and on board visiting ships, and accepted invitations to tennis and bathing parties, races at Happy Valley, polo and cricket matches. Sometimes Cantlie escorted her, sometimes he arrived late or left early, either returning later or not at all. In that small community without social recreation life would have been claustrophobic in its confinement. Boat parties to the islands broadened the horizons of the mind with scenes of beauty, where the sea and sky blended together in the distance into identical blue and the sand in the curved bays was undisturbed by footprints and the silence uninterrupted by the voices of men. Picnics to the New Territories brought glimpses of another civilisation with its ancient walled cities, mountainous peaks and strip farming in the valleys. Even on Hong Kong island the eye never lost its sense of perspective or enjoyment of contrasts, for round each corner was a vista of beauty, a glimpse of a rounded mountain or deep lagoon. To the north lay Victoria, its harbour criss-crossed by cotton-wool foam trailing the ships, to the south was Aberdeen with its busy fish market and surrounding sandy bays, whose tranquillity was interrupted only by the clang of the fishermen's rattles frightening the fish into the nets. Everywhere there were flowers, pink, white and red, and graceful blossom-laden trees growing in circles to reach the sun; and, almost obscured by foliage, wide granite waterfalls, which in the dry season were moistened by a trickle of water just sufficient to keep green the plants in the middle. Chinese art is China. It is not surprising that Mabel Cantlie found time to study painting and photography to record such scenes of beauty. Her pictures hung in the City Hall exhibitions and received excellent mention in the press but sadly not one has survived. The beauty, however, was as variant as the calm was fragile. Those bent and curved trunks of trees told of violent typhoons which whirled across the island, ripping off roofs and verandas; in thunderstorms rain pelted down upon the sand and sandstone, loosening its hold on granite outcrops and carrying landslides of rocks and earth on to the roads and into the reservoir. In the same way the happiness was punctuated by tragedy, for always at the shoulder stalked death, taking away a loved one or friend or jealously guarded patient with a suddenness that struck chill into the heart.

In 1889 a virulent fever decimated the community at Westpoint, straining the doctors to breaking point, so that a petition for an inquiry was presented to the Governor. Cantlie described his clinical experience of the disease to the Hong Kong Medical Society; Manson thought it malaria, while the other doctors thought it enteric. Fever remained the great killer. Between ten days and a month after childbirth or an operation it often set in with fatal results. Cantlie gave much attention to surgery in the tropics on which he wrote a paper and which he regarded as a branch of medicine of its own. In 1889 he performed the first colotomy operation in Hong Kong watched by a team of doctors; he also persuaded Chinese patients to have ovarsectionomies. He never underestimated the dangers of these operations; he knew that if the patients lived they would turn to Western medicine, if they died, their relations would turn back to their own. Because of the heat, operations had to be performed with windows wide open and the fact that this was possible without infection to the wound made Cantlie cautious about the totality of Lister's revolution in asepticism, a caution that was proved justified in the First World War. Care had to be taken during operations with patients who suffered from lung ailments, for opium smoking stopped a cough and disguised symptoms. Instruments had to be imported which meant delays or makeshift improvisation; needles and instruments rusted and rubber rotted. One of Cantlie's contributions to medicine was his perfection of surgery for liver abscess (often caused by amoebic dysentery), a method which Manson had invented in Amoy. For years it was described in textbooks as the standard operation, by which pus was drawn off from the liver with needles and tubes; it enabled the surgeon to operate singlehanded or with a coolie holding on to the anaesthetic mask. Without trained nurses the need to be able to work singlehanded was vital. Not infrequently Mabel Cantlie would accompany her husband to act as his nurse, perhaps walking across the island to do so, or when a note arrived one evening at 10.30 p.m. crossing with him to Macao on the last ferry. Cantlie also often escorted the patients himself, back from

Macao or to hospital in the ambulance. This laid great additional burdens upon the doctor's shoulders and in 1888 Cantlie asked Maude Ingall, whose stockbroker brother Francis later married Mabel's sister Lilla, to come out and stay with them in order to nurse. As the first trained private nurse in the colony she was at once caught up in nursing typhoid, fever of all sorts, dysentery and other Eastern diseases, as well as routine confinements and sunstroke. Sir William des Voeux, who engaged her to nurse in Government House, became a convert to the. idea of bringing out nurses from home and, the following year, a party of French nursing sisters were employed for a year in government hospitals to be followed in 1890 by a matron and five sisters from the London teaching hospitals – one of whom learnt to speak Cantonese. When Cantlie opened his hospital on the Peak, Maude Ingall became its matron and, when she returned home, one of these government civil hospital nurses, May Thomson, asked her sister Annie to come out and join her in the Peak Hospital as matron and sister.

The square, gaunt building of the Lock Hospital for Infectious Diseases was greedy for victims, and Cantlie and the other doctors on the Sanitary Board pressed repeatedly for implementation of the bye-laws on sanitation and cleanliness, believing that a step-by-step approach would lead them eventually to be able to deal with the more controversial question of drainage. Meetings were now reported in the press, and the *China Mail* hoped that 'Cantlie's views of advanced medical science, Humphrey's knowledge of practical chemistry, Francis' keen tongue and legal training and Ho Kai's thorough knowledge of the Chinese and their needs ought to keep the Board from doing that which it ought not to do and help it to act wisely'. Unfortunately however, the members who were not civil servants had little or no control over those who were, and recommendations for cleansing and destruction of rubbish were overruled so that Cantlie, Francis and Ho Kai found themselves being asked to rubber stamp decisions which they had not made. Nevertheless, Cantlie did manage to get through his proposal for filter beds being put into the water supply to cut down the ravages of disease and he also persuaded the Government to build a Vaccination Institute at the bottom of the Peak tramway for the manufacture of fresh lymph for smallpox vaccination. He started vaccinating in January 1888 using imported lymph from Saigon and by the end of the year he was also vaccinating babies, although the *Historical and Statistical Abstract* gives the following year as the start of infant vaccination. The Chinese, in fact, had attempted vaccination in the seventeenth century using human pustules and had introduced this to England via Turkey. They had readily adopted Jenner's discovery of calf's lymph, and the East India Company in Macao had been experimenting with vaccination for Europeans for some time, but not realising the importance of fresh lymph they had passed it from arm to arm with disappointing results. Cantlie realised that importing lymph from Saigon was a poor substitute for the island providing its own.

The Hong Kong Medical Society co-ordinated medical research and recorded the demonstrations of diseases given by Royal Navy, army, colonial and private doctors. Cantlie's main contributions were on tropical surgery, liver abscess, sprue, beri beri, cancer and leprosy, but the range of his interest was far-reaching. Sprue, which is catarrh of the alimentary canal, remains one of the most baffling diseases and still the only cure is repatriation to a moderate climate. Mabel's diary records the Governor's wife dying of sprue, undiagnosed after childbirth: 'I fear they have called Hamish in too late'. Cantlie thought it was caused by dirty, adulterated cooking oil. The usual diet was milk, but he recommended doses of rhubarb and arsenic in small quantities as an alleviative and a diet of beef juice and scraped beef (anticipating the high protein diet of liver and meat extract of today), together with hot and cold compresses. Beri beri made its appearance in Hong Kong in 1889. First known in the Straits Settlements, the standard work on it was by a Dutchman which had been translated into French. Mabel Cantlie, in a manner which is no small tribute to the education of girls of her time, now translated this work into English and at her wish it appeared under her husband's name.[2] Hook worm was often present in beri beri and Cantlie demonstrated this relationship to the Medical Society, pointing out that it was common in hot places with poor sanitation. There was a belief among Hong Kong doctors that the Chinese, because of their vegetarianism, did not suffer from cancer. This he demonstrated was false, and time has proved him right. Whether, in his demonstration of epitheliorinden (now epithelioma), it was realised by Cantlie or any of the other doctors that this was cancer of the skin from eye to mouth, it is impossible to judge from the minutes, but he drew the attention of the doctors to an epidemic form of glands in the neck which may, in the light of modern knowledge, have been a sign of nasopharyngeal carcinoma common in South China. He also demonstrated something he had noticed in treating the Chinese after accidents; they carry their ascending frontal or parietal convolutions further forward in the skull than Europeans and can therefore sustain more brain injury in certain parts without loss of function. The doctors played the devil's advocate, never wanting a disease to be accepted as 'new' which was only a manifestation of one already in existence. Both measles and scarlet fever were virulent in Hong Kong and Cantlie wanted this 'tropical measles' classified separately; the doctors said 'No', but time has proved Cantlie right. In his turn, he turned down a suggestion that Hong Kong enteritis was a disease on its own; and his interest in sprue led him to study 'morning diarrhoea', which was prevalent and intractable.

At about this time, Mabel Cantlie not only tired of attending social functions on her own but began to be increasingly concerned about her husband's health. Looking at the formidable list of other diseases about which Cantlie lectured or wrote pamphlets – disseminated sclerosis, influenza (which in Hong Kong was not infrequently a killer disease), virus warts, tuberculosis, dysentery, triple cardiac bruit, haemotemesis and melaena and cheloid growths, it is not difficult to be sympathetic with her point of view. The horrifying nature of Eastern disease was causing him to work harder and harder in order to stem its flood, and she soon began to work as hard as her husband, partly to save him, partly to be at his side. There was between them the deepest of bonds, each knowing the breaking strain of the other, and when that point was reached everything was subordinated to nursing the other back to health. Their love of their fellow men never blinded them to the greatest joy of their lives, their love for one another, while the rock on which they built their lives was their Christian faith. Sundays was almost always church and communion and this gave them, in the midst of death, stability, purpose and hope. At last Cantlie was persuaded by his wife to cut down his work load by giving up general work and concentrating only on consulting. This, however, lasted only a few days, then the diary records that they had started rising at 4.30 a.m. so that he could do his writing and research. His resolutions about not doing general practitioner work lasted the same length of time; anyone in need could count on his help. It was impossible to cage him and his wife never tried to do so again. Instead circumstances now altered which allowed her to work more closely with him. In March 1890 the two elder children left to stay with their grandparents at home in the care of the faithful Nanny Briesley who had accompanied them from London and stayed with the family all her life. To keep children in that climate in those days was to ask for trouble; one after another Eastern disease grasped a new victim. But the knowledge that the decision was the right one did not lessen the heartbreak of parting and Mabel felt very lonely and sad without them. She did not complain, but recorded her feelings in her diary and threw herself into her husband's work as an anaesthetic to forget her loss.

Cantlie had been planning how much better it would be to have his patients under one roof for treatment and observation. Now that his wife had fewer household responsibilities there was an obvious opportunity. As with the College of Medicine, so with the Peak Hospital; it was suddenly conjured out of the air. On 7 March 1890 the diary records: 'We have decided to start a home hospital next Monday. We have taken Dr. Hartigan's house and Maude is to be Matron.' When Monday arrived the diary recorded, 'Very busy with the Hospital. This is the first day of it. Mrs. Gray and a Russian came into it. We have decided to take Major Wilkinson's house and furniture too.' In the arrangements for this hospital Mabel Cantlie displayed a gift for organisation which was to be extremely useful in the First World War. She kept hens to give the patients fresh eggs, made curtains, supervised the kitchen and shopping, aided in the nursing, learnt and practised massage in which the Japanese were the experts, and planted violets on the grave of a young man who died in the hospital, at his heartbroken mother's request. By this time Cantlie was beginning to realise the efficacy of some of the Chinese herbal remedies such as aconite, which helped to bring down temperature in liver abscess; and Mabel Cantlie also started searching for wild flowers and studying botany in order to classify the plants she had found.

Into this hospital came not only European residents but patients from Eastern countries also, including some from Borneo and Japan.

The diary records that Cantlie operated on the eyes of a major-general of the Siamese army (the Prince of Siam was on more than one occasion a visitor at Government House), and that a Chinese woman, Ah Ho, was operated on for ovariotomy, with seven doctors watching Cantlie's work. Twelve days after the operation the dreaded fever set in. Night and day the Cantlies and Maude Ingall nursed her. On 28 August 1890: 'Awake all night with Ah Ho who was very bad. She is better today. Great anxiety as it so important she should get well.' The next day, 'Ah Ho has recovered.' In those days, for dread of disease, no Chinese were allowed on the Peak. The Ho family were outside the rule, but this Ah Ho does not feature in family records. Cantlie was not known for nothing as 'the licensed libertine of medicine', for there was a depth to his sympathy for his fellow men which swept regulations before it. Although by October 1890 he had opened a new ward in the next two houses so that three houses were run together into a substantial unit, nevertheless as far as officialdom was concerned the hospital did not exist. Thus if he did break a rule the facts were not recorded. The site was Rural Building Lot 79. There is no record of Lot 79 in the Land Register, nor in Bruce Shepherd's *Index to Streets and Houses in Hong Kong* where it is the only Lot in the series not mentioned. It remained anonymous until 13 December 1892 when the Government regularised its position by granting a lease retrospectively for seventy-five years. Doctors Hartigan and Stedman took it on from Cantlie but it was still not officially recorded as a hospital until 1902. Inefficiency or wisdom? Cantlie was almost always fortunate in the men he served, who understood and identified with his defence of and desire to serve those less fortunate than himself. It is clear from the diary just how much kindness, hospitality and support was given to the Cantlies by successive governors. The Cantlies' hard work, their humanity, love and loyalty to their own country and to the Chinese population of Hong Kong enabled them to waive the rules and yet retain the support of those in authority. Lady Des Voeux visited the Peak Hospital shortly after it was opened, and her hospitality and that of the Governor both at Government House and Mountain Lodge seemed bottomless. Asked to dinner, the Cantlies would be pressed to stay the night and, thinking of the Peak tram ride and the walk home, it is surprising they never accepted.

In November 1888 Cantlie had begun St John Ambulance instruction to officers and seamen on board ship and in the same month he started a ladies' class in the City Hall. Cards were sent out: 'St. John's Ambulance Lecture to Officers and Seamen. First Aid to the Injured. Dr. James Cantlie, F.R.C.S. Course of Lectures commences November 13th. Ladies Classes also. Names to Mrs. Cantlie.' This series of lectures was reported in the *China Mail* on 14 November. Three years later, after lectures and examinations successfully conducted to Europeans, the syllabus was widened to include nursing, and on 24 October 1891 the first Chinese lady joined the classes. It was an obvious way of getting the home nursing which the Chinese population of Hong Kong so desperately needed. In July 1890 Cantlie also started a series of lectures to the Hong Kong police and, although these lectures and examinations are no longer included in their records they were given wide coverage in the *China Mail* not only enabling the police to be effectively trained for emergencies but also improving their public image. On completion, the police made Cantlie a handsome presentation.

Upon his arrival in Hong Kong Cantlie had joined the Volunteers as Surgeon Captain and while training stretcher bearer units he particularly directed his work to the Chinese medical students who provided four bearer units which were present at all the Volunteer demonstrations. The first mention of this ambulance work was in June 1888 when Mabel Cantlie presented the prizes at a Review of the Ambulance Section, inspected by the Surgeon General; and at the Jubilee Review on 23 January 1891 Cantlie's Ambulance Corps of Chinese students was said by the *China Mail* to have 'formed a conspicuous feature of the review'. On 24 October 1891 Major-General Barker, Acting Governor, distributed certificates to St John Ambulance pupils including seventy-five members of the Police Force. 'St John's Ambulance Association,' he said, 'the modern representatives of the ancient Order of the Knights Templar of Jerusalem, is now a flourishing body doing very great good in aiding the alleviation of human suffering . . . The members of the Chinese Medical College . . . can do an immense amount of good in teaching others how to help the injured as well as doing so themselves, thus ameliorating the distress which must necessarily exist owing to the want of surgical aid in the Chinese Empire.' Cantlie's demonstrations of first aid and ambulance work again brought him into close contact with the military doctors who started to call him in for consultations. This caused temporary ill feeling until, as the diary records, Cantlie called upon the General and pointed out to him the importance of preserving the vital link between these two parts of the profession, a link which has made a major contribution to the alleviation of suffering in peace and in war.

Increasingly, now, Mabel Cantlie was becoming concerned about her husband's health; only one week after the opening of the Peak Hospital he had been taken ill with Hong Kong influenza and kidney trouble. They therefore took a short holiday in Japan, her description of which was published in the *Elgin Courier* on 2 December 1890:

We drove and walked through beautifully cultivated country, with crops of bright green paddy, masses of flowering yellow rape and, above all, here and there a cherry or peach tree, one mass of lovely blossom. The blossom of these trees is the largest I have ever seen and the beautiful climate keeps it on the tree for some time. At last we came to the rapids and got into long deeply built boats. One Jap took his place in the bows with a long pole, three men stood at one side and rowed and another man steered in the stern. Now began a most exciting journey. The water was high so it was more dangerous. I must confess we were a little astonished at the second rapid, for it looked impossible to get down without being smashed to bits and our men in the bows had a look of great anxiety. We dashed down it at a fearful rate and had no wish to do it again. We had plenty more but not quite so bad. The foliage on either side of the towering hills, on either side of the river, was so beautiful as to defy description. The young maples were out, some dark crimson and some golden yellow, and these mixing with pink and white blossoms made an unforgettable picture. At Arashyma there were some hundreds of Japanese quietly enjoying themselves and worshipping the beautiful blossoms. Some of them were in little mat booths, eating their tempting looking food, others were rowing on the river, some playing musical instruments, a number sketching, but all were happy, very quiet and intensely polite to each other. They all bow to each other when they meet, even the tiny children and they do just the same to Europeans.

They then went on to see the snow-clad mountain of Fuji, the great bronze figure of Buddha ('a wonderful image and the face inspires one with great respect'), then to the temples at Kikko with their beautiful rainbow-tinted marbles and the soft red colour of lacquer, then to Kobe and the end of the holiday.

Unfortunately the tour had been too strenuous, for no sooner had he returned to Hong Kong than Cantlie again had to take to his bed with high temperature and kidney trouble, followed by a badly strained eye. 'I am terribly anxious about him,' was his wife's comment, 'I wish our time here was over.' There and then she decided that if her husband did not get well soon, they would return home in two years. She reckoned without her husband. His answer to his ill health was to unpack the bacteriological appliances ordered from home and, while he dashed out to see patients, Mabel Cantlie found herself setting them out for him and preparing soup, potatoes and bread paste on which to breed germs in the kitchen. He then sat down and wrote to Sir Joseph Fayrer, Chairman of the Leprosy Commission, suggesting that he visit all the leper colonies of China. So much for his kidney trouble and the idea of going home; there were things to do in Hong Kong. From the start the plight of the lepers had been one of his chief concerns. The official policy of Hong Kong towards lepers was described by Mr Hugh MacCallum, Sanitary Superintendent, as 'gentle persuasion with money compensation to return to the mainland'. The method sometimes worked but there were, nevertheless, lepers in Hong Kong whose numbers hid a higher unrecorded total since the lepers, fearing deportation, hid their disease. Cantlie did not think it just to return to the mainland those whose disease had been contracted in Hong Kong, and said so. The first mention in the diary of his working on the disease was in June 1889. In his demonstrations of cases to the Hong Kong Medical Society he pointed out that it was impossible to say there were no lepers in Hong Kong, since in its early stages the disease was undetectable; also all the lepers who went to the Chinese Tung Wa Hospital were unreported. In the two and a half years since the opening of the Alice Memorial Hospital, 125 lepers had been treated as patients. Cantlie pointed out that leprosy was contagious during incubation which could be spread over months or years, and that prolonged intimate contact passed the disease on at all stages. Once the disease was apparent the Chinese shunned the lepers for fear of contagion. Though the disease was popularly classified into two types, wet and dry, Cantlie stated that the cases he had seen were mixed, tubercular and anaesthetic. He argued therefore against this classi-fication, saying that lack of sensation was present almost always initially and that, if it was not, it quickly appeared once the swellings had started. Although there were no reported epidemics, he observed that it struck certain houses and quoted the XLV Book of Leviticus, which spoke of houses needing cleansing. Although not hereditary, Cantlie believed that it could be contracted prenatally.

In December 1890 the Cantlies set out on a tour of leper villages round Canton, taking Sun Yat Sen with them as interpreter. Mabel Cantlie's diary records how 'they had happy looks inspite of the terrible disease . . . Gave them plenty of cigarettes and five dollars. Poor creatures, how pleased they were.' They went on to a leper island, 'It was very sad, for the men and women were parted poor things'. Back in Hong Kong they went out on a launch with Mr MacCallum to look for an island suitable for the isolation and treatment of lepers and, while a decision was pending, Cantlie inoculated those in Victoria with Koch's fluid, used in the treatment of tuberculosis. It is known now that TB serum does give some protection against leprosy, but the lepers' first reaction was to develop fever, and the Cantlies started visiting them regularly and taking them presents on Sundays, beginning at Easter. On 27 June the *China Mail* 'blew' the story, describing how they had visited lepers on the island of St John. This must have been Chung-chau island, ten miles from Hong Kong, which had finally been chosen for a leper settlement, and this is corroborated by Dr Skertchley in an address to the Royal Society of Queensland on 6 March 1897; but why the press referred to it as St John remains a mystery. The diary only refers to it as 'leper island'. Probably Cantlie hoped that St John Ambulance Association might interest themselves in the lepers which would not have been possible, as he was shortly to find out. Years later a hospital called St John's Hospital was receiving tuberculosis patients on Chung-chau island. Coincidence or the end of a story? No one will ever know. The press reports of June described how Cantlie had taken specimens from the lepers for analysis to send them home. The publication caused a flurry. The wife of a British merchant said that if Cantlie visited the lepers she would not consult him as a doctor. Her fear was understandable but, by curious coincidence, she later sent to him for examination an amah who was attending her children and who had lost sensation in an arm and had leprosy in the early stages. The last mention of leprosy in the diary was on 17 July. It was now im-possible to continue with these visits. Meanwhile, however, the Cantlies were working round the clock to complete a paper on leprosy which was to be submitted to the Leprosy Commission in a competition. It was a monograph of monumental length which won first prize and a request from the judges that it be expanded and published as a book.[3]

Four years had now passed since the Cantlies had arrived in Hong Kong and at last Mabel Cantlie persuaded her husband to take a proper long holiday in India where their friend Evatt was stationed in Quetta. Calling at Colombo they went to Bombay and Madras, seeing temples and palaces and a procession in which elephants walked on their knees, while at the same time Cantlie broadened his medical horizons, calling at the medical colleges at Bombay, visiting hospitals and being given research specimens. Many of the doctors they met had been Cantlie's students at Charing Cross. In Quetta they were entertained by Evatt to balls, reviews and races. They made an expedition through the newly-made Kojak tunnel to the Fort of Chaman and another to the top of the Trojak mountain. Then they went to Lahore and Delhi, saw the Taj Mahal, and thence to Cawnpore and Lucknow, crossing by train to Calcutta through scenery enhanced by moonlight. At Darjeeling they walked twelve miles before breakfast to climb a peak to see Mount Everest. Renewed in health, refreshed in mind and impatient to commence work once more, they returned to Hong Kong. Here they found a letter from Manson saying he was thinking of returning to Hong Kong and would once more like to take back his place in the practice from Cantlie. Although she wanted to return home, Mabel Cantlie pressed her husband not to re-sell his share in the practice for less than he paid for it, and on 1 June the diary records, 'A letter from Manson to say he is writing articles for a book on Oriental Medicine. Poor Hamish. I am afraid this will end his scheme for one.' Cantlie's book on leprosy had been for him only a beginning; he had already been planning to turn all his previous papers and research into a published book. Two weeks later a second letter arrived saying that Manson had decided not to return to Hong Kong. It was a decision which was to influence Cantlie's life.

CHAPTER SIX

Medicine in China – the Bubonic Plague

In July 1892 the first two students completed their training successfully as Licentiates of the College of Medicine. One of these was Dr Sun, who passed with high distinction. Arguments that he used medicine as a cloak for revolution are based on writings at the end of his life, when disaster and disappointment had darkened his viewpoint, for these hardly accord with the very great effort he put into his medical studies. Examinations at the College were stiff, and Professor Lo Hsiang-lin records that by 1901 the School had produced only twelve graduates, with twenty students either failing or dropping out. If revolution had filled his mind, Sun could have joined these ranks or been content with a pass. Temperamentally a gentle man, if the reform of China had been possible by any means, Dr Sun would have been a reformer, never a revolutionary.

The academic results of the College were produced by unremitting labour on the part of the unpaid staff. 'Dissaffection and apathy,' said Cantlie in his address at the prize-giving quoted in the *China Mail* of 23 July, 'have robbed us of many excellent men and caused us to stagger under a load which at times threatened to crush our hope and our existence. As usual the men of will and purpose have won.' The doctors, he said, were still instructing free of charge in a course of study intended to be identical to that of British medical schools, and Mr Belilios had offered a new site and building if the Government would match his generosity with 40,000 dollars. 'At this moment,' he continued,

we remember the words of the Chinese proverb that the gem cannot be polished without friction nor man perfected without adversity. Steadiness of purpose is perhaps the most constant characteristic of the Chinese. Time shakes them not from their intent nor weakens the ardour of their understanding. The passing away of one generation but endows the theme with the sacred fire of heredity. We have taught them without pecuniary reward or extraneous help and freely we hand our offering to the great Empire of China, where science is as yet unknown, where the ignorance of our own medieval times is current, where the astrologer stalks abroad with the belief that he is a physician, where the art of surgery has never been attempted, and where thousands of women suffer and die by the charmed potions of the witchcraft practices of so called obstetricians. The general effect of work done will stretch beyond this small island. Here and at the Treaty Ports suffering can be relieved by the most advanced methods. It is only at the door of this huge Empire that science knocks. Respectfully, for she honours the occupants. What hope has she of entrance? Will she be asked to approach at the back door? Not so, for the Emperor himself has succumbed to her influence. No other than Li Hung Chang, the Bismark of China, is her patron, one of the graduates of the College of Medicine at Tientsin. 'Give us science first,' Li Hung Chang wrote, 'and all the rest will follow.'

Turning to the students he again called on them to carry forth the message of modern science, but also to bring back knowledge of herbal remedies and plants for Western botanists, chemists and physiologists to catalogue, reduce to chemical formulae and test their potency on nervous and vascular systems, thus blending old and new. Cantlie realised that on Li's attitude to the new medicine the future of the young Licentiates would hang. Although the modernisation of science and medicine in China took years to fulfil, towards the end of the nineteenth century beginnings had been made and by the 1920s modern surgery was being undertaken in many missionary hospitals; while the barefoot doctor in the paddy fields today treads the path of first aid in tropical medicine which Cantlie was soon to envisage for him. In return Western science has recognised the significance of acupuncture and the efficacy of some herbal remedies. From whence, asked Cantlie, would come the motor power for this undertaking? 'From the inspiration of King and country . . . The crest of the College is a dragon with the quarterings of the Royal Standard of Britain.' Idealism shone through the Governor's tribute to the medical profession with its qualities of 'pity, sympathy and love'. 'No ministry,' he said, 'is so nearly connected with Christianity.'[1]

At a dinner that evening given by Cantlie at the Mount Austin Hotel, Mr Stewart Lockhart, Colonial Secretary, took up the Governor's theme:

At the start the difficulties seemed insuperable, but men came from a country not recognising difficulties as insuperable. Cantlie is possessed by a love of a profession second to none, unselfishness is characterstic of the profession, but in him it is very marked. Everyone present will bear me out when I say that it is to a great extent owing to Mr. Cantlie that the College is in existence today. I think I am not wrong in saying that it was at his suggestion that the College of Medicine first became a quantity worthy of consideration. It was at his suggestion that the meeting was first called to consider the matter. Dr. Cantlie is like all Scotchmen, he does not care to hear his praises sung.[2]

In his speech of reply Cantlie suggested that an agreed period of study should qualify students from the College to enter a medical school in Great Britain. He also gave a warning about the intentions of other nations, jealous of the special friendship between the Chinese and British peoples, and particularly of Russian intentions in the area. Dr Sun also made a prudent prediction as to the extent the College would be able to influence medicine, sanitation and hygiene in China, for he knew the mind of the Manchus and suspected their determination to resist reform. 'A wise ruler,' wrote Cantlie when Sun assumed the Presidency in 1911,

would have seized the opportunity to inaugurate some of the re-forms that China stood in need of. But the Manchu dynasty, of Tartar origin and resented as foreign by the Chinese, was in the hands of the Empress Dowager, the former concubine Yehonala, whose cruelty was later to deny medical assistance to her dying son and drive her pregnant daughter-in-law to suicide by electing another infant Emperor. Demoralised by the corrupt eunuch sys-tem, with the Mandarins in Peking withdrawn and remote, the Government was unable to respond to the anarchy and lawlessness in the country as the crying need for reform was pressed daily stronger upon them.[3]

It is reported that following the first graduation, Cantlie tried and failed to arrange a meeting between Li and Sun. Had this meeting taken place the future for both of them and for China might have been different. The position of Dr Sun and his fellow Licentiate was there-fore precarious. They were not equipped with a British diploma and, although allowed to practise in Hong Kong, could not give birth or death certificates, nor have the same protection in law as the British doctors. Having failed to get the College incorporated, which would have meant recognition in law, Cantlie suggested a shorter course at the College, qualifying students to enter a British medical school. This was not accepted either and it was not until 1896 that the Governor recommended that the College be recognised by ordinance and the Licentiates given equal status with British doctors. Still it was ten years before this advice was acted upon. Dr Sun, therefore, in 1892 was faced with the choice of returning to China to practise Western surgery, which his country did not recognise, or staying in Hong Kong with a diploma which did not receive full recognition from the country awarding it. He decided to compromise; to go to Ching Hu Hospital in Macao where the Chinese offered him a wing in which to practise Western medicine and surgery. Macao with its Portuguese traditions, ornate balustrades, cobbled streets and verandas dating back to the seventeenth century, gave Sun a very different picture of European life to the squares and gardens of Hong Kong, which as a young man he had so admired. But it was near to his home in Kwantung, and he was in sympathy with the work that had been done there by the London Missionary Society and others in setting up free dispensaries for the poor at which Cantlie had sometimes helped, and following these examples he decided to set up his own dispensaries as well as conducting surgery and medicine in the hospital. His diploma conferred both titles on him but, wrote Cantlie, 'When major operations had to be done I went on several occasions to Macao to assist him, and there in the presence of the governors of the hospital he performed important operations requiring skill, coolness of judgement and dexterity. Why did I go this journey to Macao to help this man?'[4] Cantlie explained his reasons in terms of Sun's personal magnetism and qualities of leadership, but he modestly did not mention what must have been the key reason for going, the expertise that he could provide in the battle to save the life of the patient and therefore the future of Western medicine and surgery in China. In spite of all efforts, however, Dr Sun was to experience problems in his practice in Macao. Indeed because of his very success the Portuguese physicians may have seen in him a professional threat, for he could have been the first of many Licentiates from Hong Kong, and after six months they persuaded the authorities to bar him and other Licentiates from the College of Medicine from practising in Macao.

It is unprofitable to ask whether Sun would have devoted his life to medicine if his qualification had been fully recognised in Hong Kong or Western medicine accepted in China, because if the latter had been the case there would not have been so pressing a need for reform. Lindsay Ride, in an essay on Sun Yat Sen, asked what his foreign medical education contributed to his political achievements and answered by saying that medical training was a link in a chain of events. 'It kept him in touch with the masses whom it was his sole aim to help, it trained him in the sphere of human relations. He began his adult career as the saviour of the sick and finished as the saviour of his people.'[5] Sun now moved to Canton and combined his knowledge of Western medicine with the old methods of herbalism; he was nearer to his relatives and started making contact with Chinese youth to discuss political reform. He describes in his book *Kidnapped in London* how he first became acquainted with a political movement called the Young China Movement:

> Its objects were so wise, so modest and so hopeful that my sympathies were at once enlisted in its behalf, and I believed I was doing my best to further the interests of my country by joining it. The idea was to bring about a peaceful reformation and we hoped by forwarding modest schemes of reform to the Throne, to initiate a form of government more consistent with modern requirements. The prime essence of the movement was the establishment of a form of constitutional government to supplement the old-fashioned, corrupt and worn out system under which China is groaning.[6]

Comparison between the justice and order in Hong Kong and the lawlessness and anarchy of his own country had always struck Sun during his student days where, as so often at universities, there had

been much discussion among the Chinese on how improvements in the
government of China could be brought about. 'After my lectures,' he
wrote years later,

> I used to stroll the streets of Hong Kong. The city impressed me a
> great deal, the orderly crowds, the artistic work at every turn and
> look. During vacations I returned to my own country home in
> Heungshan. Every time I left Hong Kong I felt the difference. Each
> time I arrived home I had to be my own policeman, my own pro-
> tector. The first thing I had to do was to look after my rifle to see how
> much ammunition was left. I had to prepare for accidents at night. I
> began to compare both places. It was not very far to my home, which
> was fifty miles away; I thought of the beautiful streets, the artistic
> parks and wondered why Englishmen could do such a thing on this
> barren rock within 70 or 80 years. Why could not China in the last
> four thousand years have a place like this?[7]

All through his years in Hong Kong, as well as winning awards in his
medical studies Sun had been continuing with his studies of Chinese
classics until late into the night, undertaking this intensive work for two
reasons – first, to be able to present a petition for reform and, secondly,
to be able to communicate with the gentlemen reformers of Peking,
who understood no other language.

There is no record of any contact between Cantlie and Sun during
Sun's years in Canton nor is it likely or possible that there would have
been, for the sad truth was that by now Cantlie's health was suffering
considerably from the climate and years of overwork, leaving little time
for extra duties or leisure. In the autumn of 1892 he was suddenly
struck down with what was probably acute appendicitis. The doctors
clustered round his hospital bed and agreed that if it was an appendix
they dared not operate although he, the surgeon, could have operated
on them. Mabel Cantlie's diary records how she shared the nursing
with the sisters and that, in spite of morphia, the pain was so great that
he was growing slowly weaker. Once he seemed to have turned the
corner, but hope was short lived, 'My darling gave me a bad fright with
one turn of intense pain. My spirits are gone tonight. I feel very
unhappy. I dare not think for my strength is giving way.' In spite of
Cantlie's robust constitution and Mabel Cantlie's optimism his heart
was slowly growing weaker. Then suddenly the entry, 'Hamish slept
naturally.' He was out of danger. Mabel Cantlie was seven months
pregnant and the strain had been great. At the end of November her
third son, Neil, was born, and his happy and lovable temperament was
one of her greatest joys during the rest of her stay in Hong Kong. No
sooner was Christmas past than Cantlie succumbed to another attack of
pain, but mercifully less violent. Also taking their time and constrain-
ing their activities was the state of their finances which, like their
health, was suffering from the unpaid work that they were doing. To
save money they let their house and moved into the hospital. This

arrangement lasted until a typhoon gave them a hideous night, with wind and lashing rain, and Cantlie realised that it was not fair to ask his wife to undertake the responsibilities of a hospital if he was attending patients elsewhere. 'Today,' the diary reads, 'we heard the typhoon coming. The wind rose at 12.30 p.m. From 6 to 10 we had a terrific typhoon and the house was nearly pulled to pieces. Fortunately there were only six patients in the hospital and we got them all into two rooms. I was terrified. Hamish saved much of the dispensary by making a hole through the floor and getting the boy cook to hand down the bottles.' Cantlie realised that he was imposing too great a strain upon his wife and in order that there should be no repeat of this disastrous night he now appointed Mr and Mrs Ewens as cartaker and matron and moved his family into a hotel. This meant that Mabel Cantlie's commitments were reduced but their financial anxieties continued.

Nothing could curb Cantlie's generosity. There were foreign communities in Hong Kong and, amongst them, Cantlie, with his readiness to answer every call, was in special request. He also won favour with the poorer classes whose ailments he treated either for nothing or next to nothing, while with more affluent patients his habit of not charging or under-charging continued unabated. The rich Chinese, however, learnt a way of countering this by arriving with presents and the diaries speak of the generosity of all rich patients in Hong Kong, both to Cantlie and his wife.

In all these circumstances Cantlie would have been wise to cut his public life to the minimum. But, as at Charing Cross, he played an active part in running and raising societies. Shortly after his arrival in Hong Kong he started a successful Reel Club, was much in demand as a speaker at Burns' dinners, was an active member of the St Andrews Society, a popular Father Christmas at Garrison parties, and three times re-started the defunct literary society with the intention of one day turning it into a Reading Room and library. There were two existing libraries in Hong Kong: the Morrison Education Society which had 5,000 volumes, a number not increased since 1865, of which only certain volumes could be borrowed and the Hong Kong Club library which was available to members only. Cantlie's idea was a library which would be both public and circulating on the same lines as in his village of Dufftown.[8] In 1893 he abandoned his attempts to revitalise the Literary Society and formed a successful new society called the Odd Volumes Society, which was literary, scientific and debating. Again he had as his prototype the evening debating societies of the north-east of Scotland, held in the parish schools and organised by the young men of the village, in which the minister and schoolmaster took part and in which the standard of debate was high — 'Do you think Nelson or Napoleon the greater leader of men?' was a typical subject and clearly one involving research. Cantlie believed that good communication was an art, and one that was vital to the proper functioning of any society. 'The art of speaking,' he said on the opening night of the Society on 3 March 1893, is still behind that of writing. By the pen the poet, novelist and dramatist can produce marvels of beauty and wondrous flights of rhetoric, whereas the art of speaking is in its infancy. The first requisite in debate is that of self control – he that ruleth his speech is better than he who ruleth a city, self control is the truest, grandest monarchy, readily acquired in debate. We must first conquer ourselves, if we aspire to greatness.

He then outlined his plans for a Public Library and on 21 April, in the City Hall, the Governor was present at an exhibition attended by 300 people, dressed as books, held in order to promote interest in the scheme.

At the outset the press was excluded from the meetings of the Odd Volume Society and therefore invented stories about what had been said. When Cantlie drew attention to the need for a university in Hong Kong, the journalists reported that he wanted a university in Hong Kong for Europeans. So on 17 March 1894 Cantlie published his text in the *China Mail*. 'The only means that the Chinese have of gaining a European education,' he said, 'is by learning a foreign language. Teach English. What is wanted is a residential College for Chinese where English alone is spoken to make them bilingual.' Cantlie's hopes were of course to be fulfilled, for out of the College of Medicine for the Chinese was to grow, in the course of time, the University of Hong Kong. Among the interesting lectures which Cantlie delivered to the Society was one on 'Athletics in the Tropics', how to keep fit and healthy in hot, humid climates. (Unfortunately neither of the Cantlies followed the advice given so successfully to others.) He spoke of the importance of evening exercise and siesta, saying that in the morning when body temperature was low it was better in heat to ride, which was good for liver troubles. He gave pride of place to the dancing of reels and polkas, which caused an increased natural intake of air; climbing hills or stairs did not stimulate this natural increase in the same way, but he outlined a technique for doing both without becoming short of breath. The Governor, a constant visitor to the Society, said in his speech of thanks that it was indeed an unselfish doctor who would explain ways of not becoming ill – the beginnings of preventive medicine.

By now it was the Cantlies and not their patients who needed preventive medicine; both were suffering from blood poisoning, Mabel Cantlie from a mosquito bite which had become a chronic boil and Cantlie from a hand which he had cut during an operation and which caused acute pain and high temperature. This time it was their friends who insisted on a holiday, one of whom offered to look after 2-year-old Neil in her home on the Peak. On 2 May the Cantlies set off for North China and Japan visiting Shanghai, Tientsin and Peking. 'We started from Tientsin', runs the diary, 'on ponies for Peking. Went twenty miles and lunched at a Chinese rest-house and on again to another where we tried to sleep but the noise was awful from the Chinese carters and their ponies. Nothing to see but mud villages.' In

Peking Cantlie recounted how his guide explained that the guns in the forts were painted pieces of wood. 'The war god,' said the guide, 'is a very simple person and thinks these guns are proper guns. Consequently Peking is quite safe.' This story brought home to Cantlie the influence the idols had on the Chinese and how they believed they could escape retribution so long as a pretence of reverence was made. After falling under the spell of Chinese art in Peking – bronzes, lacquer, blackwood and porcelain – they started for the Great Wall. 'Up at 4.30. It was a lovely morning fresh and a delicious breeze. The pass has many fortifications, also a fine gateway with an arch with carvings of the god of war and seven different languages on it, to prevent the Tartars going through. The Great Wall is very wonderful, very high and wide and made with much care of stone and huge bricks. The view from it is very fine; rode thirty five miles.' The next day, after visiting the Ming Tombs they rode thirty-eight miles back to Peking and, instead of retiring early, dined and danced in the home of Sir Robert Hart of the Chinese Customs. Mabel Cantlie brought back a brick from the Great Wall which afterwards reposed in a blackwood frame in their London home to prove that she had fulfilled her childhood dream of sitting like her grandfather, James Bayliss, on the Great Wall of China. Next they sailed to Japan, and thence to Korea, Vladivostok and back to Nagasaki where, on 5 June, they were greeted with the news that the bubonic plague had struck in Hong Kong.

Although in the previous January of 1894 cases of plague had been reported in Canton, Hong Kong had so far escaped unharmed. Dr Mary Niles had published an article in the *China Medical Missionary Journal* saying that rats had died in infected houses and that the Chinese who escaped the disease lived in upper stories, on the water or in foreign settlements. They were, of course, out of the range of rat infection but, as with the mosquito in malaria, the facts were recorded but the connection not made. In six months in Canton 40,000 people died. In Hong Kong, where the disease struck on 10 May, only 3,000 died. But the island reacted in a manner very different to its earlier decimation by disease, not only because of the terrible sufferings of the black plague but because its effects were exacerbated by the custom of ancestor worship, causing the Chinese to try and protect their stricken dead from the authorities. Macabre stories circulated of Mah Jong parties where the living members of the family propped up their dead members at the table to escape the notice of visiting inspectors. Dr J. Lowson's Report on the plague in Hong Kong, published in 1895, gives a horrifying description of entering one such plague-ridden house:

On a miserable sodden matting soaked with abominations there were four forms stretched out. One was dead, the tongue black and protruding. The next had muscular twitchings and was in a semi comatose condition . . . In searching for a bubo we found a huge mass of glands extending from Poupart's ligaments to the knee joint. This patient was beyond the stage of wild delirium. Sores covered the teeth and were visible between the parted and blackened lips. Another sufferer, a female child about ten years old, lay in the accumulated filth of apparently two or three days, unable to speak owing to the presence of enlarged glands. The fourth was wildly delirious and was constantly vomiting. The attendant – the grand-mother of the child – had a temperature of 103F and could only crawl from one end of the cellar to the other. She was wet through, and was herself doomed.[9]

At the outset the only staff upon whom the Colonial Surgeon could call for help were the superintendents, wardmasters and nurses at the government hospitals. The hospital ship *Hygeia* was commandeered, but in the first few days many of the attendants had slipped over the side and disappeared. The police, under Captain Superintendent F. H. May, and the Army Medical Department came forward to offer their services. Four more hospitals were opened, including one at the police barracks and one in the slaughter house. The Shropshires and the Engineers volunteered their help and, with the police, did valiant work entering the plague-infested houses to cleanse and limewash. Many succumbed to the plague, many lost their lives, for 'they were exposed to a concentration of contagion. The houses were of the vilest kind of habitation, small, windowless, reeking with filth and excretions. The soldiers had to use spade and shovel to dig down into the accumulated layers of dirt on the floors of the houses and throw it into the street.'[10] The Governor later presented survivors with gold medals specially struck in Britain to honour their work. Closing orders were put on severely infected houses by the Sanitary Board, from which Cantlie had resigned early in the year.

On being informed on their arrival in Nagasaki that the plague was raging in Hong Kong the Cantlies telegraphed and while waiting for a boat on 7 June they visited the beautiful scenery of the inland sea. On 18 June the diary records: 'Arrived in Hong Kong. Streets very deserted as plague is very bad. Hamish rushed off to Hospital at once to see the Black Plague. I began to make soup for plague germs to grow on. Neil and I did so enjoy each other. He is so sweet.' One of the Cantlies' gifts was that in the midst of death they could see life, and this shines through all their writings. However grave a crisis or heart-breaking a tragedy they always seemed able to look beyond, to notice the beauties of the world and the goodness of their fellow men; not only was there always tomorrow, which brought hope, but also some-thing for which to give thanks today. Since the resident doctors were stretched to their limit to cope with the immediate crisis and had no time for research, a Japanese team of doctors arrived in Hong Kong to try and discover the bacillus. Dr Yersin, a French doctor from the Pasteur Institute in Saigon, also arrived to undertake research and on his return Cantlie threw in his lot with him. 'Everyone welcomed us back', the diary records. 'Hamish is beginning to find bacillus. He is always working at the plague with Dr. Yersin. We lent him our im-mersion lens as he had not one.' Dr Simpson's *Report on the Plague*[11] records that the bacillus was discovered on 14 June by Dr Kitasato, a Japanese, and that later Dr Yersin made an independent and like discovery. On 24 June Cantlie entertained the Japanese research team to luncheon, together with four other doctors including Dr Lowson, whose work during the outbreak brought him the task of writing the report for the Governor.

By this time both the Governor and the Sanitary Board were being criticised for not enforcing the recommendations of the Chadwick Report of 1882, which had included provision for pure air, water and light, the necessity of removing excretia before it putrified and entered wells, the keeping down of subsoil to three feet and the laying of drains. Although the Report recognised the dangers of the scavenging system it had accepted it subject to these restrictions, because it knew the outcry that would follow amongst the Chinese if it was prevented. What the writers of the Report did not appreciate was that even the enforcement of these requirements would cause an outcry among the Chinese and that the Sanitary Board, being only advisory, had no powers to overcome the resistance that it would meet. This had been the comment in the diary within a few weeks of Cantlie's appointment. The European population of Hong Kong blamed the insanitary conditions for the outbreak and spread of plague, and this opinion was backed by many of the doctors who regarded them as the prime cause. On 6 July Cantlie therefore caused a storm with a letter to the *China Mail* pointing out that insanitary conditions were not the direct cause of the plague.

At a period when sanitary blame is being bestowed broadcast upon all and sundry, it is well to consider what evidence we have before us as to the sanitary conditions of the colony. The epidemic of bubonic plague is ascribed by public opinion to be due to the bad sanitary state, or in other words had our sanitary conditions not been defective we would not have had the plague. This will scarcely bear the light of commonsense or scientific investigation. The epidemic is put down to overcrowding and bad drainage systems, choked drains, evil smelling drains and so forth ... Bad drainage causes a train of diseases, diphtheria, tonsilitis, drain throat, diarrhoea, typhoid. We had had none of these present in epidemic form before May 1894. I am not of the opinion that plague is a product of evil drainage. It is caused by a specific poisoning imported from Canton city as yet unknown. That bad drains may aggravate the disease once it is set agoing everyone believes ... The second cause of plague popularly assigned is overcrowding. The diseases arising from overcrowding are pthisis, typhus, diarrhoea, dysentery, septic pneumonia ... Typhus fever is directly caused by overcrowding. We have never in this colony had evidence hitherto of the prevalence of typhus by overcrowding ... For 8 or 9 months of the year the windows and doors are shut but draughts from ill fitting tiles etc. whistle through the house. Plague is an imported pest.

It was an outspoken letter, the contents of which were later to be proved true, and it defended the Government as vehemently as did Cantlie's officially-commissioned inquiry and report on the graves of the victims, in which he gave details of the depth of burials and the amount of quick-lime used and fully endorsed the measures taken by the Government regarding both, which he felt to be sufficient. Never one to trim his sails to the wind his defence was all the more effective, but he came in for much criticism. Nevertheless, on 10 July the *China Mail* commented, 'It may be the strenuous exertions of the cleansing corps, it may be the weather or it may be the joss-pidgin, or floods of debate or Dr. Cantlie himself, but the death total is falling, three figures have dropped to two.'

Instead of directing its energies towards discovering the bacillus, the colony had been caught up in controversy about the cause and spread of the disease, thus necessitating the calling in of foreign research teams and causing fresh arguments afterwards as to why this was necessary. The truth was that the Hong Kong doctors were over-stretched, that laboratory facilities were inadequate (hence the germ culture, plague, leprosy and other bacilli in the Cantlies' kitchen), the Sanitary Board had insufficient powers and there was no Medical Officer of Health. The casualties among the teams of doctors, nurses, police, soldiers and other helpers were very high. Three of the Japanese doctors working with Kitasato contracted the disease and were sent to the hospital ship *Hygeia*, where Cantlie visited them daily. One died, but the others recovered and attended a dinner given by Cantlie on 3 August which ended characteristically with the Japanese and British joining hands and singing Auld Lang Syne. On 18 August 1894 a report appeared in the *British Medical Journal* of specimens submitted by Cantlie which were microscopic preparations of the softened material taken from the liver and spleen of a mouse infected with plague. On 25 August the *BMJ* printed the first of many articles and booklets by Cantlie on plague. It described its signs and symptoms, the incubation period of five to eight days, ideas on methods of contagion and suggested remedies. These observations were included and expanded into his lecture in 1896 to the Epidemiological Society published by the *BMJ* in January 1897, and into his book on plague in 1900. 'The intestine,' he said, 'is the means of the poison finding exitus.' He noticed and recorded in the *BMJ* of 25 August 1894 that the soldiers infected were those digging out the filth on the floors and not those inspecting, whitewashing or fumigating. 'The poison emanates from the ground, according to the Chinese.'[12] It was here that the rat flea dwelt, amongst the filth accumulated on the floor, but although Cantlie's attention had been so closely drawn towards the rat, he had not yet understood the significance of the flea in its fur. 'The height of the animal from the ground,' he went on, 'affects the order of the seized . . . a man being the tallest . . . is the last to be seized.' 'Rats,' he added, 'may be the actual carriers of the disease to human beings.' Cantlie later recounted how, during that deadly summer in Hong Kong, a Scots missionary came to see him and drew his attention to the First Book of Samuel which, in the fourth, fifth and sixth chapters, contains references to the plague. 'And the Philistines took the ark of God and brought it from Eben-ezer into Ashdod.' (Chapter V, Verse 1) 'but the hand of the Lord was heavy upon them of Ashdod, and he destroyed them and smote them with emerods.' (Verse 6). The ark was then moved from Ashdod to Gath, and again in Verse 9, 'the hand of the Lord was against the city with a very great destruction, and he smote the men of the city and they had emerods in their secret parts.' In the following Chapter VI the Philistines decided to return the ark to Israel, returning also a 'trespass offering' of 'five golden emerods and five golden mice'. Understanding broke in Cantlie's mind, the emerods were the buboes of the plague and the mice were sent also because the Philistines knew that mice or rats were associated with plague. Cantlie reports how he went to Yersin and told him what he had read. 'He was inclined to be sceptical, but I made him listen, and he at last realised that the biblical association of rats and plague was no phantasy, but fact.'[13] A report in the British newspaper *The Globe* in 1896 paid tribute to Cantlie's work during the plague. It described him 'hurrying along through death haunted streets, fearlessly going into the worst places and houses, into the most filthy dens of disease where pestilence was raging with dreadful potency, to tend poor penniless people, from whom he would accept no fee, whom he helped out of his own purse and provided with medicines. Very few know the extent of his noble and high minded magnanimity and unselfishness.'[14]

CHAPTER SEVEN

Turmoil and Tribute

Three strands at this time interwove to change China's destiny. Where there had previously been stability now there was stress. While in Hong Kong controversy continued about blame for the epidemic, the sentiments expressed by the Japanese in their singing of Auld Lang Syne were only on the surface. In August the diary recorded, 'The Japanese and Chinese have been fighting and the former have won so far.' China's weakness under the Manchu Government was now painfully obvious. Dr Sun, who had set off in 1894 for Shanghai, Tientsin and Peking to present his petition for reform to Li Hung Chang, now Grand Secretary of the Empire, had been met with excuses and procrastinations. Why should so important an official receive a humble messenger at time of crisis, for war was then threatening between China and Japan? Thus ended years of dedicated study of matter and presentation, which was in Mandarin Chinese. The petition combined the liberal ideas of John Stuart Mill with those of modern Western scientists and economists. Dr Sun stated that the source of Western wealth was not based on guns or armaments but on the maximum use of land, resources, human talent and the unrestricted flow of commodities. Sun saw that at the heart of China's problems of anarchy and lack of welfare lay not only the corruption of the Manchus themselves, but the equally corrupt and antiquated system of land taxation and holding and the almost total lack of transport. Li Hung Chang's abrupt refusal to receive the petition marked the end of a road for Sun Yat Sen and the beginning of another.

On 23 October Mabel Cantlie wrote, 'The Japs appear to be marching on Peking. If they get there the war will be over. The Chinese are in a bad way. They cannot get any more soldiers to join the army at Canton. The men refuse. 5,000 men are wanted in Formosa but no recruits come forward. The whole nation seems upside down.' The Chinese people had quite simply had enough of repression and were not going to help the Government to defend itself. Mabel Cantlie records as the last entry for 1894. 'The last night of a very trying year. May the next bring us good fortune in taking us home.' Alas, 1895 was to prove yet more trying. For one thing the plague was still alive in Canton and the Governor started two inquiries lest it strike again in Hong Kong. One was into the reconstitution of the Sanitary Board, which was criticised for not modernising the housing and drainage of Hong Kong; the other, to which Cantlie was appointed, was to inquire

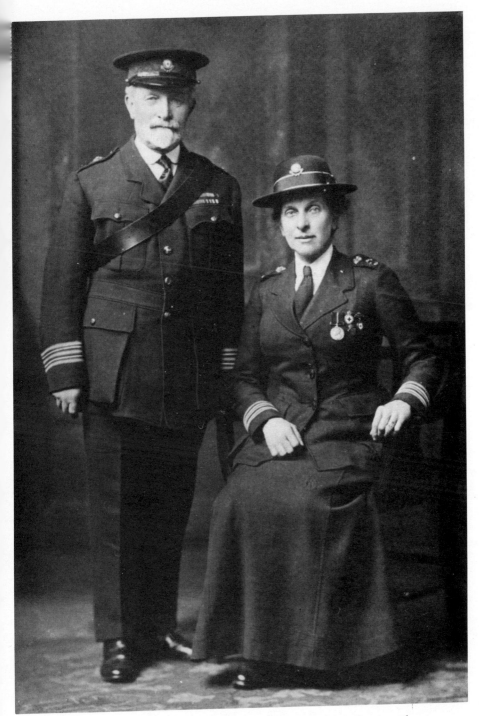

Sir James and Lady Cantlie, the first British Red Cross Commandants.

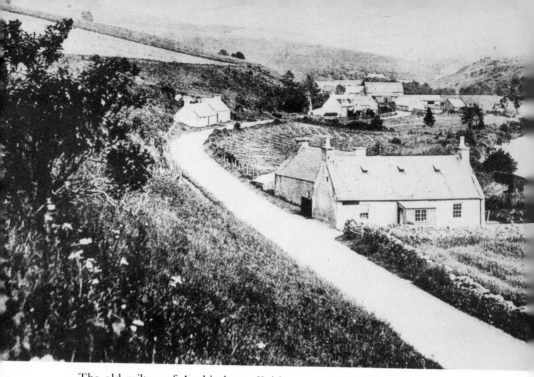

The old milton of Auchindoun. Keithmore on the hills to the left. (*Moray District Council*)

The High Street, Fochabers. (*Moray District Council*)

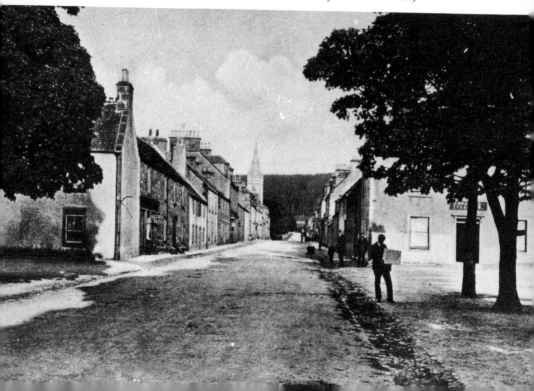

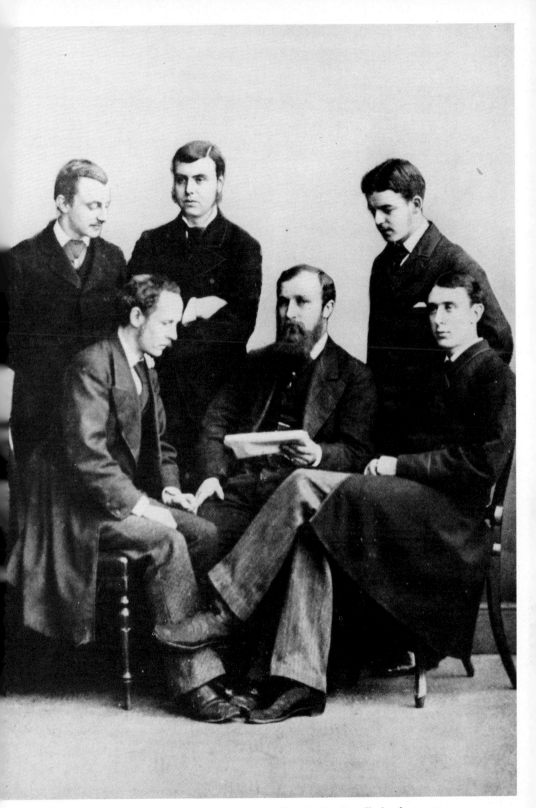

Members of the staff of Charing Cross Hospital – Cantlie in the centre.

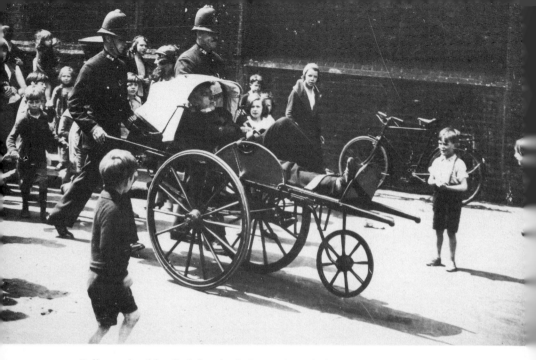

Police trained by St John Ambulance Association transporting a victim of a street accident to hospital on a Furley litter, with his leg in splints. (*Scotland Yard*)

Charing Cross medical students, the first members of the Volunteer Medical Association (later the Volunteer Medical Staff Corps). (*Charing Cross Hospital*)

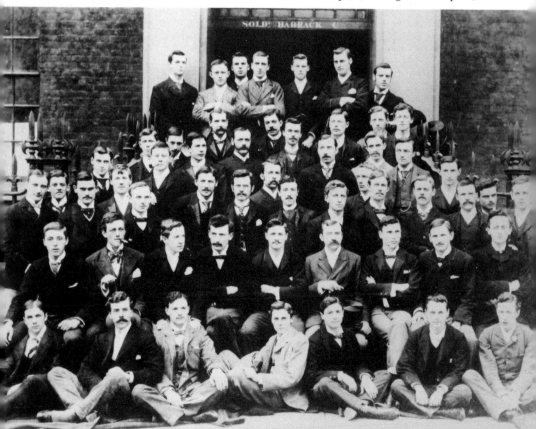

into the work of the Medical Department, which had not been able to research into the cause of plague without foreign help. While these inquiries were reporting, the Government implemented existing regulations on overcrowding and insanitariness and on 14 March 1895 the registration of lodging houses for coolies was debated in Council. Mr Francis backed the Governor in his proposals, while Mr Stewart Lockhart was more cautious and wished to consult the merchants first. The merchants were in an awkward position, and anxious to protect trade they thought it prudent to support both sides. Laid before the Council in its discussions regarding the reconstitution of the Sanitary Board was a letter to the Governor from the General Chamber of Commerce which set out necessary housing improvements: proper drainage, cleansing, limewashing, closing orders on houses unfit for habitation and the prevention of overcrowding. The letter claimed that the Sanitary Board had sufficient power to carry out these measures and had been ineffective; but now that the regulations to prevent overcrowding for which they had specifically asked were to be applied, they shrank from the consequences. This was hardly surprising for, as the Sanitary Board had anticipated, application of the regulations meant that the Chinese took to the streets in mobs. On 23 March the coolie strike broke out in Victoria and spread four days later to Aberdeen. The crisis was reported graver than the plague and a public meeting was held in the City Hall, where it was claimed that the guilds were behind the men and the island would be held to ransom. Some said strength must not be met with weakness, 'We must combine against combination'; others, including the merchants, were conciliatory and wanted the strike ended at once. Mr Keswick of Jardine Mathieson and Dr Ho Kai suggested a compromise, that the landlords should register instead of the tenants who actually gave the coolies lodging. This would have ended the dispute, for what the Chinese feared was that registration would lead to the hated poll tax and rumours to this end were already circulating. The Governor and the Colonial Secretary felt, however, that it would be seen by the Chinese as a climb down and decided instead to threaten those who had circulated the rumours with prosecution. The situation was grim indeed; the island was paralysed with uncertainty. Suddenly, on behalf of the merchants, the police recruited 350 coolies on 1 April at one dollar a day. People were too relieved to ask how. Two days later the strike collapsed.

The overcoming of this first hurdle of preventing overcrowding did nothing, however, to strengthen the powers of the Sanitary Board or to help them to implement the other yet more controversial regulations. Ever since his arrival on the island Cantlie had repeatedly pressed upon the Governor the weakness of its advisory position and the need to appoint a Medical Officer of Health whose recommendations would enable the Board to act whenever there was a threat to health. The plague was once more coming closer, spreading from Canton to Macao. Mr Francis therefore decided to press for more powers in a letter to the Governor published in the *China Mail* on 29 April.

The letter pressed for immigration and periods of isolation during incubation and stated that when the Board had previously asked for these, no one had listened. 'If the Sanitary Board,' he said, 'is to be responsible for sanitation, then its powers must be enlarged to embrace the management of public sewers, supply and distribution of water and provide it with a staff, including a Medical Officer of Health.' Mr Francis ended his letter by saying that, if these powers were not forthcoming, he would resign. The Governor was in an awkward position, and an open letter commits the writer to a course of action. Had Mr Francis waited a few more days Cantlie's Committee would have reported. His resignation was followed by those of Doctors Hartigan and Ho Kai. In their places Mr May, Captain Superintendent of Police, was appointed head of the Sanitary Board, and Mr W. E. Crow became Acting Secretary of the Board and Captain Superintendent of Police. It was a pragmatic move; the police, having been successful in breaking the strike, were now in a position of dual control and well positioned to put through the controversial housing regulations. Floors were to be made of concrete to prevent filth accumulating underneath and attracting rats and there was to be house-to-house visitation to disinfect the night soil and cleanse infected houses. Owing to the crisis the influence of the police was spreading imperceptibly across the colony.

Ten days later Cantlie's Committee reported on the government medical profession of Hong Kong. It stated that the profession was overstretched; that the doctors' hours of work were too long and they should not be required or allowed to undertake private work to augment their income; that nurses should be trained locally; that drugs should be dispensed at nominal prices to the Chinese, and that some free dispensaries should be set up. Cantlie's questions to Mr Mac-Callum, then Superintendent of the Sanitary Board, regarding sanitary regulations and the threat to health appeared in the Report of 26 February 1895 and in Appendices B and C the Committee recommended that a Medical Officer of Health should be appointed to perform all duties legally imposed on him by any bye-law of the Sanitary Authority. Cantlie, just as had happened in London with the cartoons in *Punch* lampooning his crusade for better housing conditions, was now coming in for criticism in the press over his crusade for the appointment of a Medical Officer of Health and his defence of the Governor and the Sanitary Board. The press, in a snide remark, inferred that he had no right to sit on the Committee at all. Cantlie's reaction was characteristic. In his next communication to the press, signed together with the other members of the Committee, he removed the letters Diploma of Public Health from after his name, the letters which, in addition to his wide medical and sanitary experience, gave him the obvious right to sit. It was typical of a man who once said that coming top of a list of examination candidates made him feel ashamed, and who at a recent dinner of the Sugar Boilers, when given the place of honour, immediately relinquished it to Mr Keswick of Jardine Mathieson. He did not like to be placed above his fellows. Thus, while Mr Francis returned a silver inkstand sent by the Governor as a commemoration for his work on the plague, hurt by its inadequacy, Mabel's diary records two days earlier, 'The Morgans sent us a lovely silver inkstand. We are playing a lot of croquet.' They did not seek honours or wish to be top or have letters after their names, although they understood the feelings of others who wanted recognition and did their best to obtain it for them. As they grew older and their health suffered from overwork, into Mabel Cantlie's diary does sometimes creep a wish that the reward would come Cantlie's way that his own temperament simply did not want.

By now his whole attention was focused on the formation of the Public Library, seeing it as a race against time before he went home in July. The Odd Volumes Society had collected 800 volumes for a library, and on 13 March 1895 Cantlie appointed a Committee to draw up a constitution. The Library, to be registered under the Companies Act, was to have a Board of Trustees, two to be appointed by the Governor and six to be elected at a public meeting, of whom Cantlie was one. It was to be opened free as a reading room and to charge a small fee for taking out books in order to pay its expenses. During the summer Dr Cowie, who was coming back to Hong Kong to take Cantlie's place in the practice, wrote asking him to stay until early 1896 since he could not return in June as planned. Cantlie's decision to fit in with Cowie's plans was to have lasting consequences, for the year 1895 was charged with events for China and the world. The controversy about medical and sanitary matters in Hong Kong has to be seen against a backcloth of turmoil in China, where the Chinese were being dramatically defeated by the Japanese so that national collapse seemed imminent. 'The Chinese,' said a Hong Kong newspaper article, 'have made it impossible for any European nation to help them out of their difficulty. There does not seem to be any solid ground in Chinese affairs to stand upon.' Rumours of rebellion in China had reached Hong Kong, and on 15 March 1895 these were reported in the *China Mail*:

> We do not attach much importance to secret societies, such as the White Lily. This is a survival of Ming sentiment. But apart from secret societies disaffection of a general and unorganised kind very widely prevails. There is corruption of official life . . . The storm at the moment is subterranean, but it may become volcanic. Has China no patriots? Can none forget their own gain for the country's good . . . If she is to be saved from the wreckage, if one spark of nobleness is left in her it is time for her people to awake and to say, 'no more of this' . . . It is time for those who love their country to come forward and serve her with faithful service . . . and if need be die that she may live.

One such man there was who now, owing to the obduracy of the Manchus towards reform, was turning his mind towards political changes of a more sweeping nature. The Grand Secretary's curt refusal to allow Dr Sun an audience, thus shutting the door in the face of the young man's diligent efforts to reform his country peacefully, meant that he now turned to what he saw as the only alternative, the stony path of revolution. Li underestimated the genius and qualities of leadership of this gentle-mannered young man. From 1894 onwards Sun 'searched for a combination of forces' that would take his party to power so that his country could regain her position of honour and standing in the world. After returning from his abortive journey he went first to Honolulu to rejoin his brother where he started a new society called the Hsing Chung Hui, the Revive China Society, later known as the Kuomintang. Then he set off for Yokohama where he organised a local branch and later returned to Hong Kong where he started co-ordinating all existing groups into a comprehensive movement. This Hong Kong branch was widely diverse, including gentry interested in reform, monarchists who sought only a change of dynasty, and extreme groups with whom Sun had previously had no connection, such as that run by Yang Chu-yun.

Meanwhile on the mainland there was mounting unrest. Kwantung province, under the rule of Li Hung Chang's brother, had reached a degree of corruption rarely surpassed and soldiers, disbanded after the northern treaty with the Japanese, roamed the country pillaging. On 11 April 1895, it was rumoured that the Japanese were to attack Canton, yet the British Vice Consul there wrote to O'Conor, the British Minister in Peking, on 16 April:

> there is no sign whatever of revolution in the Western sense, the bold prophecies of one of the Hong Kong papers in regard to such a rising are simply moonshine. It appears, indeed, that the Chinese Government, though practically unarmed and helpless against a serious foe, is strong enough to keep peace at home – to keep the great Chinese cow steady while foreigners extract the milk, of which it is to be hoped that the Japanese will only be allowed their fair share.[1]

It was a cynical remark which took no account of Chinese feelings; a supine cow was what they were no longer prepared to be. During the summer O'Conor's communications from Peking to the Foreign Office dealt with the war, loans, concessions, trade conventions, the price of rice, and plans for railway construction – a crisis seemed nowhere on the horizon. Meanwhile in Hong Kong realism prevailed and people wondered how long the present Government of China could survive. The *China Mail* reported on 13 May that her collapse seemed imminent, and in the same month the Hong Kong press published a proposed new constitution for China drawn up by Dr Ho Kai – who was not a member of the Revive China Society. It was based on a change of dynasty and proposed an emperor and British-style prime minister and cabinet. The country would be divided into four administrative divisions and subdivided into districts in which the people would elect their representatives who would nominate delegates to the National Parliament. There were to be judicial reforms, modern education, religious tolerance and free trade although, as a concession to the merchants, maritime customs were still to be in the hands of foreigners.

The British Government was faced with a complex problem. Sun Yat Sen, growing restive, had already designed a flag, a white sun against a blue sky, and had secretly set a date for the Canton plot. The whole reforming movement was pro-Western, and pro-British and American in particular. But Britain could not be seen to be interfering in the internal affairs of another nation, nor could she risk hostility with the Manchu regime on whom she depended for trade and the lease of the New Territories. On the other hand, well aware of the unpopularity of the Manchus and the extent of corruption, she equally did not wish to give the Empress aid against the Japanese. So Britain sat on the fence while, as Cantlie predicted, the Russians, taking advantage of her inactivity, concluded a massive loan with the Chinese. No increase of trade with Japan could recompense her loss of trade with China, for even in those days Japanese trade tended to be one-way. What the British Government appeared to lack was reliable information and thus, not for the first time in history, the service chiefs may have been anxious to acquaint themselves with the facts. This may explain the entry in the diary in March 1895: 'H wrote to Sir Guyer asking him if he should go to Honolulu on his journey home.' This was Surgeon General Sir Guyer Hunter of the Army Medical Department. Honolulu was then the headquarters of the Revive China Society. Were the service chiefs aware that the Minister in Peking was telling the Government what it wished to hear, not because of any wish to deceive, but because O'Conor did not trust his instinct and only relied on proven facts? By the time facts become results it is always too late.

The event that should have fully informed the British public was the massacre of British missionaries at Foochow. An anonymous letter in the *China Mail* on 6 August said, 'let us hold a mass meeting and say what we think and what we are ready to submit to in vindication of our rights; a just and terrible retribution must be exacted for this outrage. Let the whole colony rise up and give voice to their sentiment, so as to strengthen the hands of those in authority. There is no hope for China from within.' On 7 August, according to the diary, Cantlie was asked to get up a protest meeting, held the next day. 'All the leading men and women were present, Sir Fielding Clark, the Chief Justice in the Chair.' Bishop Burden spoke and so did Mr Francis, who asked the meeting to join in a representation to the Home Government that it was the opinion of those present that 'every Government official in China from the Viceroys downwards was cognisant of what is going on and in sympathy with the anti foreign movement. The Officials took no precaution to protect the helpless people in the treaty ports.' He wanted to warn the British Government of impending revolution. The meeting wholeheartedly supported the sending of a telegram to Lord Salisbury condemning the actions of the Chinese Government and demanding stern measures against those responsible for the massacre. It rejected Sir Fielding Clark's alternative of expressing indignation against no one in particular. The telegram was to be sent through the Governor but the press inferred the next day that he had not dispatched it.

Certainly, during the subsequent debate in the House of Lords their Lordships seemed unaware of the true facts, stating that the Chinese Government was earnest in its wish to measure out justice, while the same ignorance seemed to prevail in the House of Commons, where it was commented that the missionaries should conform to the general customs of the country.

Five years later, when the Boxer Rebellion backed by the Empress Dowager threatened the lives of hundreds of Europeans in the Treaty Ports, the British Government awoke to reality, but in 1895 it was on the horns of a dilemma. Certainly if a pro-Western revolution had been successful throughout China political and economic stability would have been secured, but if the British supported an unsuccessful revolution or one which divided China into north and south, the future would have held great risk, for another power would have backed the Manchus, with consequent bloodshed and civil war. The Chinese have always been supported by the British, Americans and Japanese in their aim to keep China undivided, whereas France, Germany and Russia wanted then to see her divided. Nevertheless, British indecision reaped its inevitable harvest, for not only had the Russians confirmed a £16 million loan to the Chinese to be handed over in London (although Britain was able to extract from the Chinese a promise that there would be no special conditions), but by the end of the year the Russian fleet was anchored off Shantung.

All through the autumn of 1895 the Hong Kong papers attacked the Manchus referring to their despotism, the helpless misery of the people, the chronic disorder, legalised anarchy and rottenness among all classes. One editorial almost inferred that Britain should herself try to topple the regime. In September O'Conor was told of his transfer to St Petersburg and this unleashed his tongue. On 23 October he reported that 'a movement . . . has been inaugurated within the last few weeks in Peking, having for its object . . . reforms on Western lines. A number of the rising generation of officials and of prominent literary men, disgusted at the state into which the country has fallen, have formed themselves into an association and issued a manifesto stressing the urgent necessity for reform.'[2] The manifesto warned that whereas formerly China had been the centre of a vast civilisation, the outlying portions of which provided a ring of defence, now these had fallen prey to foreign conquest so that she stood weak and isolated, surrounded by powerful nations, and without strenuous efforts her fate could be read in the history of other nations brought into contact with European civilisation. The reform movement planned to issue a newspaper to publicise the advantages of railways and other foreign inventions, the military, naval and educational systems of the West and the advantages of its science, thus paving the way for future sweeping reforms. The proposals were similar to those of Sun Yat Sen, but they were a year too late. He was by now laying plans of a more far-reaching nature. Perhaps O'Conor guessed this, for he reported how he had also told the Reform Party's spokesman, who was a member of the conservative Hanlin Academy, the extent of official corruption, the mistrust of the regime for any foreign ideas or new teaching methods, and above all the urgent need for speed. O'Conor saw a lack of practical application in the plan and an uneasiness on the part of the reformers as to whether they could survive the opposition they would meet, and commented, 'My visitor did not strike me as being imbued with the fervour of the born reformer, but of his earnestness there can be no doubt . . . I hinted to him that the party, if it failed to compass its objects in time, might find itself swept away by a movement of a more revolutionary character.'[3] The words were hardly out of his mouth when the dam burst. Three days later, on 26 October, Sun Yat Sen made his attempted coup in Canton. It failed because a leak in Canton pinned down revolutionary soldiers in Swatow, and because the Hong Kong police had infiltrated the movement. Having built up a reputation for courage during the plague, for subtlety during the coolie strike and for forcible persuasion in enforcing the controversial sanitary regulations, they were now in a sufficiently strong position to deal with the insurgents. The *China Mail* of 27 November referred to the betrayer as a 'prominent Chinaman who seemed genuinely reliable'. Who the betrayer was remains a mystery. Those in charge at the Hong Kong end, one of whom was the extremist Yang, were far from efficient. First they sent Sun a telegram saying that the 'goods' – 200 revolvers hidden in bags of cement – could not be sent in time but would arrive a day later. The delay and telegram were dangerous enough, but when Sun, knowing there had also been a leak in Canton, wired telling them to cancel, the reply came that it was too late, the 'goods' had already been dispatched. An inspector, searching the boat, said he found nothing and allowed it to sail, but he reported afterwards that he was told there were arms on board and wired to Canton so that the boat was met by Chinese Government officials. The conspirators were rounded up in Canton and sixteen out of the eighteen leading men were beheaded. Sun fled to friends in Macao and then to Hong Kong where he sought Cantlie's advice and help. Cantlie advised him to see a solicitor and sent him to Mr Dennys, who advised Sun to leave the island immediately and wisely did not tell Cantlie where he had gone. On the one hand the police had prevented colonial territory from being used as a base for revolution; on the other – while the Foreign Office was commenting on newspaper and College of Commerce suggestions that Hong Kong extend its boundaries: 'Can the Governor have so lost his head that he wants to annexe Canton?' – they had destroyed for ever the possibility of a British or American-style constitution being set up in China instead of the Russian-style one which was eventually forced, through economic necessity, upon the Chinese people.

Li Hung Chang, with characteristic duplicity, appreciated the strength of the new movements and changed sides. It would appear that O'Conor did not receive official confirmation of the uprising until notified by Brenan in Canton in a report dated 1 November, but two days before this Li was in conference with O'Conor, asking him to use his influence to remedy 'the deplorable state of things' into which the Empire had drifted, and which Li saw as 'so pregnant with danger'.

The following day O'Conor had a conference with Prince Kung, one of the Manchu moderates, and told him that unless the Government acted promptly the Empire was doomed. 'I told the Prince that the main burden of responsibility lay with him and that future generations looking back on what may prove to be the last days of the dynasty and Empire would single him out as a man who might have saved his country.'[4] The Russians meanwhile were pressing to obtain the right to construct a railway to Port Arthur, Nerchinsk and Vladivostok, just as Jardine Mathieson were preparing to extend theirs, and on 31 October O'Conor had another interview with Prince Kung in which he warned him of the dangers of these proposals by the Russians, combined as they were with the Russian fleet anchoring at Port Arthur and the Germans taking Chusan, and advised him that the Chinese should reorganise their army and navy with all speed. 'I said that they need not look further for a motive for my advice than the great interest of England in China. We had 80% of their foreign trade'[5] and hundreds of thousands of British people depended on this for their livelihood. On the same day Li Hung Chang thanked O'Conor for his help but left him with the impression that there was no real hope of reforms being carried out and that Li was deeply anxious as to the consequences. It was too late. The once reforming Dr Sun was now a hunted conspirator with a price on his head, each failure driving him further on his revolutionary course. No wonder, the diary records, that Mabel Cantlie was summoned to Government House to meet Sir Nicholas and Lady O'Conor on their way home from Peking. No wonder one of the subjects discussed was the necessity of securing a lease of further territories beyond Kowloon to protect Hong Kong from the rising state of unrest in China (a lease secured shortly afterwards).

By this time Mabel Cantlie was taking as much strain as she could from her husband but, like him, she too had had a gruelling summer. On a brief holiday in Japan she had been given by Professor Kitasato plague specimens and cover glasses for Cantlie's research, and she had spent August making soup for germs. It was more than even her robust constitution could manage. She was twice poisoned with the smell and sick with food poisoning. Cantlie, meanwhile, was succumbing to recurrent bouts of fever with very high temperature, the diary recording how he returned to work the day after running a temperature of 104°. The climate of Hong Kong had played its trump card; like many before them both Cantlies were now running daily increased temperatures which flared up with sickness or strain. Sadly, when at last Cantlie's beloved library was opened, the child of his hard work and dreams for which there was now a catalogue of 2,000 books and more coming from home, he was too ill to attend the meeting in the City Hall at which the Governor promised financial help. Hopes were expressed at the meeting that one day the library would be joined with that of the City Hall, which was now run in a manner 'opposed to all reason and commonsense . . . repugnant to the wishes of those responsible for the original collection'.

On 5 February 1896, after further weeks of illness interspersed with periods of work, a presentation was made to Cantlie on the eve of his departure for home which was reported in the *Hong Kong Telegraph* and *China Mail* of 13 February:

Rarely has there been a more enthusiastic meeting in the City Hall than that which was convened for the purpose of giving Dr. Cantlie, whose proposed departure from the colony is deeply regretted, what is generally termed a good send off. Every nationality in the colony was represented. The Governor, who was prevented by illness from attending, sent a letter to the Chairman which ended with these words, 'Dr. Cantlie has for many years and on many occasions, devoted much of his valuable time and his great ability unhesitatingly and ungrudgingly to the service of this community. That he will be missed goes without saying, and I should be glad if you would assure him that on public, as well as on private grounds, I deeply regret his departure.' Mr. Francis spoke on behalf of the presentation from the community, 'My dear Dr. Cantlie, when I first came to this colony I was given to understand that there was only one disease recognised by the medical faculty and that was liver; and that they only had two prescriptions, one a blue pill and the other a P and O liner. Among the many medical men who practise in this colony there has not been anyone who was your superior, or who came here more specially qualified for the very trying work, which the medical profession have to contend with at this distance from all seats of learning and consulting physicians, and where every medical man has to devote himself to the practice of every branch of his profession. Not content, Doctor, with the very fatiguing practice of your profession here in Hong Kong, you have devoted yourself, your time and your attention to many matters, some medical and some public, in the interests of the colony, and you have given time to these things which probably you ought to have devoted to rest and recreation. You became a member of the Sanitary Board and you gave the best possible advice to that institution while it existed. You joined the Volunteers as Surgeon-Captain. You trained men in ambulance work and first aid to the wounded. You established a small Ambulance Corps of which you took the lead. You established, greatly to the advantage of the residents of Hong Kong, the Peak Hospital, through which over a thousand patients have passed, and you took upon your own shoulders, I understand, the expense and the risk of the institution for the first two or three years of its existence. You were the first to bring out here trained European nurses and I need hardly add that no one who has the knowledge and experience of the attention to the sick by nurses in the colony before that date but must thoroughly understand how much we benefited ... Before your arrival the supply of lymph for vaccination was both irregular in quantity and inferior in quality, and with your accustomed vigour you pressed the subject upon the Government and successfully established the Vaccine Institute and now the supply of lymph is regular and abundant, and of the very best quality. You gave your

time and your labours to the work of the Alice Memorial and
Nethersole Hospitals. You have not merely aided and restored to
health many among the Chinese, but you have by your exertions and
kindness aided very considerably in however small a degree, to
diminish the prejudice entertained by the Chinese against European
medicine. I believe it was primarily your idea that an attempt should
be made to train Chinese students here in Western medicine . . . I
may say without hesitation that, however great the benefits you have
conferred upon the Alice Memorial Hospital and on the College of
Medicine and on the students, you have also conferred a very great
benefit indeed on the colony in so far as you have induced the
Government to train Chinese students in Western sciences and so
lessened the prejudice of the Chinese against the introduction of
European medicine into the colony. One would have thought that in
these varied occupations you had found enough to do, but you spent
many an hour in giving useful, instructive, as well as entertaining
lectures to the members of the Odd Volumes Society and to the
public who were invited to their rooms. I am afraid that the Odd
Volumes will not survive your departure. But I honestly believe that
the Public Library, which you set upon its feet, will succeed and I
heartily congratulate the colony upon it. In addition to all this work,
you have devoted yourself in the interests of general science and to
scientific research and at one time to cultivation of innumerable
quantities of microbes which you had stored at your house at the
Peak. You have also investigated with very great care the terrible
disease known as leprosy as it manifests itself amongst the Chinese
and you have contributed to the scientific journals many valuable
papers on that subject and on beri beri which makes such ravages in
Java, the Straits and Japan, besides devoting much time and care to a
most valuable work by the members of the Dutch Commission . . .
But Doctor, it is not for your labours that your fellow citizens value
you so highly. It is for your independence of character, for your
outspokenness, your constant cheerfulness, your kindness of heart,
your generosity and your readiness to assist any one in need. No
matter who it was, no one ever applied to you in vain. We respect you
and esteem you because of that superabundance of life and energy
that has enabled you to carry through almost everything you proposed. If an idea is suggested to you you say, 'Let us do it,' that has
always been your plan and you have succeeded in 99 times out of a
100. On behalf of the members of the community, I, simply as their
spokesman, express to you the high esteem in which they hold you
for your personal qualifications, your high character, your scientific
ability, your devoted labours for the past nine years in the interests of
the colony. Of course you will probably tell us that you acted only
in your own selfish interests. We will not believe that. You were
animated by much higher sentiments and feelings and the entire
community express to you their sincere regret that you are leaving
and still more that you are leaving on account of ill health.

Mr J. Stewart Lockhart, Colonial Secretary, Rector of the College of Medicine for the Chinese, ended a similar address with these words:

It is said that forgetfulness soon obliterates the memory of those who go from our midst, and this is perhaps an unavoidable tendency in a Far Eastern Colony where the population is very changing, but the memory of you and your good deeds in connection with the College and Hospitals will be green for many years to come . . . and it will always be remembered that in no small measure is their success due to you. You are, indeed, a son of whom your alma mater, Aberdeen University, may well be proud, and I trust that, before long, that University will take steps to fittingly recognise your services. We wish you and Mrs. Cantlie every prosperity. For your sons we can wish them nothing better than that they prove worthy of their father. We envy the land which is to enjoy the charm of your personality and the geniality of your disposition and we feel sure that the varied abilities and versatile gifts which have excited our admiration and affection will gain for you in the old country a still greater reputation than that which you already possessed there.

The simplest and perhaps the most moving address came from the students of the College:

Dr. Cantlie, we thank you for all your kindness to us, your patience with us, and your willingness to help us in all circumstances. We ask you to accept from us this cup, accompanied by a small gift for Mrs. Cantlie, that you may have before you a standing reminder to you of our gratitude for the many favours we have received at your hands. We promise you that we shall do our best by diligent efforts to relieve the sick and suffering among our own people, to prove ourselves worthy of all the labours you have so generously bestowed upon us. We wish you a good voyage, a speedy restoration to health and strength and all prosperity in your future life.

Cantlie was so overwhelmed by the laudatory remarks showered upon him that he was at a loss for words. His anxiety was only for the continuation of the work he had instigated. His Vaccine Institute was still in competition with imported lymph; instead he wanted to see Hong Kong lymph carried by every medical missionary free of charge across China 'to protect the human race against the ravages of the terrible scourge of small pox. Were Great Britain,' he said, 'to supply free vaccine to the Chinese it would be a greater blessing to them than the abolition of slavery to the blacks.' He spoke of the difficulties still faced by the College of Medicine, but reminded his audience that the medical colleges of India had faced the same difficulties and now had four universities and medical schools of which they could justly be proud. He spoke of the way in which the College had extended his Deanship in order that he could be its advocate in the United Kingdom. 'I mean to fulfil that mission to the best of my ability.' Returning to one of his favourite themes – that of medical and sanitary organisation – he asked once more that the position of the Medical Officer of Health be clearly defined, and that the Department of Health should not be part of the Medical Department – 'Health and disease are conditions as wide apart as the poles'. The message with which he left his audience in his closing remarks was that they should never be frightened by failure:

> Failure should never deter a man with right on his side. I have made so many failures that I have ceased to blush for them . . . Obstacles act but as stimulants and criticism is either useful in suggestion or I treat it with the motto, 'They say, what say they? Let them say.' Many a time . . . I got in reply, 'Don't bring any more schemes forward, we want a rest.' Ladies and gentlemen, my departure will favour that end, but until I myself am at rest, I will cherish the remembrances of this day . . . I can only thank you, I can only tell you how I appreciate all your kind words and handsome presents.

Cantlie's fears for the future of the College were far from groundless, for after his departure it was under considerable pressure. One of his last acts as Dean was to recommend a register of Licentiates to the Government and in 1896 the report of a Committee appointed by the Governor to inquire into the best organisation for the College of Medicine was presented to the Legislative Council. The Committee sat under the chairmanship of the Colonial Surgeon but, fortunately for the future of the College, Cantlie's old friend Evatt took the chair at the second meeting. The Colonial Surgeon and one other member were critical of College standards, claiming that Licentiates were not able to practise without supervision. But the Committee as a whole accepted present arrangements regarding the five-year course entitling graduates to practise as Licentiates, although it recommended that lecturers in future should be appointed by the Government and receive salaries. On 31 July the Governor asked Mr Belilios to give his promised site and building if the Government also played a financial part in running the College. Belilius replied on 4 August,

> Circumstances have changed completely since my offer was made. That offer was made to an institution then struggling for existence but warmly supported by Dr. Cantlie and carefully administered by Dr. Thomson. The former has left the colony, the latter is relinquishing his hospital work and the other medical practitioners are too much occupied to take any keen interest in the institution. My interest was largely made up of sympathy with the gallant efforts of the two doctors above named to found a College of Medicine for the Chinese. The situation is now wholly changed.[6]

Mr Belilios ended his letter by saying that since the outbreak of the plague the work of education of the Chinese in sanitation and Western medicine should be undertaken by the Government. 'I will not extend my offer.'

Belilios's feelings were understandable. For the College it was nevertheless a setback, although mercifully only a temporary one. Cantlie, with his extended appointment as dean, was by this time raising funds in Britain which, together with public support in Hong Kong, helped to bridge the gap until 1901 when the Government granted its first annual subsidy. What had changed the course of Mr Belilios's generosity? His letter reflected a genuine sadness. Perhaps the poet was right – the seas on to which the magic casements opened were after all perilous and the lands forlorn. The doctors had become deeply involved with their most important and beloved of patients, the suffering and teeming millions who lived under the rule of the dying Empire of China. They had helped to light a candle to alleviate the suffering of the Chinese by trying to bring to them the benefits of Western medicine and science. Perhaps, who knows, because of their very closeness to the problem, they and the service chiefs, the Hong Kong press and the merchants knew by instinct that the days of the Manchus were numbered; and although successive governors also felt sure that the regime could not survive they were powerless to convince the Government or Parliament of Britain. In the circumstances it is not surprising that they had to rely more and more on the police who enabled the island to be run. It seemed that for the moment medical progress among the Chinese stood still. The following year, Mr May, Captain of Police and now Head of the Sanitary Board, proposed a resolution to the effect that a branch of the Tung Wah Hospital should be opened for plague patients where all Chinese suffering from plague would go and where they would have the choice of Western or Chinese medicine. In vain did the doctors oppose the scheme and argue that the recognition of Chinese medicine would be a retrograde step. They pointed out that in 1894 when the Chinese doctors were allowed full scope mortality among the Chinese from plague was 93 per cent, whereas when the treatment was under the Colonial Medical Department it had been reduced to 74 per cent. They accused Mr May of merely wanting to humour the prejudices of the Chinese. The trouble was that the Medical Department was still over-stretched, with the result that only the previous year the Hong Kong Government had had to accept an invitation of help from a visiting ship of the German Imperial Navy whose doctor had treated 300 cases of plague. The doctors and the police represented two separate threads of colonialism, the one visionary and idealistic, the other pragmatic. In 1902 Mr May, who completely survived the inquiry into police corruption in 1897, became Colonial Secretary and in 1912, after two years in Fiji, he returned to become Governor in Hong Kong. The date was significant for the history of China.

CHAPTER EIGHT

Kidnapped in London

The Cantlies' departure from Hong Kong was a scene of tremendous ovation. The steam launch was decorated, a band of the Hong Kong Regiment was playing and the jetty was crowded with hundreds of people. Thus, laden with gifts and congratulations, they set sail for America, calling at Japan and Honolulu, where they were met by Dr Sun in the street while they were out driving. Neither of them recognised Sun at first as he stepped forward out of the crowd to greet them, for he was dressed in European clothes, with no *queue*. Cantlie gave him his address in Britain suggesting that Sun came to London to continue his medical studies and fully qualify as a doctor. The Cantlies then re-embarked for San Francisco, where they were given a telegram from Mitchell Bruce saying that Charing Cross Hospital was offering Cantlie the post of assistant surgeon. In spite of continuing bouts of fever, Cantlie wired acceptance. Then they started a train journey across the United States, over Salt Lake, with its spectacular change of colour from one side of the railway to the other; into Salt Lake City, heavy with snow; across the sandy deserts of Central America, with its spectacular outcrops of rock, stopping now and then at wooden stations where groups of Indians clustered on the platforms. At Chicago they were met by Cantlie's brother, George, who worked there in a music shop, and by his cousin James Cantlie's two sons, George and Frank, who took them home to Montreal. Here they stayed with James Cantlie and his wife Eleanora (formerly Eleanora Stephens, sister of Lord Mountstephen). James had by now built up for himself a thriving cotton and textile business as well as a dry goods trade. He was President of the Montreal Board of Trade and Vice President of the Dominion Trading Company. They dined with Lord and Lady Strathcona, also like Lord Mountstephen of Canadian Pacific Railway fame, and cousins of James Cantlie. Returning to the USA they went sightseeing in New York and then, in company with their cousin George, they took ship for England. During the voyage a further telegram came from Bruce asking Cantlie to hurry home, for the post at Charing Cross could not remain open long. Cantlie's health did not, however, improve as a result of the voyage and four days after his arrival in England he told Charing Cross that he must withdraw his name. The bouts of fever were less, but even a walk on Wimbledon Common brought him back 'pale and done up'. A teaching post at a London hospital would have given his health no time to recover. As soon as they had been re-united with the family they left for Fochabers with the boys where the magic of the clear, bracing air, golf and fishing and walks among the hills at Keithmore, and a journey to Garmouth, where he was the only one of the family fortunate enough to catch a fish, all served to restore him to health and happiness.

On his return to London Charing Cross offered Cantlie the chair of applied anatomy which he accepted. All that mattered to him was that he was back at his beloved Charing Cross Hospital. He now began to take up the threads of his old life. First there was the presentation of prizes at the new headquarters of the VMSC: 'Princess Louise asked to see Hamish after the Ceremony and he went and spoke to her and she was very gracious. All the Officers we knew welcomed Hamish back.' Then there was the re-commencement of his nursing and first aid lectures in the evenings. The Furleys, Sir Guyer Hunter, the Maclures, and many other names well known in the service and civilian ambulance movement, together with names revered in tropical medicine such as those of Sir Joseph and Lady Fayrer, flit in and out of the pages of the diary, calling, lunching or dining. For relaxation there were dinners with medical societies and city companies; theatres with their friends Henry and Lawrence Irving, and concerts and musical evenings at which Cantlie's voice was now beginning to make him in demand as an after-dinner singer. In August the family took Flatford Mill, where Constable was born, and Mabel Cantlie spent her time painting while the boys fished and swam and enjoyed their father's company, when he was not with patients. By now rest and the climate had restored them to health, and walks before breakfast and rowing expeditions in the afternoon were part of the norm. While there they decided to master the new method of transport, the bicycle; it was to become the alternative to the train for expeditions down to the country from London. So enjoyable was their holiday that Mabel Cantlie bought as a present for her husband the Old Kennels at Cottered in Hertfordshire, which remained their country home until they died. No doubt they looked forward to a life of peace and contentment, with the turmoil behind. How wrong they were. On 3 October a thunderbolt hit them from the blue.

On that date the diary records, 'Dr. Sun here.' Sun Yat Sen had taken Cantlie's offer and arrived on the *Majestic*, probably not aware that he was being watched by detectives hired by the Chinese Government, and certainly not aware that the Chinese Minister had made an application to the British Government for his extradition, which had been refused. Although a banishment order had been placed upon Sun in March in Hong Kong, it did not apply to other territories, and in Britain of course he was free to come and go as he pleased. The Grand Secretary of the Empire Li Hung Chang's triumphal tour of Russia, Germany, France and Britain during the summer, which had been arranged as the result of a letter to the British Government from Sir Halliday McCartney, the British Secretary to the Chinese Minister in London, had been commented on unfavourably in the Hong Kong press. Whether this visit influenced the events which followed cannot be known, but certainly Li's reputation for intrigue was well earned. Cantlie found Dr Sun rooms with his former landlady, Miss Pollard, at 8 Gray's Inn Place, from which lodging Sun disappeared on 11 October. At first Miss Pollard was presumably not anxious, for there is no record of it in the diary. Cantlie had jokingly remarked to Sun that the Chinese Legation was just round the corner from Devonshire Street and that he had better go and pay them a visit. His wife warned severely against going anywhere near the building. Some biographers of Sun Yat Sen appear to find this story strange and insinuate from it that the initiative in the ensuing events came from Sun. They forget the north-east Scot brand of dry humour, which keeps a sense of cheerful optimism in any trying or dangerous circumstances.

Every time he visited the Cantlies, which he did daily, Dr Sun could not avoid coming into fairly close proximity with the Legation. Reliance on British law and order meant that fear of kidnapping in the open street was anyway in those days minimal. On 17 October the Cantlies' calm was shattered. Written across the ordinary diary entry for the day are the words, '11.30 p.m. Got a note to say that Sun Yat Sen has been taken prisoner by the Chinese Legation, an anonymous note from European housekeeper. Hamish went off to Scotland Yard, Sir Halliday McCartney and Police.'

> A ring at the doorbell [wrote Cantlie] brought me from my bed. I found no one at the door but observed and picked up the letter which had been pushed in below the door . . . As usual a woman had come to the rescue. The wife of one of the English servants in the Legation heard from her husband of the piteous plight of the imprisoned Chinaman and sent me the following letter. 'There is a friend of yours imprisoned in the Chinese Legation here since last Sunday; they intend sending him out to China, where it is certain they will hang him. It is very sad for the poor man and unless something is done at once he will be taken away and no one will know it. I dare not sign my name, but this is the truth, so believe what I say. Whatever you do must be done at once, or it will be too late. His name is, I believe, Sin Yin Sen.'[1]

This woman has remained, as requested, anonymous. Sun in his book *Kidnapped in London* calls her Mrs Cole, the wife of his gaoler and later benefactor. Cantlie and Seaver in their biography of Sir James call her Mrs Howe. That she was a female European housekeeper employed in the Chinese Legation is all that is known for certain.

Cantlie relates how he went at once to the Marylebone Police Station and to Scotland Yard. No one believed his story and the inspector on duty told him to go home and keep quiet, taking him for a lunatic or a drunk. In his letter of Monday 19 October to the Foreign Office Cantlie recorded how he then went to 3 Harley Street, home of Sir Halliday McCartney, Secretary to the Chinese Minister in London, and was told by the constable on duty that Sir Halliday was out of town for six months. Sun, in his book, adds that Cantlie was told that there had been a burglary in the house three nights previously. Sir Halliday was a controversial figure and his part in the kidnapping borders on the bizarre. A military surgeon with service in the Crimea and India, Sir Halliday had joined General Gordon in quashing the Taiping Rebellion and later held a post in the Nanking arsenal, assuming his diplomatic duties in London in 1877. On 17 October 1895 a letter signed Mickey had appeared in the *Hong Kong Telegraph* asserting that as Dr McCartney of the 99th Regiment he was attached as surgeon to a mission in North China, but that after an alleged disagreement with a superior he left the army and attached himself to the Chinese who put him in charge of the arsenal of the Viceroy of Nanking. Speaking Chinese fluently he became to all intents and purposes a Chinese subject and married an official's daughter by whom he had a family.

The following day, Sunday 18 October, the diary records:

> What a day of hopes and fears. Hamish went first thing to see Judge Ackroyd. Then Mr. Hughes – the I.M. Customs of Chinese. But got no satisfaction about doing something for Sun Yat Sen. Met us at church . . . Then Hamish went to see Manson and see if he could find Sir Halliday McCartney. Manson took our side and was wroth against the Legation. A man who turned out to be Sun's gaoler turned up and brought 2 small cards beseeching us to rescue him. I sent the man on to Manson and Hamish was there. Heard from the man all about poor Sun. They went to Foreign Office and Scotland Yard again. This night Hamish is out trying to do more for the prisoner. It is awful.

This man, whose name was Cole, had finally taken pity on Sun and decided to risk his job and consequent lack of references in order to see him rescued. Sun recounts in his book how for nearly a week after his imprisonment he had pleaded with his gaolers, two in particular, Tang and Cole, to let Cantlie know of his whereabouts. Each time they informed Sir Halliday. Then he tried to throw notes out of the window weighted with coins. He was spotted by the Chinese and his notes were recovered. On Friday he despaired of his life and prayed that he might be saved. He was filled with a feeling of calmness, hopefulness and confidence that assured him that his prayers were heard and all would be well. When Cole came into the room he said, 'My life is in your hands. If you let the matter be known outside I shall be saved. If not, I shall certainly be executed. Is it good to save a life or to take it? Whether is it more important to regard your duty to God or to your master? To honour the just British or the corrupt Chinese Government?'[2] When Cole came back he pointed to the coal scuttle in which there was a note which told Sun that he was being watched through the key hole and that he must write on the bed and not at the table where he would be observed and that he should put the note into the coal scuttle for Cole to take away. By this method notes went to and fro, and Cantlie was able to tell Sun, 'Cheer up. The Government is working on your behalf and you will be free in a few days.'

Sun's first note described how he had been kidnapped and taken forcibly into the Legation: 'I was kidnapped into the Legation on Sunday and shall be smuggled out from England to China for death. Please rescue me quick . . . A ship is already chartered by the Chinese Legation for the service to take me to China and I shall be locked up all the way without communication to anybody. Woe is me.' Sun's first thoughts were for the man who had helped him: 'Please take care of the messenger for me. He is very poor and will lose his job.' Indeed, so great were Cole's fears that when he arrived at 46 Devonshire Street he thought he had been betrayed, seeing a life-like model of a Chinaman in the corner, so that Mabel Cantlie found him trembling with fear beside it. Cole related a number of other matters to Mabel Cantlie and to the doctors, including the fact that Sir Halliday, although officially not in London, had called at the Legation every day and had instructed Cole on 11 October to clear out a back room to which he had conducted Sun, staying ten minutes and them coming out and locking the door. This accords with Sun's version of the incident in his book when he says that on the morning of 11 October two men started to talk to him in the street and half led, half pushed him into the Legation where the door shut behind him. Sir Halliday then led him to an upstairs room and locked the door. Cole also related to the doctors that a Glenline steamer had been chartered by the Chinese for Tuesday night, two days hence. Sir Halliday had informed the Legation servants that Sun was a lunatic who was to be taken back to China. Cole had by this time appreciated that far from being a lunatic Sun was a well educated, responsible person. The two doctors again proceeded to Scotland Yard where they were told that the police had no control over Foreign Embassies in Britain and that it was not a police matter. The official note reads that it was a matter for diplomatic action 'to ascertain the truth or untruth and that no action should be taken by the police without the consent of the Home Office'. Thus the doctors went off again to enlist the help of the Hon. G. A. Curzon, an under-secretary for Foreign Affairs. It was, however, Sunday, and no one was available except a clerk, whom they saw at 5.00 p.m., and who told them that they would have to wait until the next day. Sun comments humorously in his book, 'Can no trouble arise on Sunday in England? . . . Sunday I should think it was, and my head in the balance.' They then decided to call at the Legation and let the Chinese authorities know that they knew that Sun was within. Manson did this, thinking that Cantlie might be recognised, and was met by Tang, Sun's other gaoler, who almost convinced the doctor that Sun was not there, so earnest were his denials. Cantlie, meanwhile, searched for a detective to watch the Legation. This proved difficult, again because it was Sunday. Eventually a policeman sent him to Islington to contact a man who was said to have a public house in the Barbican. Nothing deterred, Cantlie set off thither and again finding him not there left a message for him to call at Devonshire Street. Cantlie then went to *The Times* and left a note saying that there had been a case of kidnapping at the Chinese Legation and that the press could publish at their discretion. Returning home he found that the detective had still not arrived and he therefore left the house again to take up stance outside the Legation. Fortunately, on his way, he met the detective and stationed him in a hansom cab at the end of the street, so that if Sun was hurried out into a cab he could be followed.

Monday 19 October was a critical day: 'Hamish at Office for Foreign Affairs most of the day. Wrote a declaration for Lord Salisbury to see. Had an interview with Cole, Sun's warder. We have detectives watching embassy. Think Sun is safe now. Thank God.' When one thinks of the thousands of words that have been written about this occurrence it is remarkable that Mabel Cantlie set out all the relevant facts in about a hundred. At the Foreign Office Cantlie made a written statement and left Sun's scribbled requests for help. The Foreign Office then contacted the Home Department and Sir M. White Ridley (later Lord Ridley), unpaid secretary to his father, Secretary of State for the Home Department, was asked whether it would be desirable to make inquiries at 36 Little Albany Street to see if Cole could be questioned further. But Lord Salisbury had already made up his mind on the strength of the memo describing Cantlie's visit and Sun's predicament that it would be wise to have the Legation watched by detectives and that a police officer should communicate with Cole in order that Sun should not be removed from it. The memo to Lord Salisbury, giving the facts and this suggestion, asked for his confirmation by telegram which was duly sent. The same day Cole arrived again with further information, written and verbal, which Cantlie forwarded to the Foreign Office. Sun's claims for British citizenship (his life had been spent in China, Hong Kong and Japan and he had a British colonial medical qualification) were anyway irrelevant, because a decision to intervene had already been made. The whole matter was unacceptable by any standards of international law.

Tuesday 20 October: 'A note today to say that Cole the warder will let Sun out tonight onto the roof of the Embassy. Hamish consulted Scotland Yard Police but decided not to allow the risk. It is not the right way. Lord Salisbury saw the papers today.' It was the only point on which Mabel Cantlie was wrong. Lord Salisbury had already seen the papers; once set in motion the wheels of British officialdom turn with astounding speed. By Tuesday the police reports showed that Sir Halliday McCartney was being watched, that the booking on the Glenline steamer had been confirmed and that the telegrams dispatched to Distance, the registered word for Slaters Detective Agency which was working for the Chinese, had been intercepted. The police had also arranged for all ships to be watched. The waiting game continued. For the first time the diary of Wednesday 21 October records other events first – the Cantlies had unbounded optimism and faith in British justice: 'Dr. Sun will be let out soon we think. Inspector Jarvis wants Hamish to go and swear Habeas Corpus tomorrow.' It was, however, easier to surround the Legation with police and detectives to ensure that Sun was not clandestinely removed than it was to extricate him. Thursday 22 October, 'We are still expecting Sun to be liberated. The Chief Inspector of Police took H to get him to swear Habeas

Corpus, but it could not be done for some reason.' In fact, both doctors went and made sworn statements concerning the facts in the case and lodged a writ. These affidavits were endorsed by Mr Justice Wright who hesitated to make an order for habeas corpus because he doubted the propriety of such an order or of a summons against a Foreign Legation. The Judge, however, felt that the affidavits made out a sufficient case for using diplomatic pressure to prevent the man detained from being removed until there had been time for further consideration. Meanwhile Sir Halliday McCartney was still unavailable, even to messengers from the Foreign Office, so a draft letter to the Chinese Minister was sent for approval to Lord Salisbury by Sir Thomas Sanderson (later Lord Sanderson), Permanent Under-Secretary of State for Foreign Affairs. Sir Thomas pointed out that time was pressing since *The Times* had the information and might publish at any minute, causing a scandal if nothing was done. He added in a footnote that Sun was probably not a British subject. Lord Salisbury was also shown the affidavits and the Judge's endorsement, while Sir Matthew Ridley, for the Home Office, gave the same guidance and added the comment that the affidavits were corroborated by the Metropolitan Police. Couched in diplomatic language the draft letter stated that the detention of Sun was 'an infraction of English law not covered by and in abuse of diplomatic privilege accorded to a foreign representative'. It requested Sun's instant release. All the wheels were now turning together; every action necessary for Sun's safety and release was taken at the proper time.

At the end of the entry of Thursday 22 October, after a number of other matters, are the words, 'The newspapers have got the news of Sun now and published tonight'. This was the *Globe*, which had followed the habeas corpus proceedings. Its reporter arrived on the doorstep of 46 and, according to Sun in his book, confronted Cantlie with the facts. Cantlie explained that he had given *The Times* the information on Sunday and further information on Monday and he felt bound to let them publish first. However, the information that the *Globe* had received was so accurate that Cantlie, requesting his name should not be mentioned, endorsed it as correct. The fifth edition of the paper carried the story as headline news. Within two hours, according to Sun's account, Cantlie was interviewed by the Central News Agency and the *Daily Mail*. Friday 23 October: 'We were inundated with reporters this morning and Hamish was taken this afternoon by the chief inspector of police to liberate Sun Yat Sen. There is fearful excitement all over the world over this case. He came in tonight looking thin but happy ... Thank God.' All the time, behind the scenes, negotiations had been proceeding to secure Sun's release. Sir Halliday had at last made himself available and was summoned to the Foreign Office to be told that Lord Salisbury, after consultation with the Attorney General, was of the opinion that Sun's detention was an abuse of diplomatic privilege. Sir Halliday said first that he did not know the man's true name, then that he had asked for him to be extradited on arrival but had been refused, then that Sun had called at the Legation the previous day and finally that Sun had called at the Legation of his own free will, both singularly unlikely for a man with a price on his head. Sir Halliday left the Foreign Office saying that he must telegraph to China. This story of a voluntary call by Sun was one which it afterwards turned out Sir Halliday had had the temerity to plan. Sun was told by Tang, his gaoler, that if he signed a note saying that he had not been involved in the Canton plot, and that he had called at the Legation in order to prove it, he would be given his freedom. Sun realised afterwards the stupidity of what he had done but, as he says in his book, 'A dying man will clutch at anything'. When Sir Halliday called at the Foreign Office for the second time he tried to make, as a price for Sun's release, the assurance that Hong Kong would not be used as a base for plots against the Empire. This request was refused — the British Government did not make bargains. On this occasion Sir Halliday accused Sun of stealing notes of a translation from his house. On 23 October, the day all the morning papers carried the story of Sun's kidnapping and detention, Sir Halliday called to say that the Chinese Minister consented to the release. It was arranged that a Home Office messenger and police inspector would accompany Cantlie to the Legation at 4.30 p.m. and secure the release of the prisoner. Sun was taken straight to Scotland Yard where he made a statement and then to 46 Devonshire Street, where he was given a great welcome followed by a dinner party of family and friends.

If the story reads like a true version of Beau Geste, this feeling is enhanced by Mr Bertie of the Foreign Office (later ambassador in Paris) who said in his first letter to Lord Salisbury that in spite of Sun's 'spurious plot for seizing Canton of which we have heard', Sun was said to be 'a very good fellow'. This was certainly the view of him taken by the British press and shared by the Cantlie children who woke him with their games on Saturday morning. Sun described in his book how he heard the voices of children romping on the floor above:

'Now Colin, you be Sun Yat Sen, and Neil will be Sir Halliday McCartney, and I will rescue Sun.' Then followed a turmoil; Sir Halliday was knocked endways, and a crash on the floor made me believe that my little friend Neil was no more. Colin was brought out in triumph by Keith, the eldest boy, and a general amnesty was declared by the beating of drums and the singing of 'The British Grenadiers'. This was home and safety, indeed; for it was evident my youthful friends were prepared to shed the last drop of their blood on my behalf.

The diary entry for the day was: 'Reporters and friends to congratulate Hamish all day in troops, it brought old friends to see us who did not know where we were.' Press reports, articles and letters flooded the newspapers, particularly *The Times*, in which Sir Halliday attempted in a letter to excuse his behaviour. His allegation that Sun had gone to the Legation of his own free will was treated with contempt. No one had better knowledge of the Manchus' cruelty than Sun; he had seen nearly all his friends in Canton executed and no one could have less reason to put his head on the block. 'We cannot conceal our surprise,' said a *Times* article, 'that an Englishman should have taken any part in a transaction manifestly doomed to failure and the success of which would have been ruinous to all engaged in it.' The *China Mail* took up the story on 3 December and said of Sun, 'An unassuming manner and an earnestness of speech combined with a quick perception and resolute judgement go to impress one with the conviction that he is in every way an exceptional type of his race. Beneath his calm exterior is hidden a personality that cannot but be a great influence for good in China sooner or later, if the Fates are fair.' Of Cantlie it said, 'All who know Dr. Cantlie – and he is known in many parts of the world – agree that a more upright, honourable and devoted benefactor of humanity has never breathed.'

The Treasury Solicitor was asked by Lord Salisbury to make a full investigation of the affair. He came to four conclusions: first, that Sun's story of how he got into the Legation was probably true: secondly, that Sir Halliday McCartney's story was probably false; thirdly, that Sir Halliday was probably misinformed and was repeating what he had been told; fourthly, that the Legation intended to ship Sun to China. The Treasury Solicitor stated that the cards were consistent with the account Sun now gave and with the detailed statement he made at Scotland Yard on Friday 23 October when, although excited and exhausted, there was no substantial variation. It was also similar to Dr Cantlie and Dr Manson's statement the following day. He concluded that Sun's reason for being in Portland Place was that he was visiting Dr Cantlie. Of Sun's story of his kidnapping the report said that having found Sun truthful on material points he believed his story as to the manner in which he was induced to enter the house to be probably true in substance.[3] It only remained for the British Minister in Peking to convey to the Chinese Government that HM Government believed the kidnapping to be 'an infraction of English law which was not covered by and was an abuse of diplomatic privilege'. A question was asked in the House by Sir Edward Gourlay as to whether Sir Halliday as a British subject should not be held responsible for Sun's capture and detention, but the matter was dropped. Sun wrote a letter to the newspapers on 24 October thanking the Government and press for their help:

> Will you kindly express through your columns my keen appreciation of the actions of the British Government in effecting my release from the Chinese Legation. I have also to thank the press generally for their timely help and sympathy. If anything were needed to convince me of the generous public spirit which pervades Great Britain, and the love of justice which distinguishes its people the recent acts of the last few days have conclusively done so. Knowing and feeling more keenly than ever what a constitutional Government and an enlightened people mean, I am prompted still more actively to pursue the cause of advancement, education and civilisation in my own well-beloved but oppressed country.

As stated in the concluding paragraph of his letter, Sun spent much of his subsequent nine months' stay in Britain in the Reading Room of the British Museum studying Western economic and political thought, legal systems and civil service administration, military and naval organisation, industrial and agricultural matters, as well as the development of railways, to which he devoted much of his life and which he saw as the only method of opening up and uniting China, as had recently been done in Canada. After staying a few weeks with the Cantlies, he returned to his rooms with Miss Pollard. He shared with Cantlie many dinner and lecture dates on 'Things Chinese', as well as going to Oxford and other towns to lecture on his own.

In June Sun set off for Japan, Mabel Cantlie seeing him off on the dockside. After his departure the Cantlies attended a reception for the Premier of New South Wales where they met the new Chinese Minister, Loh Fen Luh – after the kidnapping the previous Minister had been quickly replaced. The diary records how they both spoke to the Minister about Sun and a week later Mabel Cantlie called at the Chinese Legation. Shortly afterwards the detectives were called off Sun's track. Doubts have been cast on whether Sun ever repaid Cole the money he is said to have promised him. The honouring of debts is one of the deepest principles in Chinese ethics and code of behaviour. Debts not paid by anyone losing his life must be paid by his descendants. If money was promised in recompense for references lost then it is doubtful that it would have remained unpaid for very long. Such rumours are some of the bubbles blown into the air surrounding the case. There is no doubt that the kidnapping left its mark on Sun. He knew the arm of the Manchus was long; he was transformed from a youthful Garibaldi into a man who trusted very few people, who played with his cards so close to his chest that accusations of opportunism were increasingly levelled at him. He continued to draw deeply on the ancient wisdom of the Chinese classics which he now combined with far-reaching and idealistic dreams for the future. His faith in Christianity had been strengthened, his hatred of bloodshed increased, while his gratitude to the British people, and his respect for their institutions and their justice had made a tie which nothing in the future could ever alter.

CHAPTER NINE
Tropical Medicine

The events of October 1896 had far-reaching consequences, not only on Sun Yat Sen's character, but also on Cantlie. Although he was just as ready to plunge into schemes for bettering mankind, the sensitive side of his nature led him to prefer to take a lesser seat and give others the praise and recognition that came from his own hard work. Publicity now accompanied him (the style of his writing brought it to him, apart from the genius of his prolific and inventive ideas), he was regarded by many journalists and politicians as an authority on China, his name was linked with the Volunteer Medical Forces, civilian first aid and tropical medicine and surgery. The bubonic plague, having struck in China and south-east Asia, was now spreading across India, responsibility of the India Office, decimating cities and populations. On 16 December 1896 the diary records: 'H lecturing at the Epidemiological Society on the Plague. He had Dr. Lowson and others to dinner first.' On 18 December two plague cases were reported in London and on 9 January the lecture was printed in the *Lancet* and *BMJ*. On that day the diary records: 'H went up to town and telegraphed he could not come back, as he had been commanded to write a report on the Plague for the Queen and the India Office. This is a great compliment.' Many of the ideas Cantlie put forward were novel; he stated that rats were the purveyors of disease, that they were the animals most likely to be attacked by plague, that they might infect other animals, that rats were always affected by a disease similar to plague at the time men were suffering, that they might infect men but by what means was not known, and that during an outbreak of 'benign plague' (or *pestis minor*) rats did not die. Cantlie stated that the present geographical distribution of plague in India coincided with the distribution of a particular family of rats (it was, in fact, these black rats which were most likely to carry the flea, of whose deadly bite the doctors were not yet aware, so that, without realising it, Cantlie had made a breakthrough in research). 'One sub family', he said,

> that of the Nesokia, is met with reaching from Palestine to Formosa, across the northern part of India . . . This is the only animal which presents a habitation well nigh corresponding to the present distribution of plague and it is this animal above all others, which is liable to be attacked by plague. The geographical distribution of this family of rats well-nigh coincides with the plague belt as delineated . . . The

bubo is essentially the swelling of the glands caused by the entrance of the septic material in the tract of the lymphatics ... There is no doubt now that the disease in the rat and the man are identical ... The bacillus of plague has been met with in every case of rate disease of this description ... The infection of the rat is raised from mere popular belief into one of scientific precision ... Whether the rat is affected previously to, coincidentally with, or subsequently to, man being attacked is open to question ... But the rat seems to be infected before the human being.

Cantlie drew the conclusion that, since islands were infected, the poison 'must be carried by human beings, by animals, by clothing or by food'.[1] He paid tribute to Dr Lowson's Report on the Plague, published in 1895, which gave as its causes 'direct contagion from the patient or from the dust or dirt of the room', with filth, overcrowding, insanitary conditions and bad drainage as contributory factors.[2] Cantlie agreed that these factors helped to spread the disease, but reiterated that they were not the cause, and only played a part once something else had set it a-going.

The doctors in subsequent discussion – reported in the *Lancet* on 2 January – did not attribute much significance to Cantlie's ideas. Lowson repeated his belief that plague was transmitted by 'inoculation, inspiration or introduction into the stomach'; he was still treating the disease as one of direct infection and said that although the 'infection of soil' theory was by no means disproved it had as yet yielded no positive results. The *Lancet* commented, 'The question of the infection of rodents is one upon which more light is needed, as it seems doubtful whether rats are, as has been believed, infected prior to the human species or whether only the incubation period in rats is shorter than in man. In this connexion Cantlie's observations as to the similarity in geographical distribution between plague and a certain sub family of rats seems to call for further investigation.' On 11 January and subsequent days the diary continued:

H not very well. He has hard writing. Sent his [report and] map of Plague to the India Office and through them to the Queen. Surgeon General Hooper, the adviser to the Indian Government (Surgeon General Sir William Hooper was President of the Medical Board at the India Office) has been here to see H about the plague in India. Panic spreading in India with awful distress caused by plague and famine ... H had map returned from Osborne and the Queen had desired Sir James Reid to write to Surgeon General Hooper and thank him and so H for the promptness with which the map and papers were sent in. H thinks he ought to offer to go to India and help with the plague and has called on Sir Joseph Fayrer. Oh, how I hope he won't go, but I cannot say so.

Fortunately wisdom prevailed; Cantlie's home and professional commitments were too many and his health too impaired by residence in the East. A fortnight later: 'H will not go to the plague in India now I think, as he has advised the Government to send Dr. Lowson who departs immediately and will have to sign on for a year.' Instead, Cantlie was appointed adviser on Plague to the India Office and the diary continues, 'H advises Surgeon General Hooper from day to day when he comes and also writes all the articles on plague for the B.M.J.' During the year, in addition to signed articles by Cantlie there were weekly unsigned articles on plague in the *BMJ*. One of his pastimes was writing unsigned articles in his own journal and other periodicals and thus it is impossible to know whether any or what number of these may be the articles to which she refers.

The crisis in India urgently highlighted the need to disseminate knowledge of tropical medicine by means of centralised teaching premises and for a society and journal to co-ordinate research. The science of tropical medicine did not start with a single seed, it germinated in different soils and grew together into a tree of knowledge. In 1821 William Wilberforce, Macaulay and other philanthropists started the Seamen's Hospital Society, allowed by the Royal Navy to anchor a hospital ship, *Grampus*, with 181 beds off Greenwich, where the Admiralty ran its own hospital for pensioners from the Royal Navy and Royal Dockyards. On *Grampus* 3,000 merchant seamen suffering from tropical and other diseases were treated during its first three years and, as a mark of its success, the Admiralty gave the Society the right to fly the Royal Navy Union flag and pennant, its own jealously guarded prerogative. Then, in 1831, it provided the Society with a larger hospital ship, *Dreadnought*, with 235 beds and an operating theatre. By now the links of friendship between the Royal Navy and the Society were close and senior naval officers became members of the SHS Committee. With the enlarged facilities in *Dreadnought* the Society was able to teach students as well as treat patients and among those attending its instruction in tropical medicine were Edinburgh University medical students, some of whom were no doubt members of the newly formed Edinburgh Medical Missionaries Association.[3] In 1867 the Society asked the Prime Minister if it might bring the *Dreadnought* ashore into a wing of the Greenwich Hospital and three years later it was granted a ninety-nine year lease by the Admiralty so that, by 1873, merchant seamen were being treated in the spacious wards of a hospital situated beside the classical elegance of the Royal Naval College, Greenwich, on a sweep of the river renowned for its beauty. The opportunities for instruction in tropical diseases were diverse, for into this hospital came merchant seamen of all nationalities with no colour discrimination, Lascars, blacks and Europeans suffering from multifarious diseases. Soon the Society extended its teaching facilities to students of the London medical schools, while at the same time starting its own nursing school modelled on the Nightingale at St Thomas's.

Meanwhile the Army Medical Department had been teaching tropical medicine and bacteriology, first at its newly formed Medical School at Chatham in 1860 and then since 1863 at its 1,000-bed hospital at

Netley, to which the School was moved, and which provided instruction in tropical medicine, hygiene and sanitation. The army had need of instruction in these subjects, not only to safeguard the health of its troops (at Tirah for every 1,000 men dying of gunshot wounds 11,000 died from fever and dysentery), but also because of its responsibility for the health of local populations in colonies where troops were stationed. The School was independent, under the Secretary of State for War, with the Director General Army Medical Department as president of the Senate. In 1885 King's College Hospital also set up facilities for teaching tropical medicine and bacteriology and, while many London medical schools followed this example, shortage of funds made them grateful for the practical and research opportunities available to their students at *Dreadnought*. In 1890 the Seamen's Hospital Society opened a branch hospital with eighteen beds at the Royal Victoria and Albert Docks at the far end of Connaught Road, right in the heart of dockland, which was opened by the Prince and Princess of Wales and which was intended for emergency cases coming from newly docked ships. The Society appointed Manson Honorary Physician to this new branch hospital, and in 1896 consulted him about enlarging it.

Such was the picture when in August 1897 Joseph Chamberlain, Secretary of State for the Colonies, appointed Manson Medical Adviser to the Colonies. Unlike Lord Salisbury, Prime Minister and Foreign Secretary, who believed in free trade, Joseph Chamberlain wanted to see trade barriers surrounding an expanding Empire, but the ambition inherent in his radical policy was humanised by his interest in colonial, medical and welfare administration, which resulted in the founding of schools of tropical medicine. Unlike the Indian Medical Service, which trained at Netley, the medical staff in the colonies had no access to a tropical medical school and, like the doctors in commercial companies with overseas interests, their need for training was great. Manson was already instructing in tropical medicine at a number of London Schools and on 1 October 1897 he spoke at the opening session of St George's Hospital of the need for systematic teaching of tropical medicine in medical schools and quoted Dr Andrew Davidson's call for lectures on hygiene and diseases of warm climates in each medical school, for centralised examinations and for government involvement in tropical pathology.[4] He pointed out that one fifth of doctors served abroad and that figure included army and naval officers. Immediately he ran into criticism. The *Dreadnought* staff, jealous of their independence and their role in tropical medicine, had already asked Manson not to refer to himself as Honorary Physician of the *Dreadnought* – from which position he had previously retired – and they now took him up on his remarks about the ships' doctors incorrectly diagnosing beri beri, which was mostly brought into the country by P and O stokers, and entering this incorrect diagnosis upon the hospital register. They made him publicly admit that he was referring to the Albert Dock Hospital and not to the *Dreadnought*. The *Lancet*, in publishing the correspondence, said in an editorial on 30 October that the medical authorities and War Office had not been so

unmindful of their obligations as had been suggested, while many
doctors, including the Dean of St Mary's in a letter to *The Times* on
3 November, emphasised the important liaison that existed between
the *Dreadnought* and the London medical schools. Even *The Times* on
4 October was critical of Manson's suggestions, claiming that instruction
in tropical disease was available at many schools and for all medical
officers of the public services.

This was not strictly true and on 11 October an anonymous letter to
The Times signed R. N. pointed out the lack of instruction in tropical
diseases at Haslar. This letter has been attributed to Inspector General
Alexander Turnbull, a friend of the Cantlies, at whose house they
stayed for naval reviews. On the 18th Cantlie also came to Manson's
aid, with a letter to *The Times* again emphasising this need. After six
years of sending naval surgeons to the Army Medical School at Netley,
the Royal Navy had started instructing at Haslar in 1881, but when
Inspector General Alexander Turnbull arrived there he found no
instruction at all in tropical disease.

> Under no circumstances [wrote Cantlie in his letter] is the medical
> man thrown more upon his own resources than at sea, where he has
> no one to consult with . . . It would therefore seem to be incumbent
> upon the Naval Medical Officers to be fully equipped and highly
> efficient . . . The loss to the nation cannot perhaps be put at its
> commercial value but the loss to science is invaluable. The Medical
> Officers of the Navy have opportunities of observing and recording
> diseases in all parts of the world. The Naval Medical Schools have no
> laboratories for the teaching of bacteriology nor lectureships on
> tropical disease.

His letter pointed out both the need for instruction and for the
collation of presently unrecorded research which the navy had unique
and world-wide opportunities to acquire. The suggestion of instruction was for the moment met on 26 October with the answer 'No' in a
letter to *The Times* from Inspector General Walter Reid who, however,
advanced the idea of once more using naval statistics on health of
medical personnel to issue annual reports. This was the chance Cantlie
wanted, for the idea of starting a journal was already in his mind. The
diary records, 'H is anxious to bring out a new Journal on Tropical
Diseases. He wrote a letter to The Times to ask that the navy should be
taught Tropical Diseases at Haslar.' He had now caught two fish. The
following year – 1898 – he brought out his successful *Journal of Tropical
Medicine*, using service, private and commercial records from overseas,
with Professor Simpson as co-editor and Dr Turnbull, Inspector
General Hospital and Fleet, adviser and proof reader. (A few years
later he floated in its pages his next idea, a Society of Tropical Medicine.) Also in 1898 he proposed a resolution at the Parliamentary Bills
Committee of the British Medical Association (BMA) that a deputation
should be sent to the Admiralty, pointing out the need for the navy to
give instruction in tropical medicine at Haslar. Following upon this

resolution, Cantlie was asked by the President of the Council to send a letter to Captain Fawkes, asking if Mr Goschen would receive a deputation. This was met on 13 July 1898 by the answer that the Admiralty was already in agreement and there were only administrative difficulties to be overcome. Arrangements for instruction were finalised by the following year.

The other public service where no instruction in tropical medicine was given was the Colonial Service. While Chamberlain was instigating discussions at the Colonial Office as to the best site for a London school, Manson was continuing with his teaching and research in tropical medicine and writing books on the diseases of warm climates, while Cantlie also researched for and published papers on a number of aspects of tropical medicine and surgery. One of these was on liver abscess, for which operation Cantlie was much in demand as a surgeon all over the country and for which he perfected the technique and the instruments for drawing off pus. In June 1897 he crossed to Ireland to give a paper to the Anatomical Society on the gall bladder's position in relation to the liver, pointing out its position lying midway between the two lobes. He said that the central location of the inferior vena cava made the liver less likely to haemorrhage there and therefore more likely to tolerate surgery or accident if incised or torn in its neighbourhood. The diary records, 'H surprised many of the doctors with his ideas', but later photographs published in Byam and Archibald's work on tropical diseases proved the correctness of his findings.[5] In Hong Kong, when Cantlie gave evidence on the death of a Chinese prisoner who committed suicide, he noticed that the right side of the liver had atrophied while the left had increased in size. Even in the case of cancer he noticed, as well as liver abscess, it was possible for the right to atrophy and for the left to be healthy.

> The anatomical evidence seems therefore to point to a completely separate vascular supply up to the mid line of the liver [situated] along a line drawn from the centre of the notch for the gall bladder upon the anterior border of the liver to the notch for the inferior vena cava at the posterior margin . . . Perhaps in malignant disease more than in any other is it observed that the disease is confined to one lobe . . . In other words we have two lobes [or two livers] which coalesce along a mid line, giving a right and left half, the left half including the minor lobes . . . One half of the liver can hypertrophy so as to perform the function of the whole . . . In the same way that one kidney can develop so as to carry on the work of the two.[6]

Cantlie's interest in the liver and gall bladder was part of his wider investigations into the functioning of the alimentary canal and in particular of sprue. In his papers on sprue he suggested that it was caused by rancid vegetable oil and recommended the addition of whites of egg and baked bread to the high protein meat diet he had previously advocated. His interest in beri beri, on which his wife had translated the standard work, caused him to turn his attention to pellagra, which he had met in Egypt and which was now prevalent in

Europe, Asia, Africa, America and Australasia, often leading, like beri beri, eventually to insanity. Interested in the problem of lunacy in the East – the diary records the number of Europeans who had to be restrained in Hong Kong – Cantlie had already been researching into the connection between tropical diseases and nervous disorders and, consequent upon this, he accepted an honorary consultancy at the West End London Hospital for Nervous Diseases. The *Lancet* was currently carrying a correspondence on damage to brain cells by tropical sun and, although now regarded cautiously, this reinforced Cantlie's theories on the importance of wearing a topee. Although residence in the East took its toll in many ways on the health of Europeans Cantlie did not believe this was necessarily permanent and he advocated that the young men he was examining as recruits for trading companies should, after returning home, have their life insurance premiums returned to the normal level. 'Why,' he asked, 'should they have to pay higher premiums years after their return to a temperate climate?' He believed, as Manson had done in Amoy, that long periods in the East caused tropical anaemia, owing to excess of unevaporated perspiration and reduction of oxygen intake caused by heat and dampness, but he said that this could be quickly cured by convalescence, such as he had had, in pure invigorating air like that of the uplands of north-east Scotland. His articles on life insurance in the *BMJ* and the *Lancet* were backed by editorials and Sir Dyce Duckworth, chairman of the Life Assurance Medial Officers' Association, and eventually met with success.

Leprosy still featured largely in his interest and, as a forerunner to the *Journal*, he prepared a paper on the subject, delivered on 17 December 1897 to the Epidemiological Society. Reported in the *BMJ* of 1 January 1898 it was based on his prize-winning monograph and later expanded into a book. It is a remarkable document and explains the admiration Sir Joseph Fayrer had for his ability. Entitled 'A report on the physical and ethnological conditions under which leprosy occurs in China, the Malay Peninsula, the East Indian Archipelago, and the islands of the Pacific', the research covers one third of the world's surface and was based on correspondence with medical men, missionaries, consul agents, customs officials and others. It established the method for the collation of material for his *Journal*. Among his observations were the following: that leprosy bore close resemblance to tuberculosis; it arose in a leprous country, apparently independent of known personal contagium; evidence on heredity was inconclusive; it was not necessarily inoculable; and it arose independent of geological, geographical or climatic conditions but overcrowding, poverty and bad food made people more susceptible. Much of this has now been proved by scientific investigation, for instance that the Eskimos in crowded tented conditions are prone to leprosy. He called for closer inspection of emigrants from China, inspection of coolies on plantations in areas administered by Europeans and deportation of lepers back to their homeland if they contracted leprosy in a country free from the disease, since once asylums were established it became endemic. Contrary to current opinion which thought all China leprous, Cantlie said that only the Southern Provinces were badly affected, in the Middle Kingdom just under half the provinces knew the disease, and in the north only Shantung, and isolated pockets. Japan, Korea, Indo China, Siam and the Malay Peninsula were sufferers, Siberia and Manchuria were not. In the Malay Peninsula the Chinese were more prone to it than the Malays and in Sumatra and Java the belief was that the Chinese coolie brought leprosy. The only islands in the Pacific with the disease were Hawaii where it was prevalent, New Caledonia where it was rare and Fiji where it was very rare. In Borneo it was unknown before the tobacco plantations brought the Chinese coolies. In the Philippines leprosy was prevalent around Manila where many Chinese settled. The vast areas treated in the report included every type of climate except the Arctic. 'Neither climate, nor geological structure appear,' Cantlie said, 'to exercise any influence over the disease . . . The variety of rock formation bears no relation to the distribution of leprosy.' He made the same analysis of the ethnology of the area, the historical distribution of population, the ancient emigrations, the spread of Islam, the push of China south, the arrival of Europeans. He pointed out that negroid races appear to be nearly immune, as do the Indonesians. From this he drew the conclusion that leprosy was not indigenous to the Archipelago or Pacific, but had been introduced recently. The Malays certainly suffered less than the Chinese, yet in North Borneo, where the rich merchant Chinese had been settled for 600 years, leprosy was unknown. 'Wherever the Chinese coolie has settled,' he said, 'leprosy will be found . . . It is the poor starving wretches that are conveyed to the plantations, and it was when they were introduced to Borneo that leprosy appeared . . . It was not till forced labour was introduced by the European that leprosy began to spread; and on this suggestion the peculiarities of its distribution receive a natural and sufficient explanation.'

With Cantlie publishing this and other papers on tropical medicine and about to start a journal, Manson saw him as a valuable ally in the formation of the proposed London School of Tropical Medicine and, according to the diary, Manson now took him to Greenwich with the aim of getting him on to the staff of the Seamen's Hospital Society. There were three choices for the location of such a school; Netley, which most of the doctors favoured – of the leading papers published before 1888 on tropical diseases almost half were written by army medical officers; the *Dreadnought* at Greenwich, the longest established teaching hospital for tropical diseases in the country, dependent on an Admiralty lease; or the small Albert Dock Hospital, which was about to be enlarged and could be the origin of a new concept, a teaching hospital for post-graduate doctors going overseas, either colonial, commercial, missionary or private. (The number of commercial firms employing doctors and of missionary societies opening hospitals overseas had swelled considerably during the second half of the nineteenth century.) It was clear that Chamberlain's views would tip the balance, and throughout the autumn of 1897 the Merchant Navy tried to draw his attention back to his early reforming interest in the conditions of merchant seamen in correspondence in *The Times*, possibly to weight the scales in favour of siting the school at *Dreadnought*. But the concept of a civilian post-graduate medical college, as opposed to under-graduate specialist training, was beginning to take root. On 10 December 1897 the diary records that Dr Fletcher Little dined with the Cantlies 'to tell H of a new Post Graduate Scheme he had on hand. All with new schemes come to Hamish.' It was the first of a number of such visits concerning this post-graduate college to be established on Amer-ican lines, which the *Lancet* suggested should be sited at the West London Hospital, Hammersmith, and provoking sufficient interest in the idea to bring a visit from Princess Louise, Marchioness of Lorne. It was decided, however, to start the college in new premises and the following year it came into existence as the London Medical Graduates College and Polyclinic on the corner of Chenies Street. It had medical and surgical demonstrating rooms, a library and a laboratory.

By 2 February 1898 Chamberlain's ideas had crystallised and he caused a letter to be written to the Seamen's Hospital Society setting out his proposals for a school of tropical medicine which, like the Poly-clinic, was to be post-graduate.

> At present the newly appointed officers receive no special training in the diagnosis and treatment of disease ... It is advised that the experience and training to be obtained at the Seamen's Hospital would be most suitable in the present instance, and he would be greatly obliged to the Managing Committee if they could give him their valuable assistance in the matter ... Mr. Chamberlain under-stands that the Committee are about to enlarge their Branch Hos-pital at the Albert Docks and he would ask them to consider whether it might not be possible to provide the necessary accommodation in the new building for the officers whom it is desired to instruct.[7]

Chamberlain's backing for the idea of starting a school of tropical medicine in which colonial medical officers and nurses could be trained has been considered the greatest contribution he made to prosperity and his country's standing in the world; the London School was due directly to his initiative, and without this lead the Liverpool School might not have come into being at the same time. For good or ill politics had begun to weave its tentacles into medicine. Chamberlain's first interest in medical administration had sprung from his municipal background in Birmingham where his brother Arthur was experi-menting with the beginnings of a local government health service. Implicit in his proposal of 2 February was the idea of a government grant. Did the doctors see this as a threat to their independence? The first like-for-like grant for voluntarily run hospitals was not until 1921, after the recommendations of the Cave Committee, which suggests that, added to the discussion about the choice of site, the arguments in favour of Netley and the disagreements between Manson and the *Dreadnought* staff was an underlying anxiety regarding the acceptance

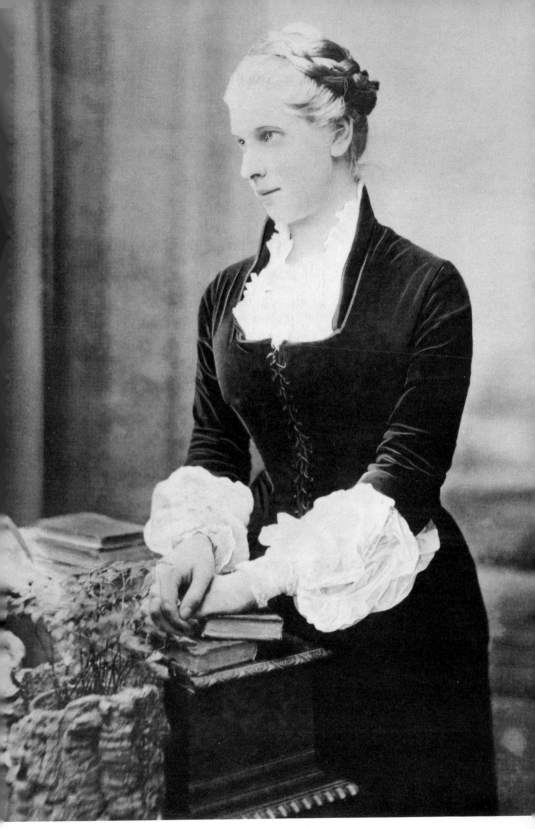

Lady Cantlie.

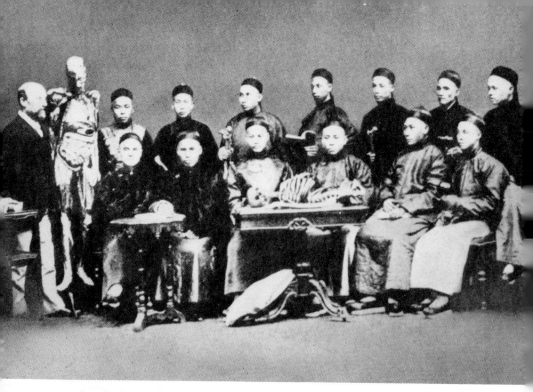

Cantlie lecturing to Chinese students in the College of Medicine for the Chinese.

An emergency plague hospital in Hong Kong; the glass works at Kennedy Town, men's ward. (*Public Records Office, Hong Kong*)

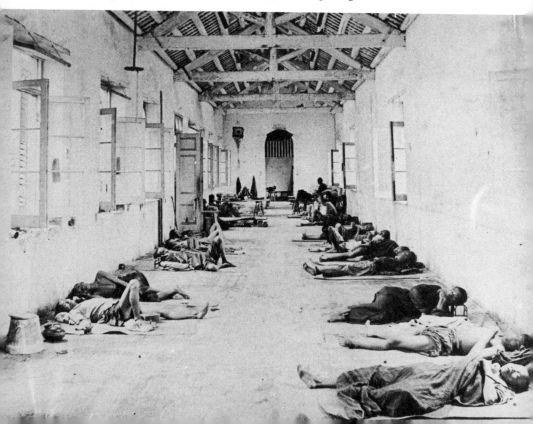

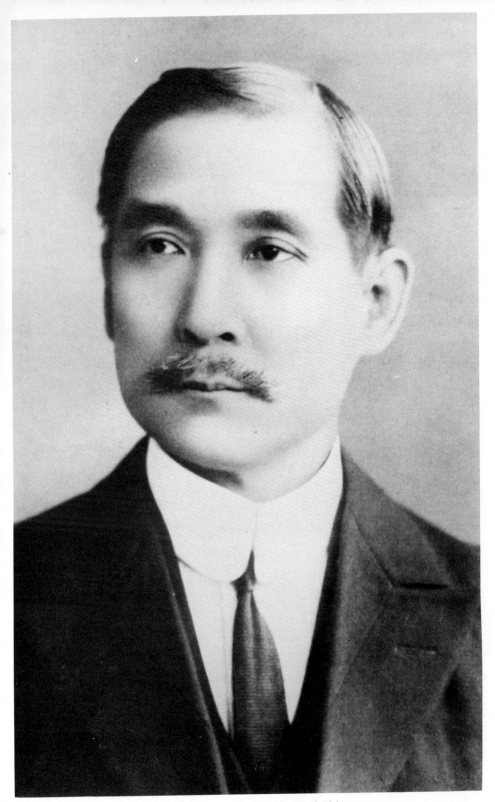

Dr Sun Yat Sen, first President of China.

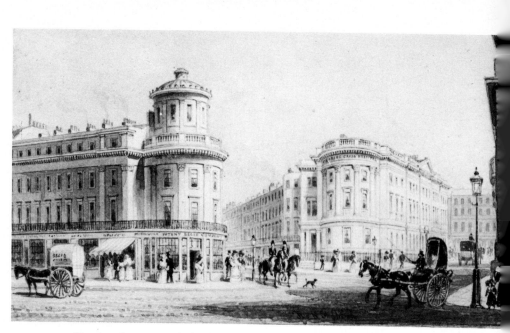

Charing Cross Hospital, nineteenth century print. (*Charing Cross Hospital*)

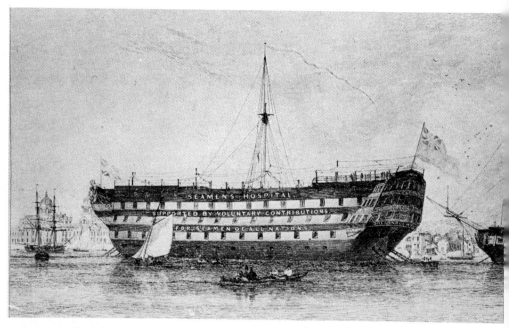

Dreadnought, the first hospital to give instruction in tropical medicine. (*Seamen's Hospital Society*)

of government money. The *Lancet* gave a stern warning to Mr Arthur Chamberlain that his scheme for municipal health in Birmingham, if extended, would destroy the medical profession.

Again Cantlie gave Manson his backing. The positive way of getting out of this problem was to ensure that the School was for medical officers in an organised public service, so that it would be no more unusual for them to receive government money than it would be for the army, the navy or the Indian Medical Service (IMS). Cantlie had seen in Hong Kong during the plague outbreak how dependent the colonial medical administration was on help from the army and wished to see it with sufficient trained expertise of its own. He therefore prepared a paper on the organisation of a colonial medical service which would give it the same advantages as the IMS, members of which received their training in tropical diseases at Netley. On 2 March Cantlie delivered this paper at a meeting at the Imperial Institute under the chairmanship of Sir Joseph Fayrer, pointing out that the colonial doctors needed not only instruction but a properly administered profession and organisation, and that the responsibility of the United Kingdom for the health of the local populations overseas applied equally to the protectorates, and to chemists and nurses as well as to doctors. (That the protectorates were later drawn into the scheme for the tropical school was due to Lord Salisbury's initiative on 12 December 1898, and the founding of the Colonial Nursing Association mainly due to that of Mr and Mrs Chamberlain.) Sir Joseph Fayrer, introducing Cantlie, expressed the hope that the outcome of the paper would be a great colonial medical service, analogous to the IMS.[8] In his paper Cantlie proposed proper intellectual and physical examinations for selection, definition of rank and a promotion ladder, with a director general of the Colonial Medical Service at the top; proper scales of pay and greater facilities for training for both colonial medical officers and private practitioners in the colonies. He remarked that Netley could not easily take private practitioners and, while leaving the issue for the siting of a school wide open, he reminded his audience that 'at the London docks ships from all parts of the world are harboured, and in connection with the docks are excellent hospitals, where it requires only the magic hand of an organiser to utilise the material to be met with there for the purpose of training medical men in tropical diseases before they proceed to the tropics'.[9] He ended on a subject always his deepest concern, that there should be an officer of health reporting to the governor, so that sanitary matters did not have to wait for an epidemic before action was taken, and that the senior medical officer be made an ex officio member of the legislative or executive council. With plague raging in India and probably about to strike again in the colonies and protectorates, it was decided to form a Committee called the Colonial Medical Association, consisting of Sir Joseph Fayrer, Sir William des Voeux (ex Governor, Hong Kong), Sir Guyer Hunter (Army Medical Department), Sir Dyce Duckworth (Barts), Surgeon General Read (AMD), Mr Osbert Chadwick, who had written the 1882 report on Hong Kong sanitation, Mr Furley (St John's),

Professor Simpson and Drs Thin and Turner, and Cantlie, who was appointed Hon. Secretary. On 21 March the Committee met in Cantlie's house and sent a resolution to the Secretary of State saying that it was 'desirable to organise the Colonial Medical Service on lines parallel to the other public medical services'.[10] Following upon this resolution Chamberlain called in 1899 for a review of all Civil Service officials throughout the Empire in order to establish a unified profession, but in spite of this initiative, and a further attempt by Cantlie in 1912 in a speech to the Royal Colonial Institute, the idea of forming a unified colonial medical service with a proper chain of promotion remained a dream until 1934.

On 11 March 1898 a Committee was set up by the Seamen's Hospital Society to consider Mr Chamberlain's proposal for forming a school of tropical medicine. The decision of the Committee was that the school should be at the Albert Docks, with a hospital of forty-five beds, teaching provision for twenty to twenty-five students, residential accommodation for ten and a laboratory, pathological department and other facilities. In their letter of acceptance the Committee stated that they had 190 cases of well marked tropical diseases annually, including Africans, Asians, Indians and Europeans and, in a memo, explained why the Albert Dock had been chosen in preference to *Dreadnought* – because it was more accessible and not dependent on a six-month Admiralty lease. The senior medical officers of the Society would be required to send their interesting cases from *Dreadnought* to the new teaching centre, but they would all be invited to join the teaching staff. In June the Colonial Office accepted these suggestions, put forward a basis of fees and confirmed a grant of £3,500, stating that the protectorates were also to join the scheme and that a representative of the Colonial Office should be admitted to the Board of Management of the SHS. In July an appeal was launched for the London School of Tropical Medicine and Mr Chamberlain agreed to attend a banquet later in the year. The appeal inferred that the staff of the *Dreadnought*, as members of the Seamen's Hospital Society, were to teach gratuitously at the new School and that the most interesting cases were to be concentrated there. Again the staff of the *Dreadnought* took up their pens saying they had never been consulted, and the *Lancet* on 16 July backed them, saying 'It can hardly be expected that the physicians and surgeons attached to the SHS can undertake any more gratuitous work than they have at present.' It may have been that, unlike the staff of many London hospitals, or indeed of the College of Medicine for the Chinese, the staff of the *Dreadnought* would have found it difficult to reimburse themselves from the pockets of richer patients who could afford to pay; but already the missionary zeal of the nineteenth century was abating, judging from the newspapers and official records which featured many requests for higher salaries.

Meanwhile on 14 May the *Lancet* had promoted the forthcoming start of Cantlie's *Journal of Tropical Medicine*, saying it was 'to be devoted to the publication of papers on tropical diseases and the discussion of subjects scientific and practical, affecting the interests of medical men in the tropical and sub tropical climates'. Cantlie's idea was not only to publish articles by doctors and surgeons on research into tropical diseases and their cures, but to collate information from all over the world, as he had done in his leprosy report, and was later to do on plague, and also to promote medical subjects for 'discussion', so that new ideas might be promulgated. In August the BMA took an historic step in tropical medicine by opening its own Tropical Section, with Manson as President and Cantlie as one of the Honorary Secretaries, and Cantlie's *Journal of Tropical Medicine* produced its first edition. 'Its object,' wrote Sir Joseph Fayrer, 'is the consideration and discussion of tropical diseases and of questions of etiology, hygiene and preventive medicine or any cognate, scientific subjects affecting a large part of our Empire. It is intended to collect in one focus the knowledge that has been acquired upon the above subjects under such varying conditions of existence and climate.' The financial cost of the *Journal* Cantlie bore himself for the first nine years, hoping that sufficient subscribers could be found to support it. These were not long in coming forward and, even by the time the first *Journal* was being prepared, he had the support of the Royal Navy, the Army and Indian Medical Service, as well as the colonial medical officers and subscribers among medical men in Europe, Asia, Africa, the Americas, the Middle East and islands in the Pacific and Atlantic. All that was being done, Cantlie pointed out, was to follow the lead of Germany, France and Holland in collating fragmentary and local knowledge together. The journalistic professionalism of the magazine, together with its lively style, explains why, in his old school at Fochabers, Cantlie is still remembered first as a writer. Appealing for public support in the *Journal* for the new London School of Tropical Medicine, Cantlie pointed out how much the owners of the shipping lines would benefit, 'for the cases are native seamen from India, Africa, China, the West Indies, and the Pacific Islands'.

It was precisely these people who had responded to a similar scheme in Liverpool initiated by Mr A. L. Jones, senior partner of a shipping firm carrying the bulk of African trade, who gave an annual grant of £350 to equip a ward of twelve beds in the Royal Southern Hospital to work in connection with the laboratories of University College Liverpool in the study of tropical diseases. Liverpool was in daily communication with the fever-haunted coasts of Africa and his generosity was soon matched by other businessmen and foreign consuls, swelling the grant of £350 to £2,000. In October Cantlie was confirmed as a member of the Advisory Committee appointed to draw up a constitution for the London School, and in November Chamberlain sent a letter to the General Medical Council setting out his intention to found a School which he hoped missionary societies, trading corporations and private practitioners would make use of as well as colonial medical officers. The letter paid tribute to the tropical work at Netley, Haslar and twelve British medical schools, but pointed out that many schools were inhibited from starting instruction by lack of equipment and funds. The letter was intended to take the heat out of the controversy, but editorials continued to point to the advantages of Netley, which handled more cases of tropical disease than any European hospital, and criticised the Albert Dock as too small, difficult of access, expensive to develop and likely to deplete *Dreadnought* of interesting cases. In December the *Lancet* re-published a letter to *The Times* from many of the leading doctors and surgeons of London (including almost every leading London hospital and many of Cantlie's personal friends), saying that even at this stage plans could be changed and Netley chosen for the Colonial Medical Service, while missionaries, corporation and private doctors could study at the London hospitals, attending *Dreadnought* for clinical practice, and go to the provincial medical schools which had facilities for instruction in tropical diseases. They stressed the long traditions of *Dreadnought* which should not be depleted of its interesting cases nor lose its links with London medical students. A letter from the *Dreadnought* staff emphasised the same points, claiming that their Admiralty lease was for ninety-nine years, not six months, and that the new scheme was too extravagant, with fees not meeting costs.

On Christmas Eve they again made a bitter attack on Manson in the *Lancet*. Certainly the proposed site was in the heart of dockland and hardly, it might seem, a propitious place to attract medical students from overseas – to the south railway lines and wharves led down to the docks, to the west streets lined with shops, pubs and shabby houses were crowded with dray horses and motor traffic. But Manson and Cantlie were used to the sights and scents of the East and the homely background of the Alice Memorial Hospital in Hong Kong and saw, as did the SHS, that the Victoria and Albert Dock was the busiest point for ships disembarking cargoes from the East and that the very absence of wealth in the area demonstrated the necessity for instruction in hygiene and sanitation. They saw also that the distance between the docks and the London hospitals was crucial to the argument, for only by shorter travelling time could vital links be forged between the new Hospital School and leading medical consultants. Whether the decision to site the hospital at the Albert Dock was right or wrong could only be known with hindsight, for it was Chamberlain's decision and the SHS fell in with it. Now, the very success of the School demonstrates the wisdom of their choice, for there is a thriving School of Hygiene and Tropical Medicine in London with which St Pancras Hospital, specialising in tropical medicine, is connected and the *Dreadnought* at Greenwich is still a leading hospital for tropical disease. Again, intending to heal all rifts, Chamberlain said that candidates such as those from King's or Liverpool who had received instruction in tropical medicine and bacteriology would be given preference in selection for the Colonial Medical Service, but that afterwards they must attend the London school for final training. On 18 March Chamberlain was reported as answering a House of Commons question on the proposed school by saying that Dr Manson considered that the *Dreadnought* offered the best opportunity for dealing with these matters. The mistaken and repeated substitution of the words *Dreadnought* or Greenwich for the Albert Dock was the last straw for the *Dreadnought* staff. They had lost the argument, and they claimed they had been treated with discourtesy and not been properly consulted. The *Lancet* on 1 April said that want of courtesy had led the Colonial Office to consult the Physician of the Branch Hospital who 'although Medical Adviser to the Colonial Office is Junior in standing to the staff of the *Dreadnought*'. The controversy can only be regretted; whether the consequences of the decision on location could have been avoided by diplomacy is a matter for conjecture: what mattered as letters to the *BMJ* pointed out was that the school was established.

The following month Lord Lister opened the Liverpool School of Tropical Medicine and tropical schools followed in Edinburgh, Aberdeen and other provincial hospitals, some being attended by nurses as well as by doctors. On 13 May Mrs Chamberlain launched an appeal to found a Colonial Nursing Association to select nurses and pay their salaries and passage overseas. The rest of the world was now following Britain's lead and by autumn Chamberlain's dream of medical colleges in the tropics in the style of that in Hong Kong was beginning to be realised. In September he was reported as founding a pathological laboratory in the Malay Peninsula to investigate beri beri and reports came back from the West Indies about improvements in hospitals there. 'As long as suffering humanity appeals to us,' wrote Cantlie, 'so long will his work endure.'

In May Cantlie was appointed Honorary Surgeon to the Seamen's Hospital Society which took him down to the docks at all hours of day and night to do emergency operations on victims of accident or tropical disease. The School was to be officially opened on 2 October. Because of the controversy surrounding its location and the acceptance of a government grant it did not prove easy to find a distinguished member of the profession to give the opening address. The *BMJ* had remained aloof from the controversy and only given details of the proposed plan and its progress towards completion. Now it reported a meeting of the Tropical Section of the BMA in which Dr Thin dwelt on the regretted resignation of the *Dreadnought* staff, likening them to men buried under the foundations and, while expressing goodwill and congratulations to the School, could not resist one last 'dig' at the need for a government grant. Cantlie, the peacemaker, circumvented the problem raised by his controversial resolution, and Manson's amendment, which might have been interpreted as giving Chamberlain too much credit for the initiative in the Liverpool School, by diverting the meeting into a discussion on sprue and liver abscess and then bringing forward a bland resolution sending their thanks to Mr Chamberlain for his starting of the London School of Tropical Medicine. Because of these problems, Manson thought it inexpedient to have a formal opening and undertook to read an address to the assembled students. The address was an eloquent exposition on the place of rats in the spread of plague. At the last moment Manson was unable to be present and Cantlie read the address for him, perhaps not entirely out of place, since his research had contributed greatly to the subject. Meanwhile, draft orders had been placed before Parliament concerning a link with the University of London and in December there was a meeting of lecturers of the London School of Tropical Medicine to discuss recognition of its training by the University.

During the first sessions twenty-eight students attended, of whom fourteen were medical colonial officers and the others were army, navy, or surgeons to railways, mines or corporations in the tropics. Two students attended from the Continent. The disputes were past, the hills climbed. That the London School of Tropical Medicine was born in dispute did it no harm. Cantlie merely aided what could be described as a difficult birth; and he started lecturing there immediately after its opening session. Now his mind was ranging on again to fresh hills and new pastures. In the same volume of the *BMJ* which described the School's opening, he was writing new ideas on tooth decay, on the fact that cancer of the ovary acted faster on younger women than on old, and on a rash with high temperature which was caused by caterpillars. All that mattered to him was that the job was done and the mission accomplished. As Sir Dyce Duckworth said in his Harveian Oration before the Royal College of Physicians in 1898:

We are perhaps too much disposed to commemorate the scientific achievements of our great men, but let us not be unmindful of their characters. We know that genius is not always co-incident with the highest moral or spiritual perfection, but when both these qualities are graciously combined in anyone we feel that we are in the presence of a truly great man, of one who becomes a power for good in his day and generation.

CHAPTER TEN

The End of an Era

The leaves of the old century were falling. The seeds of the new were beginning to spring. In it man's scientific achievements were to outstrip his spiritual stability and his capacity to live peaceably with his brother man. The year 1900 was to issue in one of the most violent periods in history that the world has ever known. The old values of individualism and philosophical liberalism were being threatened by collectivism, militarist and Marxist. Britain's large and powerful navy ruled the waves but she had a reputation for inefficiency on land and therefore had to rely on skilled diplomacy to preserve the slender thread by which peace was to hang for close on twenty years. Carried away by his praiseworthy ambition to bring progress and welfare to the peoples of the earth, Chamberlain did not see as clearly as did Lord Salisbury the inherent dangers of the powers jostling for position on the world stage. He lacked Salisbury's wisdom and gifts of diplomacy exercised as Prime Minister and Foreign Minister, and did not have the same perspicacity in seeing and trying to avoid the holocaust already on the way. While Chamberlain spoke of the dawn of a new democratic and radical patriotism and tariff reform, Salisbury spoke of free trade in a world of few barriers, for, as he said, reported in *The Times* of 10 November 1897,

> The one hope we have to prevent this competition in the instruments of death from ending in a terrible effort of mutual destruction which would be fatal to Christian civilisation is that the Powers may gradually be brought to act together in a friendly spirit on all questions of difference which may arise until at last they may be welded together in some international constitution which shall give to the world a long spell of unfettered and prosperous and continued peace.

Russian activities in the Balkans, the Czar's intervention on the side of left-wing partisans in that area, Bismarck's policy of 'encouraging his neighbours to pull each other's teeth', followed by Kaiser Wilhelm II's youthful and not altogether balanced territorial ambitions were by now all combining together to intensify the uncertainties and insecurity of the world situation. While life continued normal and relaxed on the surface, painted on the backcloth were the beginnings of the global alliances and counteralliances leading up to the First World War.

It was in this context that Cantlie's contribution in the fields of tropical medicine and first aid were made during the next decade and a half. His ambulance work, his service with the London Scottish, his raising of the VMSC made him in sympathy with the outlook of the service medical chiefs and Ministers of the last decade, so that he seemed to see as if by second sight, just as Lord Salisbury did, the holocaust that could only be averted by skill and good fortune. Time did not hang heavy on his hands. When he arrived home he undertook again the gratuitous writing of *First Aid to the Injured* for St John, which in 1901 appeared under his own name, including in the second edition two new chapters on 'The principles and qualifications of first aiders'. During his absence in Hong Kong the St John Ambulance Association had formed the Brigade, a uniformed body of men and women trained to render first aid and nursing and numbering 10,000 by 1900. At Queen Victoria's Diamond Jubilee the Brigade appeared on duty for the first time, lining the streets with the police. Cantlie went on duty with them, as he had done with his Chinese medical students in Hong Kong, and he continued to do so on occasions such as funerals at Westminster Abbey, the Military Tournament, international and service exhibitions. It may seem strange today that an eminent surgeon would do first aid duty in the streets, but it was in keeping with the spirit of the volunteer of that time, and he knew how essential it was that the Brigade prove itself as equal to the police, many of whom he had trained in first aid a decade previously. Meanwhile St John Ambulance Association was equipping new ambulance halls, manning emergency stations such as the London docks on a twenty-four hour rota and spreading their teaching to new industrial recruits including the railwaymen whom Cantlie and Mr Brazier, Chief Superintendent of the Metropolitan Corps, were now examining all over the country, and who provided a demonstration team for a fête at the Crystal Palace in celebration of the Diamond Jubilee. To promote realism in the teaching of first aid the railwaymen simulated a train smash at King's Cross. Publicity like this was the best way to get across to the public the need for a greater awareness of their responsibility towards their fellow men in sickness and accident. 'We have in civil life,' explained Cantlie on a Hospital Sunday in an address in St Peter's, Vere Street, many years later,

> exactly the same thing as in the Army. In the Army we have a front line or zone of danger, so in civil life we have our front line in our streets and factories. The front line is looked after by whom? By the doctors? No. By the nurses? No. Then by whom? By you. Very largely the public is expected to do that. This is not the work of the hospital surgeon; he is inside the hospital and says, 'You bring the injured here and we will attend to them; it isn't our duty to go out and collect the wounded, that duty is yours.' Have you trained yourselves for it? Surely it is your duty to be able to help your neighbour. The Good Samaritan sets us an example. What did he do? He first poured oil into the wounds and set the man upon his beast. What do we do in our streets? We follow his example. We first attend to the accident,

we first treat the broken leg, and then, and not till then, do we move him from the place where he fell. That is the teaching given by that wonderful body of men and women who enrol themselves in the St. John Ambulance Brigade.[1]

On his return Cantlie had reopened his session of lectures at St John's Gate, at the Working Women's College, at Toynbee Hall, at the Salvation Army, and at the Regent Street Polytechnic. The Working Women's College is now incorporated with the Working Men's College, whose origins it shared. In 1840 Frederick Denison Maurice, Chaplain of Lincoln's Inn, gathered together a group composed mainly of young lawyers to examine the causes of social unrest. They anticipated upheaval, and when it came, with the Chartist Movement of 1848, London was thrown into a panic. Maurice, in company with Charles Kingsley and others, got in touch with the Chartists and printed an appeal imploring them to distinguish between licence and liberty: 'Workers of England, be wise and then you must be free, for you will be fit to be free'. This concept, of giving people opportunities to acquire wisdom through education was the inspiration for the College which first opened in 1854 and included among its teachers Llewellyn Davies, John Ruskin and Dante Gabriel Rossetti. Technical training was not in its curriculum, its aim was to bring liberal education to the masses of people with no opportunity to acquire it, and to create better understanding between classes by bringing together those with and without academic and cultural education. The teachers were unpaid and the College a centre of service with which, from now until the end of their lives, the Cantlies identified themselves, with Cantlie lecturing on first aid, nursing, health, hygiene and sanitation.

These subjects were also welcomed into the curriculum of the Salvation Army which, starting its missionary work in Tower Hamlets under the leadership of William Booth, had by 1878 spread to eighty centres. Three years later it began its social work providing hostels, social officers and young people's meetings. The Regent Street Polytechnic had been developed on the site of the old Polytechnic Institution of Engineering and Science. The present school had been started by Mr Quintin Hogg, an unselfish and untiring young man who, since 1864, had done extensive and admirable work in bringing education to those young people of Central London whom he 'acknowledged as brothers, but whose lot was less prosperous than his own'.[2] The work began with a class of two, it grew into a night school, into a Youth's Christian Institute, and finally began to develop a four-fold purpose providing spiritual, intellectual, physical and social activities. In 1882 Mr Hogg bought the Polytechnic Institution at 390 Regent Street and when Cantlie returned home from Hong Kong he found a thriving teaching centre for young people which many regarded as home and where they were taught a variety of trades and professions. The aims of the Polytechnic were so in keeping with his own desire, to return to society some of the generosity from which he had benefited as a boy, that he started lectures there on first aid and nursing three times a week, and soon his lectures to the various societies covered many subjects, one on medicine in China drawing an audience of 700.

Cantlie continued to devote much time to fostering the link between civilian and army medicine which has proved of much benefit to medicine in peace and war. In February 1896, just as he was leaving Hong Kong, two letters appeared in the *Lancet* on the VMSC which he had raised in 1885. One pointed out that the Corps, while having various centres in the country, was not universal and that the system of regimental surgeons and regimental bearer companies continued to exist alongside it; the other criticised promotion in the Corps which was not by command but by length of service. Did Cantlie feel that his return might pose problems for the Corps? He had raised it and been its first Surgeon Commandant; would his return be an embarrassment to those now in command? It did not seem so by the warmth with which he was welcomed back but, sensitive to other people's feelings, he decided that, while maintaining the closest possible connection with the Corps and attending dinners and functions, he would for the moment rejoin the London Scottish as a Volunteer Surgeon and thus avoid any complications which might arise. There he remained until invited to become first the Honorary Colonel of the Maidstone Company of the VMSC and then Honorary Colonel of the London Companies, after which he resigned from the London Scottish, although he continued to attend their parades as a civilian. In 1898 he judged the volunteer stretcher drill at the Guildhall where the diary records, 'Scotland won again', and in the same year the St John Ambulance Brigade adopted the army medical stretcher bearer drill in which he had trained his Charing Cross medical students in the early days of the VMSC.

Although a number of important reforms had been carried out since the Crimea in the organisation of the Army Medical Department, not all had met with success and concern still centred round the question of substantive military rank for medical officers. In 1896 a correspondence in the *Lancet* commented on the unsatisfactory state of the Army Medical Department and in July a BMA sub-committee reported to the Parliamentary Bills Committee on the matter of granting medical officers military rank, with similar status to that of the Royal Engineers, the Royal Artillery and the Army Service Corps. The report was forwarded to Lord Lansdowne, Secretary of State for War, but in January 1897 Mr Broderick, for the War Office, refused the request. In November 1897 Cantlie, adding his voice to the petitioners, delivered a paper on army medical organisation to Charing Cross Medical School, pointing out the great contribution which army and civilian medicine could make to each other. The senior army medical officer, he said, was purely administrative, and never saw a patient; he knew 'how to administer a hospital, how many blankets and spoons were required, but had forgotten his clinical work', whereas the civilian medical man by the age of 60 had seen so many patients that he had accumulated a vast amount of clinical experience but, unlike his military counterpart, had no knowledge of administration and did not know 'the amount of cubic feet of air in his wards, nor the state of the drains, both necessary facts'. He criticised constant changes and consequent lack of continuity in army medical staff, and called for acknowledgement of the necessity of rank and a proper chain of command. He propounded a plan for a training school for army medical officers in London, which he wished to see them attending at an earlier age than they did the present school at Netley, which they went to for four months at the age of 24 or 25 – 'the training necessary for the Army should go with their medical education and should not be put on afterwards'.[3] His plan was similar to that adopted by the French Army, in which students, after passing primary examinations, attended an army medical school. He envisaged British Army medical students living together in London and benefiting from the experience to be gained in a wide variety of London hospital clinics. He ended by proposing a resolution to be sent to the War Office and by forming a committee to discuss the matter and report back to the meeting.

Two months later on 20 January Dr Farquharson, Member of Parliament for West Aberdeenshire, who had done so much to promote St John Ambulance work in the early days and been a loyal admirer of the ambulance work done at Charing Cross, headed a deputation of distinguished medical men from the BMA, the universities and medical schools to Lord Lansdowne, urging him that an army medical corps be formed, with military titles for medical officers expressive of army rank. Lord Lansdowne asked, if the request was granted, whether the medical profession would send its best recruits to the corps. The BMA said that it would, and on 4 May 1898 the Royal Army Medical Corps came formally into existence, with officers' ranks the same as those of the combatant army up to colonel, only the title of surgeon general remaining. Meanwhile regular and reserve nursing services had been placed upon a modern footing. The Army Nursing Service had been started at Netley in 1881 with a National Aid Society grant, accompanied with a request that their nurses be trained there, and six years later the Army Nursing Reserve was formed by Princess Christian. With the Boer War threatening, Lord Lansdowne was concerned about the readiness of the medical volunteer forces, particularly in regard to their co-ordination with the voluntary aid societies. The National Aid Society (later the British Red Cross Society), jealously guarding its independence from the War Office, directed its activities towards fund raising, making arrangements for training and sending equipment and trained volunteers to scenes of emergency. Sir John Furley, knowing that St John Ambulance was overstretched in taking on alone the role of teaching first aid and ambulance work in civilian life, wished also to place the Red Cross under the War Office on the German or Japanese model, an arrangement which would not have suited the British people as a permanent pattern for voluntary work. Nevertheless it was clearly going to be necessary in times of conflict to co-ordinate voluntary aid under one central committee and with this in view Lord Lansdowne invited the National Aid Society, St John Ambulance Association and the Army Nursing Reserve to meet the army medical staff at the War Office and discuss the formation of a Central

Red Cross Committee through which, in the event of war, offers of aid to the army medical services could be channelled.

The quarrel in South Africa grew slowly into a serious war, drawing in British volunteers from all over the Empire. According to the historian H. A. L. Fisher, 'it was suspected that President Kruger was using the wealth of the Rand to finance a wide-ranging anti-British conspiracy, and that in this enterprise he possessed the sympathy and counted on the support of the German Reich'[4] – the Pan German League, founded in 1893, was already having its influence on world affairs. The Boers resented the British abolition of slavery and saw English interests in Africa as pressing ever outwards. Continental sympathy, German, Russian and French, was mainly on the side of the Boers, whom the British, with command of the seas, eventually wore down. Lord Wolseley warned that the war, centring as it did round the relief of Kimberley, Ladysmith and Mafeking, would be the most serious Britain had ever fought. The Boer guerillas were operating in familiar bush territory with advantage of surprise, and the British expeditionary force escalated to hundreds of thousands before victory was won. At Paarderburg the sufferings of the wounded were immense; the men lay in the open for three wet days where the medical staff could do little for them because heavy transport had been left behind and there was a shortage of medical personnel and equipment, blankets and food. 'The cold on the first night was terrible'[5] and, as Dame Beryl Oliver writes in *The British Red Cross in Action*,

> Soon there appeared a far more dangerous enemy than the Boers, enteric fever, which spread with terrifying rapidity . . . The only means of evacuating the wounded was to place them in wagons which brought up the food. In these springless contraptions the unfortunate patients were jolted over the veldt . . . By day they sweltered, by night they froze, there were no blankets and the men were in their summer uniform.[6]

Demands flooded back to the Central Red Cross Committee in Cape Town for medical personnel and equipment, clothing and food. St John had 2,000 trained men in the field. The Army Nursing Reserve, starting with 100 nurses and ending with 900, joined forces with nurses sent out by Queen Alexandra and with the National Aid Society and St John in equipping and staffing field and base hospitals, two hospital ships and a hospital train commanded by Sir John Furley. Notable for their generosity were the Duke of Portland and Lord Iveagh who both equipped hospitals, the former's relations acting as nurses, the St Andrew's Ambulance Association (Scottish equivalent of St John) and countless other organisations and individuals, including ten Red Cross societies overseas. The diaries record the joy at the relief of the beleaguered cities, particularly of Mafeking, when the people danced in the streets. They also record the brave and moving tour of the Queen round London, when her people welcomed her with love and loyalty.

The Cantlies were involved in the medical organisation of the war in three ways. Cantlie examined volunteers for military service and commented in articles later published in a book on the lack of physical fitness caused by insufficient nourishment, unhealthy surroundings, overcrowding, poor sanitation, poverty, drink, tuberculosis and venereal disease. He also responded to a request for the collection and dispatch of medical equipment and stores, organised from Aberdeen for those on both sides of the conflict, while Mabel Cantlie helped at the working parties organised by Mrs Hogg at the Polytechnic, and escorted Red Cross Nurses to the boat trains and hospital ships. In this war, as in all wars and accidents, transport was the vital key to relief – Cantlie always illustrated this with the story of the Good Samaritan; in St Luke it was a donkey, at Paarderburg carts, in Ladysmith a train and in Cape Town ships. The Army Transport Corps had come into being during the reorganisation of medical services after the Crimea, and during and after the Boer War interest was focused on how best to transport the wounded and victims of accident and disease in peace and war. For nearly twenty years in Britain the Duke of Cambridge had been organising a voluntary society to provide a London Free Horse Ambulance Service, St John Ambulance was building stables for horses and wagons alongside their new ambulance halls, and the London companies of the VMSC had four horse military ambulances, when these voluntary efforts were overtaken by events, the arrival of petrol driven ambulances with which the American Red Cross was experimenting, and with which St Andrew's Ambulance was the first to follow this lead in 1906. Next year the City of London brought its motor ambulances into commission after a Home Office committee report. Thus out of the evils of war was born relief for the suffering in time of peace.

The need to find remedies and inoculations for infectious diseases was also highlighted by the War. Two thirds of the casualties died from enteric or typhoid fever and from other diseases and not from wounds. Sir Almroth Wright had already experimented with typhoid inoculations as a member of the plague commission in India, and statistics showed that inoculations were beneficial in South Africa. Major Leishman, RAMC (afterwards Sir William Leishman) was commissioned to do further experiments for the War Office after the War to confirm Wright's findings and thus Wright's vaccine was able to save thousands of lives in the First World War. The decimation of British troops in South Africa by disease re-emphasised the need to teach hygiene and sanitation which Cantlie was already including in first aid classes at the Working Women's College, the Salvation Army and St John's Gate following the pattern of Netley and the London Tropical School, and in 1905 St John started awarding certificates in hygiene and started instruction in military hygiene. On his return from Hong Kong, Cantlie was asked by Professor Smith, founder and President of the Institute of Public Health, to become its secretary. The two men had discussed the founding of such an Institute as far back as 1884 on manoeuvres at Aldershot, seeing it as a method of helping to prevent diseases related to poor sanitation, and Smith had founded it while

Cantlie was abroad. After the War, in a campaign to promote world-wide interest, Cantlie accompanied Smith, Nuttal of Cambridge, Hope of Liverpool and Lord Strathcona to Buckingham Palace to present a Fellowship to the King of Norway and then to Windsor Castle to perform the same ceremony for the King of Sweden. Smith and Cantlie then crossed to Paris to give a Fellowship to the President of France, while the Khedive of Egypt was so pleased with his award that he presented Smith with a Star and Cantlie with an Order. The Institute also held a Congress of Public Health in Folkestone and Cantlie and Smith toured the country, speaking in crowded halls on health and hygiene in all its aspects; the diary records Cantlie being entertained by the lord and lady mayoress at a number of cities including Worcester, Lincoln, Oxford and Exeter.

The movement of men and ships all over the world during the Boer War increased the dangers of tropical disease, and it was fortuitous that Cantlie's *Journal of Tropical Medicine* came out the year previously. Facts and figures poured in from all over the world; Simpson, co-editor, was back from Africa and India and was leaving for Hong Kong. For two years Cantlie sent the *Journal* to subscribers whether or not they paid: 'We are very anxious about the *Journal*,' wrote Mabel Cantlie, 'the expenses are very heavy.' He collected and published statistics on the incidence of diseases in the tropics including those on cancer and rheumatism (the latter almost unknown in the East), fevers of all kinds, surgery in warm climates and the whole range of tropical ailments. In the discussion section he led off with controversial topics, over-stated to draw replies: that Chinese and blacks living on European diets were more prone to diabetes, that breast cancer was less prevalent in the East because mothers fed their infants longer, that the incidence of cold and hot baths in different parts of the world had effects on health and disease. He was as ready to learn as to teach. He had come back from Egypt well versed in bandaging – the Egyptians were far ahead of the world in this art because of bandaging their mummies – and his first aid classes in London and Hong Kong were always preceded by an hour's bandaging. Likewise his interest in massage led him to encourage his wife to learn in Hong Kong from the Japanese, then considered past masters in the technique. He attracted readers to his *Journal* not only because of the medical research but because of the interest of present-ation and charm of style. Research was recorded in minutest detail; then, switching in technique, the editorials and articles take off into the charm and freshness of a world removed from medical technicalities. Recommending the mineral springs of Strathpeffer to recuperate from tropical anaemia he speaks of 'beautiful scenery, comprising hill and dale, woodland and water, pines, heather and bracken'. His pen encapsulates the magic of his beloved Scotland with the same ease as it did the horrors of the plague.

At the start of the new century bubonic plague struck again in Europe. There was a case in Glasgow whither Cantlie was sent by the BMA, another was reported in Liverpool and, remembering that the last time plague struck in Britain in the seventeenth century it took seventy years to eradicate, the London County Council appointed a plague officer. It chose Cantlie, for his paper of 1896 had drawn attention to the family of rats that particularly attracted the rat flea, and by 1898 Simond had proved – still not by scientific investigation – that the flea was the chief purveyor of the disease and that, as Cantlie had claimed, the disease was more prevalent in areas inhabited by that particular rat. Mr Belilios of Hong Kong, now in London, offered a prize in the *Journal* for a winning paper on 'The spread of plague by the rat flea', and Sir Lauder Brunton and Sir James Crichton Browne and others formed The Association for the Extermination of Vermin to collect and publish information on the life history of vermin and insects and the part they played in the dissemination of disease. The press, not understanding the need for the Society in spite of the decimation of troops by disease in the Boer War, lampooned it which brought it publicity. Cantlie wrote papers, collected statistics, joined the committee and lectured at teaching centres on insectology, stressing the part played by vermin, parasites, worms and insects in the transmission of tropical disease. In a later lecture at the Polytechnic he pointed out that 'Serpents are reverenced in India because they eat rats' and went on to describe the ravages of disease caused by miners' worm and guinea worm. When the Society ran into financial difficulties he held meetings in his house and persuaded the Royal Institute of Public Health to take it over, by which time it was achieving its purpose. This work proved particularly important during the First World War when control of lice, flies and other disease-carrying parasites was vital to survival.

Cantlie published a short book on the bubonic plague in 1900, a summary of his earlier articles of 1894, 1896, and 1899.[7] He paid tribute to the findings of ten other doctors. He said that plague was transmitted via the alimentary and respiratory tracts or through a lesion in the skin or by insect bite, 'The faeces of a rat or mouse getting into human food, or flies from a rat dead of plague alighting on food are sufficient to cause infection'. He paid tribute to Simond – 'Simond has lately investigated the probability of the rat proving contagious by the vermin which inhabits its body'. Simond's work had been recognised in an unsigned article in the *BMJ* in December 1898, an article which had also pointed out that Yersin, with whose research Cantlie had been identified, had noticed that plague bacilli multiply in the intestines of flies which swarm round dead rats. Cantlie gave an account of the history of plague, its etymology and its modern endemic centres and listed the inoculation attempts by Haffkine and Yersin. His division of plague into bubonic, pneumonic and septicaemic are those of modern medicine. He had acknowledged in a previous article that pneumonic plague was transmitted by direct infection, and he went on to list seven further sub-divisions, including Pestis Minor, which he had always claimed was a less virulent swelling of the glands lasting about three weeks and much experienced by men of the Royal Navy. The incubation period he always put at between three to five days, leaving it open to ten. He listed signs, symptoms, pathological anatomy and methods of stamping out the disease, including sea and railway inspection and incubation (for which Mr Francis had unsuccessfully pleaded in Hong Kong in 1894), the extermination of vermin, particularly rats, and disinfection of soil and houses with lime, formalin solution and fumigation. He recommended a host of remedies and drugs, mild purgative stimulation, including that by alcohol and food, ice packs for delirium, flying mustard packs over the heart, abdomen and limbs and such drugs as hyoscine, morphine, bromide of potassium, camphor, musk, strychnine and enemas of starch and opium.

While typhoid fever was decimating the British troops in South Africa, southern China was suffering renewed outbreaks of plague which the Empress now used to further her own ends in a manner which caused great consternation in Britain and Europe. To understand what was happening in China at the end of the century it is necessary to recount some of the activities of Kang Yu-Wei, a reformer opposed to Sun. The Cantlies had heard little from Sun Yat Sen since he had left in 1896. Sir Henry Blake, now Governor in Hong Kong, had met Mabel Cantlie at the Des Voeux before leaving for the East; Mr Stewart Lockhart, Colonial Secretary, had come to stay at Devonshire Street and Mabel Cantlie visited Lady Knutsford, wife of the former Colonial Secretary 'who was interested in things Chinese'. In Hong Kong at this time there was great concern about piracy in the New Territories and the British said that if nothing was done they could only conclude that the Empress was losing control of Canton. In 1898 Kang secured an interview with the Emperor and impressed upon him the need for reform, asking him to appoint Richards, an English missionary, as Imperial Adviser, and assuring him of fictitious English support. Kang had a military man on his side, Yuan Shik-Kai, former President of Korea, promoted by the Emperor, who had 7,000 men under the command of a Manchu princeling. But the Dowager Empress, the cruel and devious concubine Yehonala, imprisoned the Emperor who was not her son and outlawed the reformers. Kang, on board a Royal Mail steamer, was warned by *The Times* correspondent of his intended arrest in Shanghai and, knowing the Chinese were risking international incidents by searching ships, the Royal Navy escorted his launch to a P and O steamer. With a price on his head Kang made for Hong Kong where the Empress asked for extradition and sent Li Hung Chang as Viceroy to Canton with the intention, it was said, to secure him. Blake would have let him stay but Salisbury, who had refused Sun's request, would not differentiate and replied to Mr Bertie's note: 'I have no objection. I suggest Kang should be obliged to remove himself.' Kang went to Singapore where he was given protection to prevent murder on British soil. Pressed by Chamberlain to protest, but warned by Sir Claude Macdonald in Peking that only threatened hostilities would make the Chinese withdraw their reward, Salisbury refused to intervene. Not only could the Manchus retaliate against British merchants, but they could also accuse Hong Kong of providing cover for conspiracy. Sadly, the result of Kang's attempted coup was that moderates like Prince Kung faded from Peking, his grandson relinquishing rights to the throne. Queen Victoria had written, 'We do not want to see

China weakened', but already the Germans were extending their hold on Shantung – it was to them that Kang later sent his list of reforms – the Russians were dominant in Manchuria, the British and Americans had trading influence in the Yangtze and the French in south-west China.

This interference by the powers in the affairs of China meant that in 1900 the Boxer Rebellion put an end temporarily to the efforts of the Western missionary societies to spread medical enlightenment in China. Roman Catholic and Protestant missions and hospitals had been opening in many Treaty Ports, in Shanghai, Peking, Tientsin and other centres. Now a semi fanatic anti-foreign movement called the Boxers with no connection with Western-style reformers or revolutionaries and which it was said the Empress, with Russian help, secretly backed, whipped up feelings against these Western missionaries, hospitals and schools and against German railway engineers in Shantung and the French in Paotingfa, while placards accused foreigners in the plague-ridden south of causing destitution. In the 1894 epidemic 90,000 people had died in Canton where the mission hospitals had been unable to stem the tide of suffering and with plague again rampant, disaffection and resentment in the two southern provinces was at boiling point. Kang had support there, the Japanese were stirring up republicanism and the Americans were offering help to both Sun and Kang. The British Government, seeing the importance of preventing the reforming movements from acting during the Boxer Rebellion, persuaded both men to desist. The Boxer Rebellion lasted from June to July 1900. The diaries reflect great anxiety, for it was thought the Legation members had been murdered. Sun Yat Sen was in Japan at the time and in June Li Hung Chang tried to persuade him to come and discuss the forming of Kwantung and Kwantsi into a separate state. Sun's faith in the genuineness of these proposals was not sufficient to induce him to visit Li and he passed by to Singapore, where he tried and failed to see Kang. The British authorities there again told him that this was no time for pro-Western disturbances and Sun promised to hold back his men. During the Boxer Rebellion the Germans offered their services to Governor Blake in Hong Kong as volunteers and special constables. Blake turned down the first offer but May, a fluent German speaker with South African connections, accepted them into the police. In June the Empress ordered Li north to Peking, whither an international relief force was heading under Admiral Seymour which failed to get through. Twice the Empress changed her mind about sending Li north and while in Canton Li appeared to be making real or contrived plans to set up a separate South China with a Western-style police force. For the moment the press was reporting better news about the Legations in Peking, but on 12 July the diaries say, 'They fear the worst in Peking'.

On 13 July the Empress sent final orders for Li to go north, and he went via Hong Kong, with Salisbury instructing Blake that if Li wanted to see Sun, who was returning from Singapore, Sun was to be allowed to land in Hong Kong. Li's overtures to Sun included the proposal that the reformers should march north together with arms supplied by Li to see if the Emperor was alive, re-instate him if he was, and bring in reforms; if he was dead they would set up a separate South China. Sun, remembering his detainment in the Legation after Li's visit to London and the British advice, which he trusted, not to be involved in an uprising at this time, insisted on a large sum of money being laid down against his safe return. Meanwhile the British press was reporting all the Ministers dead – this was false, only the German Minister had been murdered. While negotiations with Sun were foundering Li visited Blake in Hong Kong on his way north, to whom he did not give the impression of having lost faith in the Empress (his record for changing sides was unmatched), but he wanted to know who the British would favour as her successor. He then proceeded to Peking where he received the leaders of the international relief force. Within a week of the end of the Boxer Rebellion the Americans were making offers of help to Kang. Blake advised both Kang and Sun, the latter having returned to Japan, to take no action for the moment, but Kang's supporters could not be restrained and in August there was a half-hearted uprising in Hankow which was apprehended by Consul Fraser. Sun controlled his supporters until October when there was a rising in Waichow, and a long march to link up with Sun, now in Formosa. These forays on behalf of Sun tested the people's feelings, but the Imperial forces caught up with the rebels and the leaders fell back on Hong Kong, Sun returning again to Japan. He knew now that four provinces were behind him. The Chinese are a peace-loving nation, but are warlike when roused. The Cantlies had urged Sun to avoid bloodshed, saying that revolutions do more harm than good. In his book *Sun Yat Sen and the Awakening of China*, Cantlie recounts how they pressed upon him the advantages of a constitutional monarchy, and of how Sun had finally convinced them that the Manchus were too hated for it to work in China. Ironically it was Sun's desire to avoid bloodshed and achieve parliamentary government by peaceful means if possible that led to some criticism of him as being too gentle a leader for troublesome times.

Meanwhile in South Africa the Boer War was slowly grinding to its close. Both combatant and medical volunteers had been drawn from all over the world and the war strengthened the ties of family and friends in the Commonwealth. William Cantlie of Montreal, James's second son, fought in the war as a British Gunner and arrived at Cottered, in the words of the diary, 'with a soldier servant, a magnificent hound, a silver watch and a monkey as presents for the boys and a lion's skin for myself'. Many of the volunteers in the medical services and voluntary aid societies in the war returned home anxious to start and spread the teaching of first aid to bring relief in emergencies in peace and in war. St John began a crusade for members in India, and in Canada the Canadian Pacific Railway played a significant part in spreading first aid teaching from east to west, in the name of St John, equipping a demonstration first aid railway coach. The precipitous declines and ascents of the CPR, circling inside the Rocky Mountains for thousands of feet in one of the world's most remarkable engineering feats, demanded a constant vigil on the part of trained personnel, and first aid and cutting equipment was carried in each coach. The Cantlies of Montreal had always taken the closest interest in their cousin's first aid teaching. James Cantlie was a governor of hospitals and 'renowned for his benevolence and readiness at all times to assist in any charitable project', and Eleanora Cantlie was, like her brother Lord Mountstephen, most generous in her contributions to good causes, particularly first aid. George, their eldest son, was a keen volunteer like his father and in 1885 had joined the Royal Scots of Canada which he later commanded as the 5th Royal Highlanders of Canada (Black Watch). Also in 1885 he had joined the CPR as an audit clerk, so that by the turn of the century he could exert some influence on its policies.

As always, there was criticism of regular and volunteer medical services both during and after the war. To help instruction of the Volunteers, Maclure had started the Voluntary Ambulance School of Instruction while Cantlie was in Hong Kong and, on his return, had asked him to instruct. Recruits came particularly from south-east England, Hampshire and from miners in South Wales. Lord Methuen and Mr Haldane, Secretary of State for War, attended its annual dinner. Meanwhile, the new organisation of the RAMC was having its teething troubles. Evatt was deeply concerned about its readiness to meet a national emergency and, under the pseudonym Justice, wrote a book about the state of the new Corps, scathing in his criticism, which he entitled *The Truth about the R.A.M.C.*, a copy of which he sent to the King. Reformers and men outspoken for the sake of truth were respected at the turn of the century and it made no difference to his army career, while making a contribution to bringing the Corps to a state of readiness. He and General Preston came to see Cantlie many times to enlist his help and Cantlie drew attention to the matter in his *Journal*, describing the outlook of many medical officers after the Boer War as being one of 'broken heartedness'. 'That there is something wrong somewhere, everyone seems agreed upon, but where the cause of the dissatisfaction exists it is not easy to determine . . . The magnitude of the task before them was out of all proportion to the strength of the Corps.'[8] He said the Corps had accommodated hundreds with provision for tens, that they were expected to bring up field hospitals with no transport, and provide food in barren country. He repudiated criticism levelled at the calibre of young medical officers joining the Corps, it was 'the fault of the military authorities if they mis-used the material supplied to them'. He made a plea for less red tape: the 'correctness of reports', he said, 'must be of less importance than the saving of lives. It is the system and not the material that is at fault.'[9] Arrangements for more comprehensive and integrated training were soon to be provided after the setting up of a Royal Commission, which resulted in the RAMC moving its School from Netley to London, and in 1907 the RAMC College opened in Millbank, where links with civil medicine were to be close.

The war also highlighted the need for a modern and efficient nursing service and the Royal Commission proposed that the Army Nursing Service and the Indian Nursing Service should be amalgamated into a new body, the QAIMNS, which became the Queen Alexandra's Royal Army Nursing Corps in 1949. Meanwhile training for civilian nurses, which had started in St John's House in 1848 under the supervision of a clergyman, had bloomed after the Crimea with the founding in 1860 of the Nightingale School at St Thomas's Hospital. From this the army nursing sisters and matrons of hospitals with nursing schools were orginally drawn, with the result that by 1901 nurses' schools had been established in most of the large hospitals, so that nearly half of the 63,000 nurses in the country had received some training. Against this figure, however, the Poor Law Nurses had by 1898 only 800 fully trained nurses, in spite of generous grants in many large cities and the foundation in 1879 in Scotland of the Association for Promoting Trained Nursing in Workhouse Infirmaries by Constance, Marchioness of Lothian. Discussions regarding centralised examinations and state registration had begun, Miss Nightingale believing that character qualities were more important in nursing than academic qualifications, while Mrs Bedford Fenwick, ex Matron of St Bartholomew's and founder of the British Nurses' Association, thought intelligence the first prerequisite; others again believed in a two-tier standard. Cantlie, who was drawn into the movement in 1903, believed like Sir James Crichton Browne in the two-tier standard.

The Boer War ended in 1901, but the Queen did not live to see peace declared. As the New Year was ushered in Mabel Cantlie recorded in her diary, 'What will it bring. We have much to do, that is one thing certain. God give us the power to do what we should in the coming years and especially to work for those around us and always be charitable and quarrel with no man.' On 19 January came the end of a great era. 'The Queen is very ill and there is much consternation.' Then, on the following day, 'The Queen still lingers and there is much sorrow', and then the further entry, 'Queen Victoria died today and passed away among a sorrowing people. The whole nation is shocked, for she has been the greatest sovereign that has ever lived.' 24 January: 'The wonderful effect of the Queen's death has brought forth messages from all the four corners of the earth. How she was beloved and now we all feel we have lost a dear sovereign.' St John Ambulance Brigade lined the route and thus Mabel Cantlie, now like her husband a uniformed member, was able to give an eye-witness account:

> It was a magnificent and stirring sight. Our beloved Queen's coffin covered with a white satin pall and the crown, sceptre and orb were placed thereon. Her gun carriage was pulled by her grey horses. It was very sad and very beautiful. Everybody in mourning. Immense silent crowds. It was the most stirring sight ever seen and wonderful in its simplicity. God rest our noble Queen, the mother of her people.

An era had passed. Queen Victoria was a remarkable monarch, sound in beliefs and appreciation of world problems. She took infinite pains to inform herself in the utmost detail by eye-witness accounts of trouble occurring anywhere in the world and acted upon it at once within her constitutional powers. She had an instinct for knowing how her subjects would react in Britain, India or the colonies. She avoided giving offence to foreign dignitaries and tried to see that her Ministers did likewise. She distrusted publicity. She loved her fellow men and this affection sprang from a commitment to spiritual aims which directed the purpose of the nation. Upon her death Lord Salisbury said of her in the House of Lords:

> My Lords . . . being a constitutional monarch with restricted powers she reigned by sheer force of character, by the loveableness of her disposition over the hearts of her subjects and exercised an influence in moulding their character and destiny which she could not have done more if she had had the most despotic power. She has been a great instance of government by example, by esteem, by love and it will never be forgotten how much she has done for the elevation of her people, not by the exercise of any prerogative, not by the giving of commands, but by the simple recognition and contemplation of the brilliant qualities which she has exhibited in her exalted position.[10]

In almost every field of human endeavour, scientific, diplomatic, medical, literary and many others she had inspired a Golden Age of great and distinguished men and women who served their country and the world with high endeavour.

The war had political and military results which were to influence the course of history. First it taught the British soldiers to shoot with deadly accuracy and rapidity which saved them from annihilation in the opening battles of the First World War; secondly, the magnanimous peace which followed and the constitutional settlement agreed upon were happy ones, which meant that South Africa fought with Britain during the First World War and not against her. Both results were crucial to her national survival.

CHAPTER ELEVEN

Family and Friends: Hands across the Sea

The first decade of the twentieth century was the lull before the storm. They were happy years, but the far-sighted saw the tragedy to follow. The age of greatness had passed; the statesmen Palmerston, Disraeli, Gladstone were dead; Salisbury, the last of the giants, retired in 1902. Irish politics interwove between English party boundaries and led to a Coalition or Unionist Government of Conservatives and Liberals opposed to Home Rule but split by arguments about free trade and tariff reform (or imperial preference). Mr A. J. Balfour held the Government together by compromise, but without Salisbury's gift of diplomacy its resultant ineffectiveness led to its fall in 1906. The Liberal Government under Asquith did not fulfil its hopes, however, in spite of a reforming belief in better conditions and prospects for poorer people. The inspiration of the country had gone. Tennyson, the Poet Laureate, who belonged to an age in which he had many competitors, was replaced by a poet to whom the dictionary of quotations awards only a few lines. Abroad the Government vacillated, while Germany, Britain's industrial rival, thwarted in her desire to expand in Africa, in 1898 and 1900 passed the Navy Laws, converting a coastal defence force into a high fleet, proving right Queen Victoria's reluctance to allow the mistaken cessation of Heligoland to Germany in 1885. The Edwardian age of elegance disguised these underlying anxieties by providing opportunities for graceful relaxation. Receptions at embassies, at Apsley House and Lansdowne House, polo at Hurlingham, a house boat at Henley – as in Hong Kong the Cantlies flit in and out of the pages of the press, often arriving late and leaving early owing to pressure of work. The Cantlies, as much at ease in Whitechapel as in Mayfair, might have been expected to attend a prize giving at the Salvation Army or an exhibition at the Working Women's College, but the history books do not record, as the diaries and newspapers do, that most leading people of the day were likely to be present at such functions, believing in raising standards of living and sharing culture and opportunities with everyone in order to create Disraeli's dream of one nation. This unity of aim was misjudged by Lloyd George, whose virulent attack on the aristocracy in his Limehouse speeches nearly cost him the Liberal re-election.

All Cantlie's public work had to be financed out of his work as a surgeon, yet, in company with all doctors and surgeons of his day, much of his work even in this field was given free. He was now Honorary Surgeon at the West End Hospital, the Royal Scottish Corporation, Charing Cross Hospital, the North Eastern Railway Company, the Welbeck Children's Hospital and the Albert Dock Hospital for Tropical Diseases as well as remaining consultant to the Alice Memorial Hospital in Hong Kong. At the Albert Dock Hospital he carried out one of his most interesting operations on a 16-year-old boy. A cyst had been caused by a blow from a cricket ball which had produced epilepsy. When opened, fluid escaped; on the fifth day there was a high temperature and copious haemorrhage at the removal of the gauze; the wound was repacked and the patient recovered. During these years Cantlie was turning his attention increasingly to cancer and was oper-ating on a number of patients considered hopeless. According to the diary, Mabel Cantlie assisted in nursing some of these patients who recovered quickly but many of whom died upon recurrence. In June 1904 he appealed for doctors to send home specimens of cancer from abroad as he had done with leprosy, and to furnish information as to the prevalence of the disease in their areas. If a disease was absent, 'Was it fauna, geological formation, climate, precautions taken by natives, immunity, or something else?' These requests did not apply only to cancer, but to other diseases as well. He pointed out that the absence of enteric in epidemic form in China was due to drinking tea and rice water instead of milk and fresh water, as well as to seldom eating uncooked food. The doctors put each other's ideas to the test and recorded their experiences. Following Sir Lauder Brunton's advice that a change of diet in sprue put the bacteria at a disadvantage, Cantlie suggested alternating a diet of meat jelly and pounded beef with a twenty-four hour diet of milk every fourth day. He also pointed out the beneficial effects of sea water as an enema for any form of intestinal flux – the antiseptic and healing effects of salt water were proved and used to the full during the First World War.

While the doctors wrestled with these problems of disease both at home and overseas the nurses were now pressing for a unified and improved service. In 1903 Cantlie operated on Mr Munro-Ferguson, MP for Kirkcaldy (afterwards Lord Novar), and was asked by Lady Helen Munro-Ferguson, who had taken a close interest in nursing and whose father, the Marquis of Dufferin and Ava, was one of the prime movers of bills for state registration in the House of Lords, to accom-pany her to speak at a meeting attended by 150 matrons from the London hospitals, all in favour of state registration, and all of whom had excellent nursing schools. In 1905 Cantlie spoke again on state registration at the invitation of Lord Londonderry, and in the same year his friend Sir James Crichton Browne gave clear evidence to a Committee of Inquiry which reported in favour of a two-tier standard. During the next ten years great strides were made in nursing standards abroad. The Colonial Nursing Association, started with the help of Mrs Chamberlain, sent out 238 nurses to the colonies and in Hong Kong the Governor promoted a scheme to bring out private nurses from the United Kingdom. Meanwhile Cantlie wrote in his *Journal* of the need for nurses on board ship: 'What is the use,' he asked, 'of a doctor without a nurse; he is like an engine driver without a stoker? . . . Nowhere is the doctor or patient more on his own than at sea.' There was also a need, he said, for dentists on board ship and, in the case of smaller ships, he suggested that ship's officers should take lessons in dentistry before qualifying to sail a ship.

In January 1902, with the *Journal* beginning to pay its way, Cantlie thought the time had come to float his other idea, a Society of Tropical Medicine. 'We are willing,' he wrote in the *Journal* on 1 January, 'to consider the formation of such a Society if subscribers think it desirable.' His plan was that the *Journal* would then become the official organ of the Society. On 30 October the diary describes how Manson and Sambon came to see Cantlie and suggested taking over the *Journal* from him. For once his wife put her foot down and Surgeon General Crombie called the next day and gave the same advice: 'Don't let anyone take over the *Journal* from you.' Professor Simpson, wanting that Cantlie should have the credit for his work, suggested removing his name as co-editor, since he had been so much abroad, but Cantlie would not hear of it. He heeded the other advice, however, and kept the *Journal* under his control until 1904 when he sold it to the printer, obtaining from him first a promise that he would remain its editor, which he did until 1925. In 1904 he obtained the Colonial Medical Reports which he published en bloc at the back of the *Journal* and he made a plea that the Royal Navy and Army Medical Services should allow their junior officers the freedom to publish as did the Indian Medical Service, which would enable the medical profession to benefit from the widest circulation of ideas. 'The fact that papers have to be submitted . . . before being published is apt to stifle individuality and check professional zeal.' He described this as a form of discipline calculated to lower rather than improve. 'A well regulated discipline is an elevating power . . . but when ill regulated . . . it fetters the inclination of those subjected to it, it stands over them at every turn, until the character and mind are enslaved by it, and many young spirits broken. Discipline should not imply slavery, but a training whereby freedom may be safely given.'[1]

In 1906 Cantlie replied in the *Journal* to a letter in *The Times* which criticised the giving of overseas aid when there were needy people in Britain, and pointed out that the time to spend money was between epidemics and not during them. He compared the well organised government departments of sanitation and medicine in India with the lack of facilities in China, where medical colleges and schools, medical books and nursing associations were either dependent on Western help and restricted to Peking and the Treaty Ports or just plans on the drawing board. 'In China,' said Cantlie in a speech to Livingstone Missionary College in July, 'there are no medical men upon whom the Government can fall back for immediate help, no public health department, no organised medical service, no trained nurses.' He went on to outline his idea of first aid in tropical medicine in areas where the only medical man was the missionary, pointing out that it would be assumed he had medical knowledge, whether this was true or not. The Medical Missionaries had, in fact, been among the first in the field of tropical medicine. In 1841 an American doctor, Peter Parker, had founded the Edinburgh Medical Missionary Society which ran a residency in George Square for its medical students who attended Edinburgh University and may well have been among those who went to the *Dreadnought* at Greenwich for their instruction in tropical ailments. The Edinburgh Medical Missionaries also ran a free dispensary in the Cowgate and in 1878 one of their members founded a similar London Medical Missionary Association. Nevertheless it is still true to say that Livingstone College, founded by Dr Harford in 1891, was unique, because it gave a short medical course to lay missionaries in hygiene, sanitation and elementary medicine – Cantlie once said that it should be compulsory for every missionary to have some rudimentary training in medicine. With only twenty students qualifying yearly, it was a drop in the ocean, but he urged them, as he had the Chinese students in Hong Kong, to go out and found hostels and dispensaries for Western medicine, while at the same time bringing back Eastern plants and herbs for Western doctors to analyse. He was always impressed by Chinese herbal medicine as he was by their early preventive medicine, which included peace of mind as an element of health, and there is a report that he used acupuncture in 1896[2] although there is no comment on this in his writings or any of the diaries. 'For the missionary to die for Christianity,' said Cantlie in his speech, 'is a noble aim, but there is a still nobler aim, that he might live for Christianity.'[3] He disposed of the argument that a little knowledge in medicine is a dangerous thing by saying that the first lesson a first aider must learn, in the case of accident or disease, is what not to do. 'In China, where there are no railways, factories or horse vehicles, a different sort of First Aid is needed even in accidents.' Missionaries with medical knowledge should learn

> how to deal with the sudden onset of disease which destroys life almost as suddenly as a railway engine may in this country. The disease comes suddenly, its course is short and the patient may die in a few hours. People will say we are training men for doctors. When St. John's Ambulance Association began its First Aid training people said the same thing. That dread has long since disappeared, all medical men approve of First Aid in our streets and how much more necessary when going to parts of the world where there is no doctor that teaching suitable to those in far distant parts be insisted upon.[4]

What Cantlie was envisaging was the Chinese 'barefoot doctor' of today, a man with some medical knowledge, living among the people, working in the paddy fields and ministering to their needs, but he forgot that it was the surgeons who had supported the ambulance movement, whereas now he was speaking mainly to physicians and sowing seed on untrodden ground. It was not until after the First

World War that he was able to give lectures in first aid in tropical medicine at the College of Ambulance.

It may be that this speech and its far-reaching implications had some influence upon the events to follow. In April 1906 Cantlie had called again in his *Journal* for the creation of a Society of Tropical Medicine, a metropolitan rallying point for medical men, assuring his readers that the proposed Society would work within the British Medical Association and that the idea was to co-ordinate medical work overseas. On 4 January 1907 he called a meeting of twelve men at the Colonial Office to discuss such a project, at which Manson was voted to the chair. A sub-committee met in January and February in Cantlie's house to draw up a constitution and laws for the proposed Society, with arrangements for making Fellows, and in March a further meeting was held to endorse these proposals at the Royal College of Physicians. At the inaugural meeting in May it was agreed that, as with the Hong Kong Medical Society, the Society should have papers read to it by medical men with discussions from clinical experience, and that these papers should be published in a periodical entitled *The Transactions of the Tropical Society*. Cantlie was to continue with his *Journal* as well, but was to have editors helping him although, as with Professor Simpson, the additional editors were more in name than reality. Sir Patrick Manson was elected to the chair as President and Professor Ross (later Sir Ronald Ross), famous for his clinical proofs of malarial infection, was voted Vice President. Only two surgeons were elected to the sixteen-strong Council, one of whom was Cantlie. It may well have seemed to Cantlie that this was insufficient representation, for he always regarded tropical surgery as a specialised branch of surgery. He therefore now called on doctors studying for the FRCS to attend the Tropical Section of the BMA and the meetings of the newly formed Society of Tropical Medicine. The *BMJ* of 8 June said:

> The successful foundation of the Society has in great measure been due to the approval and co-operation of the Schools of Tropical Medicine in London and Liverpool, the universities, and other teaching bodies, the naval and military medical services, and the large and rapidly increasing number of physicians who are engaged in mission work and in the practice of medicine and hygiene in tropical countries. Among the active supporters of the movement have been many eminent biologists.

In 1909 Dr Sambon, who had contributed research both towards the discovery of the tsetse fly as the cause of sleeping sickness and the transmission of typhus by louse and flea, came to Cantlie and asked for his help in opening a laboratory at the London Zoo. Sambon was currently working on a cure for pellagra, an eastern disease causing madness, which was active in Italy, Austria, Eastern Europe, Egypt, Spain and many other countries. It was thought that pellagra was caused by eating infected maize, and in June 1907 the *BMJ* reported the increase in cases in Rumania after a bumper harvest. Later opinion suggested it was caused by sandflies or midges; Sambon thought that *simulium reptans* was the means of infection and suggested arsenic as the cure. Cantlie invited Manson, Sir Lauder Brunton, Sir Charles McLaren, Mr Chalmers Mitchell and Mr H. S. Wellcome of the Wellcome Trust and Institute to dinner and these men agreed to help to get a laboratory built. Cantlie then set up a Pellagra Commission which met in his house. Members included the Italian Ambassador, the Marquis of San Ginfiano, Sir Thomas Clifford Allbut, Regius Professor of Physics, University of Cambridge, Fleet Surgeon P. Bassett-Smith, Lecturer in Tropical Medicine, Haslar, Sir T. Lauder Brunton, Consulting Physician St Bartholomew's Hospital, Mr C. F. Harford, Principal of Livingstone Missionary College, Sir William Leishman, Professor of Pathology, RAMC College, Sir John McFadyean, Principal and Professor of Comparative Pathology and Bacteriology, Royal Veterinary College, Professor William Osler, Regius Professor of Medicine, Oxford University, the editors of the *BMJ* and the *Lancet*, the lecturers of the London School of Tropical Medicine, the Secretary and Assistant Secretary of the British Museum and the Secretary of the Seamen's Hospital Society. The inclusion of Sir John McFadyean from the Royal Veterinary College helped to form a link between the veterinary and medical professions which was fostered by the London School of Tropical Medicine and was invaluable during the First World War, when much combined research was undertaken and the Veterinary Corps was able to share laboratories with the RAMC at a time when diseases such as tetanus were as much a scourge to animals as to men.

Although the London School of Tropical Medicine was attended by doctors of the Royal Navy, Army, IMS, Colonial Service, US Navy and foreign governments, and 700 students had passed through its doors, it was, unlike that of Liverpool, short of funds. Mr H. S. Wellcome and Sir John Craggs had given liberally; in 1909 classes were started for nurses and Cantlie added these to his programme of lecturing in the School; London University made the course an optional subject for MD; but nevertheless the endowment stood at only £1,000. In November 1909 the *BMJ* pointed out that room was needed for expansion, with more facilities and laboratories. It was an ideal site, said the editorial, for tropical diseases were trapped at the inlet before they came ashore and there was a duty for scientific work demanded by the flies and vermin prevalent in the dock area: 'The flower of manhood is dying in the tropics of preventable disease' – and London should arouse itself to a sense of personal interest. On 22 October 1910 Cantlie appealed for funds from the chair at the Annual School Dinner, thanking Lord Sheffield and Mr Blessig for their support, which had put the School in better shape. Competition is, however, the finest spur and while the Seamen's Hospital Society was approaching people for funds for *Dreadnought*, Sir James Porter, a former student of Cantlie's, outlined proposals at the Annual Dinner of the London School in 1911 to found a Naval Medical College at Greenwich, to which medical officers would be sent for two months from Haslar. The College would have professors of pathology and hygiene, but otherwise would depend for teaching and research on *Dreadnought* and the London School. The Admiralty, said Sir James, had appointed a Consultative Board, including Sir Watson Cheyne, Sir Dyce Duckworth and Professor Simpson. This announcement acted as a welcome stimulant upon the Colonial Office and at the Annual Dinner of the London School the following year a Committee was formed at the request of Lord Harcourt, Secretary of State for the Colonies, to raise funds for new teaching facilities and accommodation. An appeal for £100,000 was launched by Mr Chamberlain resulting in an enlarged and improved building where the School flourished until moving to its present site in Gower Street in 1920.

As well as providing funds for the London School, Mr Wellcome was active in founding Schools for Mothers for Infant Feeding and in 1907 Mabel Cantlie was approached by Mrs Simpson, wife of Professor Simpson, to join the Committee. Cantlie believed mothers should feed their babies, both for the sake of the infant and to avoid frequent pregnancies and cancer of the breast, which he thought related to bottle feeding. The first of these schools was in Euston, but they soon spread over London and to other towns in England, while Mabel Cantlie introduced the first Scottish school to Aberdeen. Like her husband she was invited to speak in many parts of the country, and women as diverse as Lady Curzon and Mrs Sidney Webb interested themselves in the schools, which attracted many clergy to its first Annual General Meeting. Mabel Cantlie gave an address on the schools to the International Congress of Public Health in London and then Berlin. Her success as speaker and organiser was preparation for her public work in the Balkan and First World Wars. Soon, under the chairmanship of the Duchess of Marlborough, a house was opened as a centre in Fitzroy Square. Mabel Cantlie was now doing what she had done in Hong Kong, standing in at his request for her husband when he was too occupied with work to fulfil engagements. She was on the Ladies Committee of Charing Cross Hospital, fund raising and making hospital jackets and other clothing, and when the Duchess of Portland visited the Hospital she took her husband's place: 'Saw all the wards. I could never bear going before because of the sadness of it.' It was the same story when the Duchess of Wellington opened new wards at Charing Cross and the Duchess of Devonshire new wards at the West End Hospital. Yet in spite of these commitments, she found time to make markers for the church and take classes in lace-making, as well as maintaining close links with the Working Women's College and remaining a uniformed member of St John Ambulance Brigade. On one day, while her husband was lecturing and doctoring, she attended Charing Cross Hospital School Prize Giving, where Princess Louise was presenting the prizes, a Royal Institute of Public Health Committee Meeting, a presentation of prizes and certificates at the Salvation Army and the opening of the London Tropical School Session.

The Cantlies' days were packed, each starting early, when Cantlie did much of his writing. He wrote fast, two articles in three hours, the diary says. As well as articles he was writing a chapter for a book on

Aberdeen professors; a new paper on 'The Health of the People'; an addendum on yellow fever for Scheube's *Diseases of Warm Countries*, which was opportune since the Americans working on the Panama Canal were being ravaged by the disease, and a book on *Physical Efficiency*, which had very good reviews: 'a mass of excellent advice', said the *Daily Mail*. His observations on physical fitness, food, clothing and exercise, now subjects of national importance, were based on his work in the Boer War examining army recruits. His extensive correspondence, much accounted for by his *Journal*, made the library a scene of intense literary activity. The shelves were stacked with medical journals, boxes of articles and newspaper cuttings which bulged from files. The leading article for his *Journal* was undertaken in a race against time and the buzzing of the telephone. Their busy life can be seen from a diary entry in 1903, 'H and I spent our first quiet evening together for many a long day and I read a book without feeling wicked'. Cantlie hated solitude and abhorred a sanctum of his own. He was happiest surrounded by his family, amid distractions which would have defeated most writers. Tea was a drawing room meal, China tea served in eggshell china cups amid Chinese surroundings, where carpets, blackwood furniture, pictures, porcelain and bronzes all gave an atmosphere of China, unusual and charming in a London drawing room. After dinner Cantlie would go out lecturing, then at 10.00 p.m. join his wife in the library where, over a cup of cocoa, they would discuss the day's work and future plans.

The Cantlies now had four sons, for Kenneth, 'round, jolly and always laughing', had been born in 1899. The elder boys attended a day school in London and, at nine, went as weekly boarders to a school at Cheshunt. Weekends were spent at Cottered, in Hertfordshire, where a farm was bought as a kindness to a farmer in failing health who wanted a partner and to supply fresh milk to the village. Soon the Cantlies were running it on their own, rearing pigs as well and adding acreage to the fields of wheat and barley. Cantlie, whose vacations were spent on the farm at Keithmore, attributed much educational value to young people undertaking physical work and was happy for his sons to be thus employed during holidays, but he did not expect his wife and the domestic staff to be caught up in the activities also. Nevertheless at harvest time, the whole family rose at 4.30 a.m., stopping in early evening for tennis, croquet or cricket. This meant that they all maintained a high standard of physical fitness which may explain their immense programme of work. On one occasion Cantlie bicycled down to London and back next day but, after a spill, breaking his jaw, straining his shoulder and damaging his eye, he returned to the train. The boys, however, did the journey regularly by bicycle and the family thought nothing of setting off one summer's day for Cambridge, 50 miles away, where they spent the night. A shooting lease was taken, for Cantlie was a keen and good shot and, while the elder boys carried guns with their father and his guests, the young ones walked in line with a dog or game bag. When Keith was 13 he enrolled at Robert Gordon's College in Aberdeen, travelling by sea like his father had done, leaving from Temple Pier. Why Aberdeen, when there were good schools in England? Cantlie gave his reasons in an after-dinner speech at the Aberdeen University Club. 'For the last three hundred years Scotland has been ahead of the world in education, since John Knox propounded his motto that all children must be educated and the poor must be helped.' He recommended north-east Scots to send their sons home to Scotland to be educated, making particular mention of the bracing air of Aberdeen. 'Why did the English choose low lying places by rivers for their seats of learning?' He advocated also the traditional Scottish day school with boys living at home or boarded out in lodgings. 'The Scots tried the monastic type of education, but found it wanting.' So Keith went north, lived in lodgings with friends and was a brilliant scholar, particularly in English and classics, although the Headmaster said his brain was so flexible that he could have applied it to any subject. He played golf, won the Rosebery Golf Championship and was a keen debater. He also learnt to play the banjo and pipes and joined the Gordon Highlanders as a volunteer. He gained distinctions in arts subjects and in zoology, which led him to make an expert collection of butterflies in Assam, on which he published a book. Versatile and vivacious, he was a hard elder brother to follow and Colin, on arrival, was given a daunting introduction by the Headmaster who said the name Cantlie was one to conjure with in Scotland. Colin did not settle happily, broke his leg in his first term, returned to Cheshunt, thence to a naval crammer and passed into the Royal Navy, working hard, achieving good results, gaining promotion and winning his colours in football. His mother marked him out early for a naval career, after 'he saw the young Navy for the first time at a Royal Naval College Christmas party at Greenwich' and, on holiday at Broadstairs, instead of playing golf with Keith, 'he walked about with glasses like a sailor'. Meanwhile Neil, who, on the sands at Broadstairs was described as 'happy with the diggers' amusing his younger brother, was developing his father's sunny temperament and beautiful singing voice – like his father 'never happier than when helping other people'. 'Neil is a wonderful boy to work,' his mother said, 'he never ceases when there is anything to do', and when he went away she felt her right hand had been taken from her. His interest was in the farm, particularly the horses, and he learnt to ride on a high-spirited mare he and his mother bought for the trap, thinking he might follow hounds. Fishing was enjoyed at Fochabers, but Colin was the only boy who inherited his father's life-long love of the sport.

At 13 Neil went north to join Keith at Gordon's. He was, like his brother, brilliant, and won prizes at school and a bursary to the University where he took Firsts in all his class subjects, joined the Gordons as a volunteer and decided to follow his father's career in medicine and to join the RAMC. In 1908 Keith came down with a First Class Honours Degree in Classics and was offered a scholarship at Oxford. This he turned down; like his father he wished to serve overseas and had applied for the Indian Civil Service, thus feeling that the dons would be displeased if he passed the examinations and could not take it up. He attended Wren's Tutors in London, passed high into the Indian Civil Service and was given a year's scholarship at Christ Church, Oxford, before setting out for India. 'No wonder it is so well thought of by scholars,' said Mabel Cantlie, 'a really lovely place.'

By this time Kenneth was also attending Robert Gordon's College and doing well. Then suddenly disaster struck. He was playing with his trains during the holidays, dismantling a turn-table with a screwdriver when the spring slipped and the screwdriver went through the iris of his eye. Day after day the eye specialists consulted and did not immediately realise how hopeless was the effort to save the sight of and latterly the eye itself. Kenneth suffered agony and his mother with him; and when a telegram came calling Cantlie to a sick patient for the first time he put his family first and sent someone else. Neil returned to Aberdeen without Kenneth, leaving him to be taught at home. After his health had improved and he had returned to school, his plight was never far from Mabel's mind. Knowing how busy her husband was and that the boys had nothing to inherit but ability, she was the parent who interviewed headmasters and thought about careers. One evening at dinner she met a Canadian railway engineer who pointed out that much of an engineer's work is done with one eye shut. Thus Ken's future was moulded by his accident and he was later to become a railway engineer, apprenticed at Crewe, following his father to the East by joining the Chinese railways. Fate seemed to be always reminding the family of Kenneth's disability; Cantlie, in his earlier fall from his bicycle (when he had refused to tell his wife how badly he was hurt), had done damage to his eye, which was later, after a further war-time accident, to turn to glaucoma; then Neil suffered from a rare microbe in his eye from the dust of the threshing at Cottered which gave him excruciating pain; and, before he had recovered, his mother developed painful eye trouble from an ingrowing eye lash. Finally Keith developed eye strain at Oxford which, although it disappeared on the voyage to India, when he entertained other travellers with his banjo and pipes, nevertheless reappeared with high temperature in Assam, when he was swept off to hospital. He was invited to convalesce by the Governor, who complimented him on his reliability, honesty and hard work and told him that he would get on. Colin's eyes luckily did not let him down, for otherwise his naval career would have been in jeopardy. Having passed his qualifying examination for Greenwich with a star, he was often coming and going through London, where he was one of four sub-lieutenants chosen to dine with 500 naval officers at the Mansion House. The diary also reports him accompanying Queen Alexandra to the Baltic, and 'dancing away until the small hours at a Ball attended by our Queen, and the Dowager Empress of Russia'. Then there is the entry, 'Colin is seeing the world, he has sent for his golf clubs', and, a few weeks later, 'Colin has got submarines'. From then on he lived up to the reputation of the Silent Service, commenting little on what he was doing and interspersing his periods at sea with fishing in Perthshire with cousins and elsewhere in Scotland.

The houses in London and Cottered were always full of guests, friends and relations of all ages and professions and often of many nationalities; the Cantlies' liberality seemed bottomless. After the annual inspection of the Maidstone Company of the VMSC they entertained all the officers in their house. On another occasion, the diary records, '43 in the house today, coming and going'. At Christmas the old people in Cottered village were given a meal and tobacco and fruit for a plum pudding. Doctors, soldiers, sailors, friends from Hong Kong, young and old, stayed, lunched or dined, as did Mabel's sister, Lilla Ingall, with her husband and sons – her brother Kenneth also with his boy, Bob. George Cantlie and his wife from Montreal were constant visitors to London with their four daughters and son. His sister Mary, married to Dr Adami of the RCAMC, was also a frequent visitor with her two children. Frank, George's youngest brother, was often at Cottered; he studied medicine on the Continent and then joined the P and O as a ship's doctor, dying young, like his Gunner brother William. James, christened after his father, visited England once; he went to Winnipeg where he made and lost a fortune, marrying and having two sons and a daughter – his son Stewart commanded the Black Watch of Canada in the Second World War.

In 1905 Dr Sun made a brief visit to London and stayed with the Cantlies. He attended the new China Society which Cantlie and a number of friends and colleagues had founded the previous year in order to interest the British people in 'things Chinese' and which was a follow-on to the Friends of China Society, started by Cantlie and Sun in 1898. This Society was non political and was attended by members of the Chinese Legation, by Sir Robert Hart of Chinese Customs, and on occasions by Sir Hiram Wilkinson, Chief Justice of HBM's Supreme Court in China and Korea who, according to the diary, expressed admiration for Sun. The Chinese Government presented the Society with a rare Encyclopaedia, now in a university museum. The Cantlies' friendship with Dr Sun in no way inhibited their relationship with the members of the Legation; they went to receptions there and were asked to attend the Chinese Minister at gatherings in London. Mr Munro-Ferguson, MP, aware of Cantlie's knowledge of Chinese affairs, was a frequent visitor at Harley Street and, in return, entertained the Cantlies in the House of Commons. When, as Lord Novar, he became Governor General of Australia, he understood, as the British Government did not understand, the depth of Chinese admiration for Sun Yat Sen. Sun's friendly contacts with people in Britain was not unnoticed by Kang Yu-Wei who was so jealous that after a subsequent visit he surprised Mr A. J. Balfour, to whom he was unknown personally, by presenting him with a piece of china, saying he was sorry he had not been able to meet him. After Dr Sun had departed for Japan various Chinese friends arrived to stay, being swept up into family activities, including chasing butterflies with Keith in the garden at Cottered.

Cantlie's professional contacts were as world-wide as his friendships. By 1905 his patients had sufficiently increased to warrant the move from Devonshire to Harley Street. Here he was consulted by a Ghurka doctor from Nepal, and then by a maharajah who, with his son, doctor and two servants, arrived in a motorcade with Sir Lauder Brunton. Cantlie's expertise on plague brought a Russian doctor to call for advice about a serum accidentally infected which had caused an out-break of disease – it was a Russian bacteriologist, Haffkine, who was leading the world at this time with inoculations for cholera and plague. The Japanese doctors who had been in Hong Kong during the plague also visited Cantlie in Harley Street and the Cantlies put on an Exhi-bition of Japanese Art at the Whitechapel Art Gallery, for which they were responsible, while Mabel Cantlie attended a garden party for the Japanese naval contingent at the Botanical Gardens, with Admiral Sir Edmund and Lady Fremantle. In 1902 Britain, although pursuing a policy of 'splendid isolation' in Europe, so that the balance of power should not be tipped, had concluded a friendship treaty with Japan to contain Russia's eastern flank should China be further weakened.

A man with world-wide connections who has not the inclination to refuse anyone anything will find himself repeatedly approached by those in need. Seven Indians, in dispute with the India Office, arrived to tea in Harley Street and with Evatt, Simpson and others were taken by Cantlie to the House of Commons; the diary describes not only the visit but also their gratitude when matters were satisfactorily resolved. In 1907 the College of Medicine for the Chinese asked him if he could raise money in London for the endowment of two Chairs in the pro-posed University of Hong Kong, which was now to grow from the College incorporated that year. Funds were being raised to start other universities and medical colleges in China – one of these was the International Medical College in Peking – and Hong Kong was anxious to maintain the position which it felt the College of Medicine had given it. Cantlie promised help, formed a Committee in 1907 and raised funds which, together with those being collected in Hong Kong, en-abled a University to be founded in the island on the same site on which it stands today.[5]

Kindness brings kindness and Cantlie's not inconsiderable ability as an amateur actor brought the Cantlies into friendship with two genera-tions of Irvings who gave them tickets for the theatre. The Irvings, Sir Henry and his two sons, were one of the most remarkable families ever to be identified with the English stage. Sir Henry, who worked to found a National Theatre, had a power and versatility as an actor which have never been surpassed, while his son Lawrence was a playwright as well as an actor, his knowledge of Russia leading to a stage presentation of *Peter the Great* as well as to a rendering of *Crime and Punishment* never bettered. The diary records his visits to Harley Street for information and background for a play he was writing on Japan. 'Whenever I think of a strong and kindly face about whom to write,' he once said to Cantlie, 'your face comes between me and the paper.' It was praise indeed. Cantlie's interest in and knowledge of music and his beautiful voice were not only bringing the Cantlies into contact with musical acquaintances but were making him much in demand as an after-dinner singer, for he had the gift of moving men to laughter or to tears.

Of Ada Dent, an old friend whose marriage had broken up, Mabel Cantlie says in her diary, 'I think she should be an opera singer'. Next year she was singing with Henry Wood's Orchestra in the Bechstein and Queen's Hall and another friend was composing one of Henry Wood's concertos. These stage and musical connections provided a sense of perspective to the world of medicine. Yet in the high professional standards set in each there were similarities. 'Excellence in any art,' said Irving, 'depends on arduous labour, unswerving purpose and unfailing discipline.'

One of Cantlie's interests which combined his love of Scottish music with that of dancing and at the same time brought him into contact with young people was his work for the Caledonian Schools. These had been started in 1815 to provide education for the children of Scottish soldiers killed in the Napoleonic Wars, and were now extended to children of Scottish soldiers killed on active service for their country. This interest involved frequent visits by both the Cantlies to the School at Bushey to award prizes for various competitions, while boy pipers from the School attended Scottish dinners in London and provided the after-dinner music on the pipes. Cantlie was at that time President of the Royal Caledonian Society and enjoyed many dinners and membership of societies with a Scottish flavour. He was an authority on Scottish music which he always saw in an international context echoing across frontiers and in which he interested his friends from all over the world. 'Scottish music,' he wrote,

> is more widespread than ever it was. There are more pipers in the world today than in the '45. I have seen the 42nd, the Black Watch of Canada, march through the streets of Montreal to the tune of 'Highland Laddie'. I have heard a native Belauchi band on the North West Frontier of India play the Edinburgh Quadrilles as the Afghan guarding his border listened enthralled. I have heard the 'Keel Row' and 'Bonnie Dundee' played as the Bengal Lancers trotted and galloped past Lord Roberts at Quetta. I have seen the Sikhs march past in the Punjab to the 'Barren Rocks of Aden' . . . the skirl of the pipers and the music fitting well with their gallant bearing. I have seen twenty pipers marching to 'The Flowers of the Forest' and 'The Land of the Leal' through the streets of Hong Kong . . . I have taken part in the singing of 'Auld Lang Syne' by Japanese in the Japanese language. Most things in the world are perishable, but Scottish music is not one of these; it will not pass away.[6]

Cantlie wore many hats in his time, said the press, but he wore them all with 'great good nature, energy and kindliness'. Many character qualities drew men to him, but none more than his musical ability and his stories rendered in Doric. One evening he attended a concert of the Aberdeen University Club in London. There was a band of seven violins playing reels and strathspeys of William Marshall, his great great uncle by marriage, in 'real Auchindoun time' – for in the area of Dufftown the bowing is different to violin playing elsewhere: 'It just

gaed roun ye're heart, like a yard o' new flannel'. He offered a prize
that night for a song from a poet and musician from Aberdeen which,
he claimed, had no one to compare with the composers of the three
surrounding counties – The Reverend John Skinner who wrote 'Tulloch Gorm is my Delight', or John Ewen, 'Mrs. Grant of Carron, Mrs.
Grant of Lagfan', or Dr Alex Geddes of Banff who wrote 'The White
Cockade'. Then came a demand for a song and Cantlie gave the
'Tinker's Wedding' which brought uproars for an encore. He sang two
more – 'Worse uproar, but I could do no more. The most eloquent
thanks came from a man who came up and shook hands and went away
a bit, came back and shook hands again and said, "Aye . . . Doctor . . .
Well . . . Lord . . . Doctor . . . Aye," shook hands and went away
greetin'.[7]

In order to appreciate Cantlie's love of Scottish music it is necessary
to understand how deeply rooted these melodies, airs, strathspeys and
reels are in the uplands of Scotland. The Strathspey comes from the
Spey valley, where it rises from the musical inspiration of the people
like the mists from the river in a Highland glen. Round this desire to
express themselves in song and dance the people have built their social
heritage. Whether the tunes are played on the fiddle, bagpipe or
mouth-organ the players, listeners and dancers involve themselves in
the music with remarkable vitality. But the strains can also be sad so
that when in lands far away the Scot hears the music and joins hands to
sing Auld Lang Syne he hears also the distant 'sough of the Spey and
the ripple of the burns'. At one time these airs were composed for the
bagpipe, but when the violin became the vehicle of composition it
enlarged the scope. There are three great Strathspey composers: Neil
Gow, the first, whose music was popular at the Regent Street Polytechnic, where it was often played by his son Nathaniel; William
Marshall, the second and greatest of the three, and James Scott Skinner,
known as the Strathspey King, who arrived one day in the kilt at
Cantlie's consulting room, seeking help in financial difficulties. He was
an itinerant player who popularised the Strathspey in Europe and the
United States, composing a few tunes of his own, one of which was the
'Bonnie Lass o' Bon Accord'. Cantlie promised to organise a concert for
him which took place in 1910 – and upon hearing this the composer
leapt to his feet, took up his violin and plunged into the 'Reel o'
Tulloch' until the consulting room walls rang with sound. (It was also
due to Cantlie's initiative that Scott Skinner's portrait was later painted
by Mr Young Hunter and hung in the Dundee Art Gallery.)

In a talk at the Scottish Corporation Hall, Fleet Street, to the London
Morayshire Association reported in the *Elgin Courier* on 29 November
1904 Cantlie made a contribution to Marshall's biography by suggesting that he had a meeting with Burns. Marshall joined the Duke of
Gordon's household in 1760 becoming butler, house steward, factor,
JP and farmer at Keithmore. He was a brilliant self-taught musician as
well as an astronomer, architect, mathematician and mechanic. One
of his inventions was a clock which almost answered the theory of
perpetual motion, requiring winding once a month, while he also laid

down a meridian line at Keithmore to correct the time. A staunch Tory and admirer of William Pitt, he had a reputation for industry, perseverance and constancy, his opinions being so highly valued that disputes ended in arbitration – he was also an excellent shot, keen fisherman and a skilled dancer, athlete and falconer. One of his sons was a major in the service of the East India Company under Lord Cornwallis, inspiring his tune 'The Marchioness of Cornwallis', while his daughter married John McInnes, brother of Cantlie's grandmother, Miss Helen McInnes, for whom Marshall also composed one of his airs. He had a gift of composing instantly to suit occasions of joy or sadness, such as 'The Marquis of Huntly's Farewell', when he took up his violin to cheer the Huntly family seeing the young lord off on his continental tour, and 'Craigellachie Brig' composed in like manner to commemorate the opening of the new Spey Bridge. He had intuitive knowledge of the rules of composition, so that his melodies flowed in a connected story, and being a very skilful player the sudden transitions of his music did not trouble him. Humble about his gifts, he was only persuaded to publish by the Gordon family and dedicated his works to Lady Huntly, 'trusting you will accept them as the only testimony of respect I have in my power to offer to your Ladyship and to the noble family of Gordon to whom, in all its branches, I feel unalterably bound by every tie of gratitude.'[8] In his talk Cantlie claimed that Marshall met Burns in Edinburgh, pointing out that in a picture illustrating the poet reading 'A Winter's Night' before the Duchess of Gordon, Marshall can be recognised in attendance. Burns certainly called Marshall the 'finest composer of Strathspeys of his age' and was inspired by his music to write 'O' a' the airts the wind can blaw' to his tune 'Miss Admiral Gordon' and 'My love is like a red, red rose' to his tune 'Mrs Hamilton of Wishaw', although later this was changed to 'Low down in the broom'.

This link between Marshall and Burns may have enhanced the admiration Cantlie had for Burns's poetry. When he spoke of the Afghan listening enthralled to Scottish music he spoke of the immortality and universality of Scottish airs, be they melodies or poems. Thus he never failed to accept an invitation (and there were many) to propose the Immortal Memory anywhere in the world, always in Doric upon which the press loved to comment. His command of Scots never left him, which was unusual in a man so much travelled and with little opportunity to use it, but he had a good ear and retentive memory. Doric is classical in origin, in the sense that the broad earthiness of local north-east Scots is disciplined by the elegance of the classics, then translated and learnt in all Scottish parish schools of the area. It is a vehicle for expressing in grammatic prose the deepest, simplest emotions and spiritual thoughts of one of the oldest heritages in the kingdom. Burns wrote in Lallans, a language so flexible that it can produce the 'couthiest' and most exquisitely lyrical poetry, and the two dialects, Doric and Lallans, blend together in Cantlie's speeches on Burns to the benefit of both.

It was the enchantment of Cantlie's personality and his gift of word painting that caused audiences to sit spellbound while he created for them scenes of Scottish life remembered from his childhood:

> The carpet below your feet becomes the green girse o' the haughs of the Nith, the Ayr, the Doon and the Logan Water. The exotic flowers you see on the table seem to be changed to the broom, the bracken and the bluebell. The tobacco smoke above our heads recalls to us the peat reek risin' frae the cottage lums, and curling in graceful circles, high in the air against the dark green of the fir woods. The walls around fade away and are replaced by the banks and braes of the rivers of our native land, transcendent in beauty, rich in lore, fit cradle for a poet and poetic thoughts. In such a setting you are to place the abode of Robert Burns, a humble dwelling, a but and ben. The 'kitchie', the living apartment, you will recognise by its earthen floor, wi' here and there a slab o' stane where it was worn doun, and serving as a sort o' steppin' stane when the damp rises or the floor gets weet frae the drappin' frae the divots, and the peat drush that serves as a theckin' to the roof.

Cantlie's gift for poetic imagery was never bettered than in this passage, nor his gift for recording the minutest observation, which was one of his greatest strengths as a doctor and writer. He spoke of a way of life which he had known intimately as a boy:

> The wa's that aince were white, but noo black frae the reek that finds its way into the kitchie instead of up the lum when the win' is shifty, and the flan carries the soot into the middle of the floor. The box bed opposite the fireplace, its door steekit in the daytime to mak' it look like a press door, for decency's sake; a dresser, wi' its shelves o' bowls and cups, plates and trenchers and underneath, the girdle and the pots and pans, milk cogs and the jellie pan, polished up to mak' it, as it is, the pride o' the hoose. The kitchie table, weel scrubbit wi' san' until its deal boards are a bit worn, showing the roistie knobs here and there, making it gey uneven. A hearthstane blue-washed a' roon, a fire o' peats and truffs, wi' the tattie pot simmering, as it hangs, frae the branks of the lum. On the tae side of the fireplace hangs the saut backit, awa' in the neuk the meal girnel, and frae the corners of the mantlepiece a freshly trimmed rush lamp sheds its rays over the trim abode, and displays the only adornment of the room, namely, last year's cliack sheaf abune the door. Such was the dwelling place of him we delight to honour and thither Burns cam' after he had suppered the kye and beddit doun the horse ... In summer he would tak' a daunder doun the watter side, listening to the sangs of the birds, the sough of the watter, viewing the 'lingering star with lessening ray', and the 'risin' moon' as she 'began to glower the distant Cumnock hills oot ower'. During such moments poetic fancy inspired him and he would wander awa' hame to get a bit o' paper to transcribe his thoughts. Jean, aifter-makin' the little anes a' snod in their beds, would help him in the search ...

Passing from this description of his house, which could have applied to any other Scottish humble abode of its time, Cantlie went on to describe Burns's methods of composition. 'What did Burns write?' he asked.

You all know that of the poets recently selected for a place of honour in the British Museum, Burns was excluded. What did these men want in the way of poetry? Was it love? I would quote:

> My love is like a red, red rose,
> That's newly sprung in June,
> My love is like a melody,
> That's sweetly played in tune.

Show me an equal to these four lines in any literature. Did ever troubadour 'neath southern skies serenade his lady love in lines to be compared with these? I have often thought that when I was born, had I been told 'You are given the option of living five minutes and writing "Auld Lang Syne" or "My love is like a red, red rose", or living to a humdrum age of ninety' I would have chosen the former, and then be content to die. What did these men want? Similes? I quote:

> But pleasures are like poppies spread,
> You seize the flower, its bloom is shed;
> Or like the snowflake on the river,
> A moment white, then melts for ever;
> Or like the borealis race,
> That flit 'ere you can point their place.[9]

With these gifts and appreciation for words and song, it is hardly surprising that when Cantlie and Harry Lauder were introduced they spent a very happy evening together to the evident satisfaction of each other and the other dinner guests whom they entertained. Lauder sang a song, Cantlie sang a song, Lauder told a story, Cantlie told a story, and they went off arm in arm down the street, thoroughly content with each other's company. But these happy times were passing away. In the next decade the poppies spread were not to be those of love, but of young lives sacrificed in the saddest war of history.

CHAPTER TWELVE

The Threat of War

The Christian purpose of the nineteenth century contained a capacity for hope and joy which perished in the mud of Passchendaele. In the first decade of the twentieth century the British Government countered the German threat to the peace of the world by a programme of ship building. The race into armaments, which Lord Salisbury had dreaded, set the prelude to the First World War. Except in its response to German expansion and ship building, the Government drifted indecisively amid the political uncertainties of the international scene. Hemmed in at home by industrial unrest, clamour for Home Rule in Ireland and the reform of the House of Lords, abroad, as crisis followed crisis, it followed events, leaving important decisions to the man on the spot. On the stage George Bernard Shaw, member of the First International, sneered at the old values with wit and sarcasm – values which the British held most dear – while the brilliance of Lawrence Irving, a playwright and actor of the old style, was lost when he was drowned, his wife in his arms, in the Gulf of St Lawrence, as the *Empress of Ireland* was cut in two before the outbreak of the First World War. In 1905 Mabel Cantlie wrote in her diary, 'The Czar has been shot over, I fear there are terrible times ahead.' Now, added to their desire to help their fellow men, fear for the future was beginning to motivate many people to work round the clock, not only to meet peace-time world-wide needs in health and sanitation, but also to ensure that if the dreaded cataclysm came, they would be ready with trained first aid to succour the victims of disaster.

The voluntary aid societies had emerged from the Boer War with their status unresolved. The Central Red Cross Committee remained the co-ordinating committee between the National Aid Society, St John Ambulance and the Army Nursing Reserve, but it now looked upon itself as a permanency, changing its status and name to Council and proposing to form nationwide branches. Naturally the NAS (or British Red Cross, as it was later to be known) felt that its position was usurped and in 1904 the controversy reached *The Times*, the Central Red Cross Council accusing the NAS of inactivity, unreadiness and lack of organisation and training, while the NAS accused the CRCC of merely being a department of the War Office. Cantlie's only link so far with the NAS had been when the Society gave a grant to the VMSC and to a lesser extent during the Boer War, otherwise all his work had been for St John. In June 1904 however he attended a Red Cross meeting at the

Mansion House and in January 1905 the diary records, 'I called on Lady Furley. H has been put on Red Cross Committee.' Those interested in first aid and nursing realised that in the event of a war in which the nation was involved, the only organisation capable of sustaining the medical and nursing staff required and providing an umbrella of neutrality was the Red Cross. Thus in March 1905 a break-through came from Buckingham Palace to which all the chief personalities in the dispute were summoned. Here Lord Esher asked the NAS representatives, as being the first in the field of organising international disaster relief, whether if the NAS remained in possession it could organise relief work on a scale that might be required in the event of a major conflict. The NAS said that it could, explaining that it wished to come under the War Office only in war time, since further involvement would affect fund raising and was not in keeping with British traditions. In March there was a further meeting at Buckingham Palace where a Council was formed and a Society organised with members and associates based on county branches. The King became a Patron and the Queen President of the BRCS which was thus able to trace its origin back to 1870 when the NAS was first formed. Many of the members of the now defunct CRCC, however, had been engaged in early first aid work in St John and when the new BRCS proposed that it alone would be responsible for co-ordinating all voluntary aid in time of war under the War Office, St John did not take kindly to the suggestion. Eventually a compromise was reached, with the authorities agreeing that the BRCS should co-ordinate all help under the War Office except that coming from St John's and St Andrew's ambulance and from the colonies. What had been gained was a nationwide Red Cross organisation to act as framework within which training could now take place, and when war broke out a Joint Committee was appointed to co-ordinate the work of the two societies in war and peace. In spite of controversy Sir John Furley's establishment of the CRCC in 1898 had been justified, although his motives may not have been understood at the time.

In the forefront of Cantlie's mind at the moment was how best the wounded on a battlefield could be swiftly searched for and transported to safety. This rescue work was particularly important during retreat, as was understood during the retreat from Mons in 1914. At an army manoeuvre on Wimbledon Common in September 1904, Cantlie was approached by Major Richardson who suggested a demonstration of how his dogs could be used to search for the wounded. This was arranged and Cantlie was successful in encouraging Major Richardson to bring his dogs with him into the RAMC (TF). In the forthcoming International Red Cross Conference the transport of wounded was one of the subjects discussed, along with the immunities proposed by the Geneva Conventions for ambulance workers. Meanwhile Cantlie was continuing with his lectures on first aid and home nursing at a variety of institutions, to which he was soon to add an invitation from Lady Esher, representing the BRCS and St John, to lecture at her house in Tilney Street and later at Craig's Court House, Whitehall. 'As the classes are being given by Mr. J. Cantlie,' said the magazine *First Aid*, 'popular author of the Association Text Book and Lt. Col Lees-Hall they will prove interesting and popular.' These classes are described in Dame Beryl Oliver's *British Red Cross in Action*. Cantlie also taught the Duchess of Bedford's classes at her house and later lectured at the Duke of York's Royal Military School at which Sir Joseph Fayrer was a one time medical officer, at the same time continuing with his lectures at the Salvation Army, the Working Women's College and the Regent Street Polytechnic.

Between the years 1895 and 1928 the Regent Street Polytechnic trained 40,000 first aid and nursing volunteers and in 1909 it formed these St John's volunteers into the first Red Cross Voluntary Aid Detachment in the country. The currents of Cantlie's life swept him into waters suiting his temperament and if they did not he created those which did. The Polytechnic, like Charing Cross Hospital School, was an educational establishment with Christian purpose which believed in learning by sharing and by living together in a full social life with numerous student societies. Charing Cross had drawn much of its inspiration from Edinburgh; the Polytechnic had a strong flavour of Aberdeenshire, for Lord Haddo, a cousin of Mr Hogg's, was a member of the Council and Lord Leith of Fyvie provided much of the generous funding for its rebuilding in 1911. At the unveiling of the Quentin Hogg Memorial in 1906 the Duke of Argyll said 'Here is the throb of life [the words Dr Johnson used of Charing Cross]. A stream of young manhood without parallel the wide world throughout. There is work here indeed. Man's work and God's work.' The memorial, he said, was a symbol of the past, present and future.

Throughout these pre-war years there are in the *Polytechnic Magazine* a series of poems summing up the inspiration and work of the College. The sequence opens with a poem by Christina Rossetti already quoted in this book, 'Does the road wind uphill all the way? Yes, to the very end'; and almost all those which follow are anonymous. There is one on the Forgotten Workers: 'Give to me a place among the workers, though my name forgotten be'; on True Nobility: 'There is nothing so kingly as kindness. And nothing so royal as truth. For he who is honest is noble . . .'; on Conscience: 'For to sit alone with my conscience will be judgement enough for me'; on Labour's Reward: 'You shall reap in joy the harvest you have sown today in tears'; on Friendship: 'But I will sit by the side of the road and be a friend to man'; on Character: 'For the ways of Fate are the winds of the soul'. In answer to questions about authorship, the editor placed above one of the poems entitled 'The Last Days of Life', 'Mrs. Hogg requests the insertion of the following lines found in an old number magazine. On inquiry learned that they were sent to the editor by Mr. Hogg, authorship unknown.' Were people asking who the poet was? Some may have been attributable to known authorship, but what of the others? Was it Mr Hogg? Cantlie composed verse quickly and some of his poems are published in the *Charing Cross Gazette*, but none extant are of this quality; he thought in prose. Then comes one reprinted from a Chicago newspaper, whence Cantlie's brother George had emigrated and worked in a music shop, sending his own musical compositions to his cousin Beatrice in Montreal:

> He kept his soul unspotted as he went upon his way,
> And he tried to do some service, for God's people day by day.
> He had time to cheer the doubter who complained that hope was dead,
> He had time to help the cripple when the way was rough ahead.
> He had time to see the beauty that the Lord had spread around.
> He had time to hear the music in the shells the children found.
> But the crowds, the crowds that hurry after golden prizes said,
> That he never had succeeded when the clods lay o'er his head,
> He had dreamed, he was a failure, they compassionately sighed,
> For the man had little money in his pockets when he died.

Then, just before the outbreak of war in 1914, there is a poem, of considerable beauty, conceived in the same vein and metre as many of the others, signed by the Duchess of Teck, mother of Queen Mary:

> If each man in his measure
> Would do a brother's part,
> To cast a ray of comfort
> Into a brother's heart.
> How changed would be our country,
> How changed would be our poor,
> And then might Merrie England
> Deserve her name once more.

Did the Duchess of Teck write any of the others and, if she did not, who did? It is sad that no one will ever know, for the spirit of the age is in them. They are what the Polytechnic stood for, what its teachers stood for, and why it accomplished so much in peace and in war.

In 1907 the Territorial Forces Act became law, and the scope of Cantlie's first aid work increased. The Act imposed upon county associations of the Territorial Army the duty of making arrangements and organisation for first aid and nursing training or delegating it to Red Cross county branches. If the Territorial County Associations delegated the duty to the BRCS, then the latter was to be the only body through which aid could be channelled, but if the Territorial Army retained the duty themselves, all aid was to be channelled through its Association, wherever that aid came from. The majority of St John's members served in the Brigade and provided only a small number of Voluntary Aid Detachments which were mainly made up from members of the BRCS. Similarly the idea of training county Territorial Companies in first aid was not really considered seriously until 1918 and even then the idea did not get much further than the drawing board. These arrangements, however, were a compromise made to embrace a variety of interests. It was understandable, on the one hand, that St John should guard the rights of the Brigade, for it had been formed as far back as 1879 by Mr Brazier from a nucleus of trained men and women in

Margate, who rendered first aid in accidents and emergencies. It was also understandable, on the other hand, that the public could not picture the barbarities of modern warfare, which people believed civilisation had long outgrown, nor therefore the necessity to try and establish immunity for the Red Cross, which was the one and only hope of crossing the frontiers of suffering. Cantlie was one of those who did understand the need for this Red Cross umbrella of immunity and he threw himself into this new work with enthusiasm, giving the date for the first meeting held to raise No. 1 BRCS Voluntary Aid Detachment as October 1908. Mr Hastings, Secretary of the BRCS, came to the Polytechnic to address St John's first aid volunteers and explain that he wanted two Voluntary Aid Detachments, a men's and a women's, to be raised as an experiment. The diary records that in the early spring of 1909 Mabel Cantlie went to discuss the question of nurses for the Territorial Army with Miss Heather-Bigg, Matron of Charing Cross Hospital which was later to give training facilities to Detachment members. Since Princess Christian's Army Nursing Service Reserve had been absorbed into the QAIMNS (R), she must have referred to Territorial or Red Cross nurses. In a further entry in May 1909 Mabel Cantlie describes how she was bidden by the Lady Mayoress to a meeting at the Mansion House, after which she went to see Sir Alfred Keogh, DGAMS, 'about a meeting for Red Cross work'.

In August 1909 the *Scheme for the Organisation of Voluntary Aid in England and Wales* was promulgated by the War Office, with a similar scheme for Scotland. This official paper stated that the Territorial Medical Organisation was sufficient to meet the needs of the Volunteer Army on the field of battle allowing for three field ambulances to one Division, but that it lacked the services behind the front line – clearing and stationary hospitals, rest stations and ambulance trains, all of which in an invasion the Red Cross could provide. 'The clearing ambulance is a mobile unit which receives the sick and wounded from field ambulances and transfers them to stationary hospitals (on the lines of communication) and to ambulance trains.' The wounded would start their journey from the entraining stations, and stop en route at rest stations, some of which would be attached to hospitals with one to fifty beds, where patients too ill to continue their journey could be nursed and fed. (In the event most of the clearing hospitals in 1914 were situated at the entraining stations.) Schemes to provide private base hospitals and convalescent homes were to be submitted to the Territorial County Associations and the BRCS and had to be complete in themselves for the treatment of surgical and medical cases. The duties of Voluntary Aid Detachments were to include the preparation of country carts and all vehicles for transport of the wounded, improvisation of stretchers, conversion of buildings into hospitals, provision of personnel to accompany the wounded, and collection and distribution of medical equipment and supplies. Detachments were to be registered at the War Office under a commandant. Men's Detachments were to include a medical officer, a quartermaster, a pharmacist, four section leaders and forty-eight men, twelve to each team, including clerks, carpenters and mechanics. Women's Detachments were to include a quartermaster, a trained nurse and twenty women, including four qualified cooks. First aid and nursing certificates which were to be kept up to date could be awarded by St John's or St Andrew's Ambulance Association, the Fire Brigade, the National Health Society, the county councils and, after December 1910, by the BRCS.

In August 1909 No. 1 VAD, with Cantlie as Commandant, came officially into being, and No. 2 VAD, the Women's Detachment, followed in January 1910 with Mabel Cantlie as Commandant. The Cantlies wished to encourage doctors and trained nurses to join Detachments, believing that first aid was a training in its own right and in 1912, following this idea through, Mabel Cantlie persuaded Dr May Thorne, a doctor in the West End Hospital, to become Commandant of No. 2 and she became a joint Superintendent. Shortly afterwards Mabel Cantlie was asked to start and become the Commandant of Detachment No. 110 in Bedford College, in order to spearhead the Red Cross movement into the universities. In the Cantlies' Detachments doctors and trained nurses took certificates in first aid alongside lay volunteers and, had this practice been nation-wide, lack of understanding between trained nurses and VADs might have been avoided. In March 1910 Cantlie, now Director of Marylebone Division Red Cross, addressed a meeting in the Town Hall to launch the raising of other Detachments, and a member of No. 2 was chosen for a nation-wide advertisement to encourage recruiting. In April Nos 1 and 2 VAD started a full training programme and in July they were ready for an inspection by Colonel Valentine Matthews, RAMC (TF), London.

Meanwhile Sir Frederick Treves, Chairman BRCS, Surgeon-in-Ordinary to the King, eminent surgeon and writer, asked Cantlie to write the Red Cross first aid, training and nursing handbooks. Cantlie was District Chief Surgeon of St John Ambulance and a Knight of Grace of the Order of St John, and not wanting to offend St John by putting his name to the title, asked that it might be anonymous. Somehow, however, his name slipped through into publication. Again, in order to accomplish the task he rose regularly at 4.30 a.m. For a man approaching 60 his day was a long one; it never ended before 10.00 p.m. and sometimes much later, since emergency operations at the Albert Dock Hospital were not rare. His sole means of support still came from fees as surgeon and consultant, and the diary records that on one day that year he had the highest number of patients ever – this meant financial security, but extra work. The three handbooks were illustrated with photographs, drawings and diagrams and at weekends at Cottered the Cantlies were busy erecting tents and photographing carts, stretchers and stretcher bearers, who were mostly volunteers from the railways.

As Cantlie said, the *Training Manual* opened up a new vista of ambulance work. Instructions from Sir Frederick Treves, who had served in the Afghan Wars and pictured the full onslaught of Prussian might, were that Cantlie should presume all regulation appliances exhausted, avoid all previously published work and create a system of ambulance methods dealing with improvisation only; in other words, evolve a system of training out of nothing. The book contains instructions on how to erect a tented field hospital, convert sheds, construct makeshift shelters from blankets and poles, improvise beds, lift and carry patients using regulation or improvised stretchers, convert wagons into ambulances with fixed or slung stretchers, and fit and load steel stretchers into railway rolling stock. There are also instructions for finding, purifying, filtering and softening water supplies; lighting fires and learning the necessities of camp life; and for the treatment of bullet and shell wounds, relief of pain, instructions in surgical cleanliness and preparation of food. Stress is laid on knot tying, not only for bandaging and slings, but also for assembling improvised stretchers, the transverse pieces of which can be carried on the back while the poles are used as walking staves, so that bearers searching for the wounded are not impeded by carrying. The *First Aid Manual* is precise and scientific. Cantlie tells the reader why, as well as how, so that the principle is grasped as well as the practice. Again, lack of materials is never far from mind, so he first explains the best method and then the method that may have to be adopted. For instance, in a fracture it is better to take the splint to the fractured leg and then tie the legs together rather than tie them together first, because that means moving the injured leg with no support; but if no splints are available then that is the best that can be done. Regarding haemorrhage, he said that the tourniquet should never be applied except in cases of absolute necessity. He starts by explaining natural clotting, then gives the pressure point method of arrest and finally the pad and bandage. In an address on bleeding, Cantlie said:

> The blood coagulates under the strapping. The clot, expanding into the mouths of the small capillaries, blocks them and arrests haemorrhage and the rushing blood causes congestion. The wound is choked full of white corpuscles which form connective tissue . . . Arteries the size of pencils feed capillaries the size of crow quills. The white corpuscles roll along the sides of the capillary walls . . . They have the power to thrust through the capillary walls like a moistened finger through soap bubbles. They seize nutriment and incorporate it. This is what they do to germs. If there are not enough white corpuscles then infection sets in . . . If a piece of skin is taken away it is never reproduced, bone heals by bone, nerve by nerve, tendon by tendon, skin and muscle heal by fibrous tissue only.[1]

The *Handbook on Nursing* caused some controversial comments, not because of its contents (Sir Frederick Treves and the BRCS praised it most enthusiastically) but because some matrons felt that a nurse and not a doctor should have written it. Their feelings were understandable, but Cantlie was already the author of an excellent article on nursing in Heath's *Dictionary of Practical Surgery* and in the war which followed conditions at the front and on communication lines were naturally more akin to those experienced by army medical personnel than by trained nurses in civil general hospitals.

All this training was put into practice at the White City on 29 October 1910 when the first Red Cross demonstration was held in the Japan–British Exhibition. 'Improvised stretchers of pitchfork handles and straw ropes, made and twisted on the spot for stretcher beds in place of canvas, the handles of the spades converted into bed posts for the stretchers to be supported on'[2] were on show along with improvised carts, tents and shelters. Cantlie had joined the BRCS Executive Committee and a Uniform Sub-Committee and this was the first time BRCS members had worn uniform. 'H had a fearfully busy morning,' says the diary:

> twelve uniforms came from the tailors and my uniform was plain blue serge dress with red collar and band. We bought black braid on the way. At the White City we waited for the carts to come and put braid round the men's hats and a safety pin for an emergency. Uniforms were blue with R.A.M.C. red facings and V.A.D. on the shoulders, with puttees, breeches and jacket. At 2 p.m. came the carts in which to put the wounded and a trolly, an operation tent, a hospital and a kitchen over which I ruled. H was wonderful, getting up the tents and we all helped hard. Then the Detachments arrived, men and women, and they all wore Red Cross brassards on the arm. Colonels Peterkin, Valentine Matthews, Dr. Sandwith and Sir Frederick Treves inspected us. Sir Frederick stopped and admired the uniform. Afterwards H showed all his original stretchers, tents and appliances.

Nos 1 and 2 VAD were now giving displays all over London to interest others in starting Detachments. Hammersmith and Hampstead followed and soon Cantlie started Detachments at the Oxford Street stores, including Debenham and Freebody's, Marshall and Snelgrove, Selfridges, Bourne and Hollingsworth, Peter Robinson and D. H. Evans. Cantlie was now in his 60th year and was increasing rather than cutting down his activities. Mitchell Bruce tried to persuade him to retire from voluntary work: 'I do not want to prompt him,' Mabel Cantlie wrote, 'but sometimes he looks very tired. But when one hears the applause which always greets his appearance one knows that he is doing really good work.' To please his wife, Cantlie told Dr Sambon that he could take his place lecturing when he retired; but already his mind was running on to fresh needs. He had always wanted to found a college of ambulance, and he confided to Sir Frederick Treves his idea of starting such a Red Cross institute for teaching first aid which (like the St John's members working in his Red Cross No. 1 VAD) would make a bridge between both voluntary aid societies uniting them in a common aim of teaching first aid.

In March 1912 Cantlie attended a levée at Buckingham Palace and, on the same day, the King and Queen went to the opening of the new Polytechnic building. 'Passing across the Entrance Hall, which Their

Majesties were kind enough to admire greatly, the Great Hall was next
visited. This had been specially set out so as to enable all who were there
to get a good view of Their Majesties. In the Great Hall, Dr. Cantlie had
been speaking upon ambulance work for nearly two hours and had
been able to so interest as well as to amuse his large audience that they
were not weary or fidgety when Their Majesties arrived.'[3] One of the
topics on which he had been speaking, according to the diary, was the
danger of broken backs in road accidents. 'Lord Esher spoke to H and
said he knew how much he was doing for Red Cross work.' The next
day Cantlie organised a demonstration of ambulance work at the
Polytechnic in which students drilled, carried stretchers and invalid
chairs, loaded and unloaded carts, improvised tents and fires. Sir
Frederick Treves was there, the Mayor, Mr Debenham, whose contribution to ambulance work was considerable, and Colonels Bedford and
Matthews: 'All spoke so charmingly of H and said he was unique.
Frederick Treves said he was the foremost man in ambulance'. Like
many others, Cantlie worked equally hard for both societies, as he had
done for the Volunteers. He lectured to the commandants, BRCS and
St John's; he examined for both societies and attended their drills and
inspections as well as the reviews and inspections of the London and
Maidstone companies of the RAMC (T) of which he was Honorary
Colonel. In June 1912 he paraded with 17,000 St John's volunteers at
Windsor, where he was the oldest serving member present. In July,
before retiring from the chairmanship of the BRCS, Sir Frederick
Treves took a party of Red Cross workers, including the Cantlies, to
Marlborough House, where they were presented to Queen Alexandra
and Princess Victoria. Princess Christian, who was a member of the
Red Cross Executive Committee, and Princess Beatrice, who was Presi-
dent of the Schools for Mothers, were also present, 'being most
gracious'.

The Balkan War was by this time threatening. In 1912 the Young
Turks began a rebellion and seized control of their country. Calling
themselves liberal they were extreme and aggressive, and the Christian
Balkan States united against them. The Austro-Hungarian Empire was
already under strain. Russia had for some time been active among the
left-wing revolutionary parties in Serbia, and in 1903 the murder of the
pro-Austrian King and Queen of Serbia made the Austrians fear the
dangers of Serbian strength. When war finally broke out between the
Balkan States and Turkey it was Serbia who gained most from the
peace which followed and who thus emerged from the war stronger
than her Balkan partners. In that strength lay one of the seeds of the
First World War.

The Queen of Greece asked Queen Alexandra to help the sick and
suffering in the war and, in answer to this plea, the BRCS sent a medical
expedition and set up a Balkan Appeal Fund. Units were dispatched to
Bulgaria, Montenegro, Serbia, Greece and Turkey, all of which had
doctors, dressers, nursing orderlies and orderlies, while some included
also a sergeant major and X-ray operator. The diary comments
'they were medical students for the most part'. First to go was the

Montenegro Unit on 20 October followed by the Polytechnic members of Nos 1 and 2 VAD who formed the second Montenegro Unit. The *Polytechnic Magazine* reported in December:

> Three of the members of No. 1 Polytechnic V.A.D. Messrs Solomon, W. D. Sheffield and W. G. Osborne volunteered to go out to the front in connection with the present war in the Balkans. Their services were accepted by the B.R.C.S. The first two went to Montenegro (together with the women members of No. 2), the third to Sofia. All passed through the Polytechnic Classes in Ambulance held by Dr. Cantlie and have been members of the Voluntary Aid Detachment since its inception four years ago. The training they received at the hands of Dr. Cantlie, whose ability and enthusiasm for imparting instruction knows no bounds, will undoubtedly enable them to render effective and invaluable service in the field in attending to the wounded, arranging transport to hospital and in many other ways.

The Cantlies saw off two units to Greece on the 27th, and two to Bulgaria on 3 November and, according to the diary and a photograph in the *Daily Graphic*, Cantlie put these units through a crash course at the Polytechnic before they left for the front. The photograph shows the unit for Turkey learning first aid at the Polytechnic before they left on 29 October. 'These men cannot stop an artery or carry a stretcher,' wrote Mabel Cantlie, 'it is awful to think of such ignorant men going out. H will lecture to them every day.'

The second unit for Montenegro left on 11 January. The weather conditions on much of the front were arctic, rough tracks and winter made transport almost impossible. In many cases the wounds of the soldiers had not been touched for over a week and were full of maggots. Whole regiments were stricken with cholera, there was typhus and gangrene. Trains were crammed with dying and wounded. On one train those who died in transit were lashed to the footboards. The Red Cross units cleaned and nursed and clothed. The total number of patients they treated was over 16,000. They behaved with heroism in the face of fire, carrying their stretcher cases to safety. The commandants of the units were men of distinction and courage: three were officers of the RAMC, two had VCs, of which one was Major H. Douglas, VC, DSO, who commanded the Second Serbian Unit from Scotland. The Turkey Director was Major C. H. M. Doughty-Wylie, CMG, and the Greece Director Colonel G. Delme-Radcliffe, CVO, CB, Sir Frederick Treves's son-in-law. While her husband taught and lectured, Mabel Cantlie advertised in the papers and set up a workshop where clothes were made and collected. She had plenty of experience not only in making hospital jackets for Charing Cross Hospital but in devising, cutting out and making pyjamas, shirts and waistcoats for her sons and husband in order to economise, and this training now was useful. Packages were sent to the Red Cross and taken to the trains to go off with the volunteers. Lady Fremantle, Lady MacKenzie Davidson, Lady Godlee, the Hon. Mrs Howard and General Evatt joined the work party and, having settled to the routine of the Balkan War, began again in August 1914. No sooner was the first Balkan War over than the victorious Balkan States fell out among themselves. This time victory went to the Serbs and the Greeks; and it was inevitable that Austria would see Serbia, friend of Russia, as a threat to her security. Members of the BRCS and St John volunteered again for the second war and aid continued from both societies. In all, sixty-three bales went from Mabel Cantlie's working party. She acknowledged all these articles herself: 'Up at 6 a.m.,' she wrote, 'not in bed till 2. or 1.30 a.m.' She exhausted herself in the task, but the methods of organisation and the contacts she made proved of infinite value in the First World War to come. In her final letter of thanks to her workers she asked them to act again in any future emergency, and at a committee meeting suggested setting up an auxiliary corps for the supply of clothes, bedding and medical equipment. General Evatt also spoke of the need for an organisation for the supply of materials and of the excellence of the Marylebone work party. At a council meeting of the BRCS Princess Christian made a point of saying to Cantlie how much kind help his wife had given. It was during the Balkan War that Mabel Cantlie began to suffer the pain which four years later led to a cancer operation. Without revealing the extent of her suffering, she sacrificed health and eventually life itself for the service of her country.

While these conflicts were going on abroad, conditions at home were far from easy. In March 1912 the diary records: 'The strike continues, 14 London Stations shut. Food shortages feared. Greatly fear country will be in dire need. Dr. Garrett Anderson has two months hard labour for smashing windows. H is delighted. She deserves it.' 22 March: 'Two million men idle, trains stopped. Mr. Balfour came back to help against the Coal Strike. Weak Government.' 26 March: 'Mines protected. Coal Conference given up. Men back to work. Trades Unions exhausted.'

In February 1914 Cantlie astonished the medical world with a new method of diagnosis. He was asked by the Committee of the Polyclinic to help them raise funds. He did this by demonstrating his use of the tuning fork in diagnosing liver abscess, which could, in fact, have been applied to other diseased organs. The magazine *First Aid* recounted how 'Cantlie found that when a tuning fork was set vibrating and the shaft held against the body wall and moved about, a note, which varied with the density of the organ immediately beneath it, was transferred to a stethoscope placed over the organ.' This method, said the article, was particularly useful in the discovery of localised pleurisy and to gauge the area covered by the liver if looking for enlargement; it was a 'valuable contribution to medical science'.[4] Among the newspapers taking up the story were *The Times*, the *Globe*, the *Daily News* and the *Leader*. Cantlie's idea was the forerunner of the scanning techniques of today, in which an electrical wave is sent out and, by studying the note it makes on meeting the organ and returning, it is possible to gauge the healthiness or unhealthiness of the tissue. Cantlie's discovery required a good ear to detect which sound was 'true' and which 'false'. He said that he found the note G the most reliable in diagnosis.

The Chinese Minister in London was interested in the discovery and this again gave publicity to Cantlie's founding of the Hong Kong College of Medicine, so that he was asked to help with the starting of a tropical agricultural college in Ceylon. His support for this venture, for which Mrs Harcourt gave a reception at the Imperial Institute, led to a generous donation during the war from the Governor of Ceylon for the King Albert I Hospital in France, which the Cantlies were instrumental in starting and running. Cantlie's interest in the use of herbs in treating disease had been well known since his return from Hong Kong, as was also his interest in vermin-carried disease, but he was now researching further into the relationship between diseases in people and animals such as glanders in horses, and lecturing at the Polytechnic and other centres on this transmission, and the link in diagnosis and treatment. The First World War was the last time the army went to war with horses. A number of leading bacteriologists of the time were veterinary surgeons and, as well as sharing some bacteriological facilities and research, every hospital arrangement made for soldiers had its replica in the treatment of horses, with rest stations on lonely roads where they could be cared for before entraining, and which were inspected by royalty and leading men and women.

War was now imminent, and with the international situation fast worsening and disharmony growing among the nations on the Continent, Mr Asquith had combined the Secretary of Stateship of War with the Premiership. In March 1914 army officers in Ireland, faced by a policy they thought would lead to crushing a Protestant rebellion in the north in order to force through Home Rule, sent in their resignations. It was against this background of growing anxiety that 662 members of Chertsey Division of Red Cross Surrey Branch staged one of the largest demonstrations of Red Cross work ever seen, at which an invasion was envisaged and a battle simulated by the East and West Surreys. The display took place on 20 June 1914 and was attended by Queen Alexandra and the Empress of Russia. A week before, the diaries record, 'To Brooklands to see Major Lindsay Lloyd and arrange for Saturday.' On the 17th, 'To Brooklands. Mrs. Locke King, Surrey Branch drove us.' (Mr Locke King had provided much finance for Brooklands Race Course.) 'Saw beds needed for Base Hospital and got tents pitched. General Evatt came in the evening to discuss.' On the 19th, 'Brooklands again. Worked hard and got the tents right.' On the 20th, H on ambulance train early in the morning. Queen Alexandra and the Empress of Russia arrived and went to Base Hospital, which H had filled with patients. General Evatt in charge of Base Hospital. A large party of us, led by Lord Roberts and Sir Frederick Treves, greeted the Queens. H and I kept in the background, as Surrey County Day. Home. H so tired he fell asleep with half his clothes on.' Both Sir Frederick Treves and Mrs Locke King were warm in their praise and thanks. Sir Frederick wrote at once, 'My dear Cantlie, a thousand congratulations. The whole demonstration was perfect. The details were most complete. It was the best Red Cross Display I have ever seen and should show the country that, in the unhappy event of invasion, there is a competent body of well trained volunteers of which you may well be proud.'[5] Mrs Locke King wrote at the same time:

Dear Mr. Cantlie, You'll have heard that I called up your house to try and find for sure that you survived yesterday and that Mrs. Cantlie was also not dead. Had I been able to speak to you, I wanted to pour out to you a very small part of the immense gratitude I feel to you for what you have done for us. As Sir Frederick Treves said, nobody but you could do it and nobody in the world but you would do it in the extraordinarily generous way you do, giving your whole self to the job, inciting and inspiring everyone who comes in contact with you. I am told that Mrs. Cantlie also worked like a brilliant slave and that the Stationary Hospital would have been nowhere without her. I wish I saw any possibility of being able to do anything comparable for you and her. Sir Frederick Treves tells me he believes it to be by far the best display of the sort that there has been. That is entirely thanks to you. Indeed I hope it has done neither you or Mrs. Cantlie harm.[6]

What was this display of medical services organised by Cantlie, and what was its significance in the light of events to follow? Within the three mile area of Brooklands Race Course a mock battle was staged; the line of communication was the motor race track and along it the ambulances travelled, bringing back the wounded. Aeroplanes of the Royal Flying Corps and Major Richardson's dogs sought out the wounded. 'There was a Clearing Hospital of 50 beds, 4 Rest Stations of 20 beds each, a Stationary Hospital of 50 beds (which represented one unit of the usual 200) and a Base Hospital of 50 beds (also forming one unit of a base hospital which might contain 500 to 3000 beds).'[7] The tented clearing hospital was as close to the front as safety allowed. It consisted of four large tents equipped as wards, an operating tent, camp kitchen and accessory tents. The four rest stations each had two tents, with wards and back-up tents containing kitchen and stores. The stationary hospital had four marquees, an operating theatre, X-ray, dispensary and chief officer's tent, as well as supporting tents including kitchens, laundries and so forth. The base hospital was situated in the Members' Enclosure (within months the Epsom Grandstand was to provide a similar war-time emergency hospital) and the motor ambulances plied between. All the equipment had to be brought and erected, temporary beds had to be made of straw, faggots cut for hospital fires; everything that could be had to be improvised, such as packing cases for operating tables. Detachments in charge of individual units were left to decide on their own initiative what to do within the limit of their responsibility, and their efforts and achievements showed individual resource and thought. The stationary hospital was erected and all its equipment found locally within twenty-four hours, showing efficiency and ingenuity. The base hospital was in the charge of Camberley Division and demonstrated high standards of order, cleanliness, air, light and up-to-date equipment, which would have been a credit to any military hospital.

Three weeks later on 9 July, the members of Nos 1 and 2 Voluntary Aid Detachments went into camp. 'To Eastcote,' says the diary, 'Got tents up. H and I slept there.' On the 10th, 'Lit fires. Men finished getting up 18 tents. 50 or 60 in camp. Colonel Valentine Matthews and a Major inspected us. Severe scramble. Served tea.' 'At this time,' wrote James Taylor, Assistant Commandant and Quartermaster of No. 1,

> the Detachment had already a history extending over five years, during which time the members had qualified in the usual subjects and under the able and enthusiastic leadership of their Commandant had progressed beyond the limits set by the text books. On the ground were advanced dressing stations, clearing hospitals, quartermaster's stores, canteens, sleeping quarters for orderlies and nurses, officers' quarters, etc. The actual field work was made to approximate as nearly as possible to those conditions which a state of war would be likely to produce and no detail which could be foreseen was omitted. It was the best Red Cross camp the members of V.A.D. 1 had up to that time experienced.[8]

Apart from the usual inspections and practice in first aid and nursing there were lessons in signalling in order to maintain contact with the front line, training in camp life, laundry work and sanitation. On 13 July the diary runs, 'Still in camp, cooking. Up early, lighting fires. Women woefully ignorant on how to do stove and clean up.' On the 15th, 'H not down, very wet night. I went out and slackened guy ropes all round the camp.' Many of the men were travelling to and from London, doing jobs as well and, as James Taylor described, 'sitting under the instruction which poured forth from their respected Commandant' at weekends. Cantlie was also employed seeing patients for part of the time and much of the responsibility for the camp fell on his wife, who was Commandant-in-Charge. It was hard work, 'Packed up and finished camp today. Hard work carrying heavy pails of water.' That entry was on the 25th. The next day Austria declared war on Serbia. The training had not come too soon. 'While yet our camp fires, though cold, were visible,' writes James Taylor, 'while yet the sunburn of the camp was on the faces of those members who had participated in it, an astonished nation realised that they were face to face with one of those cataclysmal events in the world's history.'[9] On the evening of 26 July Dr Harper, now Colonel RAMC (TF) of the Corps which Cantlie had raised thirty years earlier, came in to Harley Street for notes to make a speech on the raising of the Corps. On the 27th the diary records, 'Neil to War Office to be interviewed. Passed. Age 21.' The following day Mabel and Neil Cantlie went to Aberdeen University for his graduation. 'Everyone spoke so well of Neil. They say he will succeed because he has much quiet determination. He is a wonderful fellow to be so well liked. Dr. Williamson said, "Neil is the most promising Officer in the University Training Corps".' He had won the

Gold Medal in Surgery, had Firsts in all his subjects and passed his finals with a star. Then on 2 August comes the entry, 'War is declared by Germany against Russia. What an appalling state of things. Germany must be absolutely mad. What are we going to do. I know not. God have mercy on us all.'

CHAPTER THIRTEEN

Sun Yat Sen: First President of China

Meanwhile events on the other side of the world were contributing in no small measure to the balance of power in the West and the alignment of nations. On 18 August 1909 the diary records, 'Sun Yat Sen to stay. The Chinese reformer, our old friend, came to stay yesterday. He played some croquet. He told us about his cause which has made much progress. It rained all day. Sun reading from morning till night.' 21 August, 'Sun went away. He is very silent this time and he seems to read and think a great deal. He has £80,000 on his head. An enormous sum.' Sun came to see the Cantlies again in October and left at the end of the month for America. Nearly two years passed with an occasional postcard, photograph of himself or letter; and then on 8 January 1911 Sun Yat Sen called on the Cantlies again and the following day arrived to stay. On 10 January there is the entry, 'The papers tonight have much about China and talk of revolution, so Sun is interested. We spent a quiet evening and enjoyed the peace.' The following day Sun left for the United States and towards the end of the month Lady Stewart Lockhart, whose son had been Colonial Secretary in Hong Kong and who was now in China, said in a letter that there might be great changes in China which would affect the world.

In October 1911 Mary Adami, Cantlie's Canadian cousin, telephoned to say that her son had an acute appendicitis at school in East Grinstead. Cantlie, not free to go himself, asked a leading surgeon to operate who pronounced it the worst case he had seen and saw little hope of recovery. Mabel Cantlie spent the night at the school keeping in the kitchen fire for the nurses she had brought down and records how she 'saw little need for all his dreary comments. I cannot understand why the nurses are so depressed. Donald had a quiet night and seems comfortable. Mary wants a doctor to stay all day. I said it was not possible, but H is coming down to East Grinstead for the night tonight.' Then in a footnote, 'Great revolutions in China. Wuchang has been taken.'

On that day the newspapers were reporting that Chinese revolutionaries were arrested in Hankow where a bomb was found in the Russian concession. By 11 October Wuchang, Hankow and Hanyang were in the hands of the revolutionaries. Jordan, the British Minister in Peking, reported that the movement was anti-dynastic and not anti-foreign and that injury to foreigners was forbidden on pain of death. What sparked off the immediate trouble was a Government decree stating that trunk railways built, building or to be built were the responsibility of central government and this annoyed provincial governments who had taken loans from foreign finance houses and sometimes could not account for the money. On Sunday the diary records, 'Went to Church and prayed for Donald and Sun Yat Sen.' It was typical of the Cantlies' priorities. Donald's life was in greater danger. Elsewhere in the diaries are two lines of poetry, 'How small of all that human hearts endure, The part that Kings and laws alone can cure'. Nevertheless, the weakening of the Pax Britannica was to bring changes all over the world, undreamt of by those who had helped to build it, changes in which the common man was to become the innocent victim of violence and warfare in a world uncontrolled by law and justice. During the next year a drama was enacted in China in which all the leading European powers were involved and about which, because of the strains in Europe, they could come to no agreement or decision, interfering sufficiently to alter the balance, but with insufficient knowledge and integrity to stabilise the confused situation.

In the aftermath of the Boxer Rebellion some improvements in medical care had taken place in China. The Americans gave a lead in spending the Boxer Indemnity Fund, to which the Chinese paid crippling fines, on welfare and reforms in China and the rest of the powers followed suit. St John's volunteers had been involved as medical orderlies with British troops at the time of the Rebellion and this may have helped to interest the Chinese in first aid. The London Missionary Society and the American Missionary Society opened the Peking Union Medical College in 1901; in Shanghai St John's University founded a School of Medicine attached to St Luke's Hospital, and in 1908 the Western railway companies opened hospitals for their employees. Schools for nurses started and a Nursing Association was formed. There were also beginnings of public health work and the foundation of a School of Hygiene. Much impetus for these medical improvements came from the medical missionaries – French Roman Catholics, American Methodists, British Protestant societies and many others. But the Chinese were weary of being milked by foreign powers and the days of the Manchu Government could be counted; the reforming Emperor had died in prison to which he had been committed by the old Empress, who died in 1908, and was replaced by an infant Emperor and a reactionary Prince Regent. What was going to happen when the Manchu Government fell? That was the question troubling the powers; the event was regarded as inevitable. In the circumstances, particularly the woeful ignorance of the Chinese concerning medicine, nursing and sanitation, it is not surprising that the man to whom the nation turned in its hour of crisis was a doctor.

On 14 October Mr J. Ellis Barker, who knew Sun, called on the Cantlies and two days later wrote to Mr Asquith[1] telling him that the reforming movement had right on its side, was popular, worthy of sympathy, likely to succeed and that the Chinese people would not forgive European nations who supported the corrupt Manchus. On the 16th Jordan reported rebel claims to have constituted a government which would respect international treaties, but Sir Edward Grey refused to acknowledge it, except on a *de facto* basis, for the Manchu Government was still trying to save itself, and the same day appointed Yuan Shik-Kai, a Manchu official and former President of Korea, who had supported the revolutionary Kang and then reaffirmed his loyalty to the Empress, Viceroy of the two Southern Provinces. Unfortunately Jordan relied on the advice of Morrison, *The Times* correspondent in Peking, who saw himself as Yuan's personal adviser after his rise to power and said that Yuan would support the Manchus, whereas he was out to further his own ends, as his son warned. Bankrupt and tottering, the Manchus approached the powers for a loan and suspension of Boxer Indemnity Fund payments. The Hong Kong Shanghai Bank did not want to lend without British Government backing and Sir Edward Grey was not in favour of giving this, although he feared the implications if the other powers lent and Britain did not. Meanwhile anxieties about Yuan's personal ambitions were highlighted by his refusal to go to Hankow to fight the rebels unless given direct command of the troops. Jordan, possibly at last seeing the danger of Yuan as a dictator, considered trying to save the Manchus, but the next day the Imperial Army was again in retreat and the British press reported a Chinese Parliament meeting in Peking. The Secretary of the Chinese Legation in London said to the Cantlies that the Manchus were done for and that he expected a peaceful change over.

In view of the worsening situation, the powers decided to guard the railways built with foreign loans in the last twenty years, but could not agree who should guard which stretch. The British, anxious to keep political temperatures cool, hesitated about moving the Royal Inniskilling Fusiliers from Hong Kong, but the Germans landed in Hankow on 23 October, to British displeasure, ostensibly to protect their settlement, and the Japanese sent infantry. Inevitably, tensions rose. The Germans were not popular in China; the Kaiser's instructions to his troops, leaving to put down the Boxer Rebellion, did not earn respect or love: 'Give no quarter. Take no prisoners. Even as a thousand years ago the Huns under King Attila made such a name for themselves as still resounds in terror in legend and fable, so make the name of Germany resound through Chinese history a thousand years from now.'[2] The situation was delicate and the Japanese asked the British Admiral to stay in Hankow so that they would not come under German orders. Meanwhile, the Chinese Senate, seeing the dangers of their railways as rivers down which would flow foreign troops, impeached the Transport Minister. The Hong Kong and Shanghai Bank besought the British Government to ask Jordan to mediate between the two sides, but Jordan replied it was impossible. On 28 October the Manchus appointed Yuan as High Commisioner and, seeing this as a sign of possible recovery, a Franco-Belgian group, with some British backing, said it would lend money to the Imperial Government. The people, however, were behind neither the Government nor Yuan; 4,000 Imperialist troops refused to entrain for Hankow and Grey finally ended arguments about lending money to the Manchus by saying 'This is no time to lend to the Chinese Government'.[3] He was right. The British press were reporting that Yuan had seen the rebel leaders and that fighting had ceased. On 30 October an edict was issued in the name of the baby Emperor, confessing mistakes. On 3 November Jordan reported the issuing of a decree ordering the drafting of a new constitution by a National Assembly and on the 4th the rebels took Shanghai and set up a government there, backed by influential Chinese. The same day, the diary, based on press reports, records that Yuan refused the premiership under the Manchus and, on the 6th, Jordan explained how hopeless his position was, with city after city falling to the rebels. On the 7th came reports that Peking had fallen and on the 9th official communications confirmed the revolution successful. On 13 November Jordan, realising the Manchus were doomed, saw the two-fold dangers of Yuan as personal dictator and the powers taking advantage of Chinese weakness to intervene on opposing sides. Already, seeing the Chinese Army withdrawing from Northern Manchuria, Russia was planning to send troops to replace them and guard the railways, while Japan gave notice that if her stretch of railway was used to transport Chinese troops she would regard it as an overt act. Jordan, beginning to comprehend the extent of Chinese sympathy for the new regime, told Grey that if the British did not allow the rebels to use their stretch of railway the Chinese would think they were favouring the Manchus.

The Japanese now reported that Sun was in Europe, stirring up trouble among German students. Nothing could have been further from the truth. In October he had sent a postcard to the Cantlies from Colorado and on 10 November the Cantlies received a letter from him written on board the liner *Adriatic*. On the 12th two cypher telegrams came for Sun, one at 11.30 p.m., so the Cantlies sat up till midnight waiting for him, but he did not come. On the 13th Cantlie went to see a patient in Ockley and, during the day, as the diary records,

A double telegram sent from the Legation was brought by the porter Andrews thinks. It was addressed to Sun and sent to the Legation. I copied the numbers in the cypher and the Chinese characters, which evidently the Embassy Secretaries had written against the numbers, so that Sun could read them and then sent the telegram back and said Sun was not in the house. Sun and General Homer Lea came in about 3 p.m. Sun looked so well. The General is a hunchback and very tiny, but evidently very clever. [He wrote *The Valor of Ignorance*.] He says Lord Roberts has been with them and Lord Charles Beresford and several other important people. They dine with two bankers tonight. Sun does not want the papers to know and calls himself Nakayama. General Lea and Sun looked at the telegram. It was asking Sun to return to Canton to take charge. General Lea says he must be Premier. I looked at Sun and wondered if he thought he could take it on his shoulders. It seems difficult for us to realise such a huge change. I had no opportunity of speaking to Sun alone. He promised to come back after their dinner tonight with the bankers. I gave Sun all the telegrams and told him that I had telegraphed to San Francisco that he had not arrived, so he was to telegraph again that he had done so. I have always been so fearful of doing the wrong thing.

The following day Sun and General Homer Lea arrived after lunch with Lord Charles Beresford. At a dinner party that evening, which included Manson and General Evatt, Sun said that if no one better could be found to be President he would take on the job. He said he had already chosen his Cabinet. Meanwhile, through the Legation, he heard that a cruiser built for the Manchu Government had started out from a British yard but had been ordered to return. The British Government was uncertain what to do about these ships and Sun was already trying to get help from the Royal Navy to build and train a Chinese navy. Next day Mabel Cantlie wrote to Admiral White on Sun's behalf, asking if he could help. He courteously replied that he was too old, but promised to call the following week. She then wrote to Captain Barrett, who feared losing promotion if he went to China in this way, but Sun was apparently more successful with the War Office for, after he had gone, Colonel Maude called at Harley Street and said he was going to China to help remodel her army. Mabel Cantlie also went to see Mr Whitehead of the Chartered Mercantile Bank of India, China and Japan, who was an old friend, and told him that Sun was in London. Meanwhile Sir Trevor Dawson of Vickers called on Sir Edward Grey and tried to convince him that Sun was pro-British and pro-American and that he was confident of a loan of $1 million if the British Government would agree, giving the names of two American senators who would confirm this.[4] Jordan's recent reports to Grey, however, had been conflicting, first that Yuan had been asked to be President – his son repeating the warning that he would make himself Emperor – and then that he was trying to save the Manchus by heading a party favouring constitutional monarchy, offering to move Parliament from Peking to Tientsin or Shanghai, if the rebels were uneasy about going to Peking, and saying he would conquer the south by force if it would not co-operate. Although Grey admitted that these reports did not coincide with Sun's story, he stressed his confidence in Jordan's judgement and said that Britain could not take sides in internal Chinese affairs, beyond saying that there must be a government strong enough to secure order and deal with foreign nations. On 19 November Colin, home on leave from the navy, drove Sun in the morning to see his likeness in wax at Madame Tussauds; in the afternoon General Homer Lea and Sun went to see Lord Roberts and Earl Grey and the following day Sun left for China. 'We felt sad to say goodbye. God knows what is in store for our old friend, but we will pray for his success with all our hearts.'

Two weeks later, on 2 December, Nanking fell to the reformers and the Prince Regent abdicated, but Yuan merely saw this as an opportunity to bring forward another Empress Dowager as regent, throwing the blame for conditions on to the Prince. This made even the Manchus uncertain of Yuan's intentions and they deposited their treasure in the Hong Kong Shanghai Bank. With far-sighted duplicity Yuan then committed himself to a British-style constitutional monarchy with an Assembly, from which Manchus would be debarred, and a Council of Regents for the young Emperor, consisting of a Manchu, a Chinese and the new Empress Dowager. He promised reforms and the abolition of eunuchs. Time, however, was running out for the Empire. On 7 December Mongolia declared its independence, noted by the Russians whose presence in the area the British feared, and the next day the Russians threatened to fire on the Wuchang forts opposite Hankow, which were in the hands of the rebels. The British Admiral interceded, but had the threat not passed foreign lives would have been at stake. The Russians said Chinese shells were endangering their concession, but Admiral Winslow was scathing in his criticism of their discourtesy in not informing the other powers; 'The rebel leader,' he said, 'has in all his dealings with us behaved in a most correct and humane manner'.[5] Throughout the uprising Western naval surgeons had operated on the wounded on both sides of the conflict under the newly formed Red Cross branches in Shanghai, Peking and Hankow. On 9 December Shantung Province declared its independence, later to be withdrawn, and now, impatient for a decision, the French decided to lend to the Chinese Post Office; the Germans were also in favour of a loan, although agreeing not to act without the other powers. Grey, however, remained adamant; no money must be lent without the sanction of the reform party and in this he was supported by Sir Claude Macdonald in Tokyo, who said that the Chinese did not want the Manchus to remain at any price. Also on the 9th the Chinese declared a fifteen-day Armistice and three days later the rebels said they would not agree with a loan to Yuan.

The Cantlies were overwhelmed by a stream of visitors calling to have their views on the confused Chinese situation. Two of these were the Changs, a Chinese couple from Aberdeen, who claimed to be friends of Sun's. Mabel Cantlie arranged with Mr Munro-Ferguson for them to visit the House of Commons, but a journalist who called elicited from Mrs Chang that Yuan was the adopted son of her grandfather, whom the latter had later come to distrust. On 16 December the British press reported that Yuan was to be President, Sun Vice President and the dynasty was to go. On the 18th, however, the north and south could not agree at a conference at Shanghai and the south set up a Military Government of its own in Nanking. On the 20th Wu, the rebel leader, called on Jordan and told him the Chinese would not forgive the powers if they refused to support a republic, but Jordan pointed out the military strength of the Northern Imperialists and the Imperial Guard, three-quarters of which was now loyal to the Manchus, and pleaded with him to put the country first and compromise, since more fighting would only leave it weaker. Wu promised to exhort the people, but said the Chinese wanted a republic which should embrace the old Chinese Empire of Manchuria, Mongolia, Turkestan and Tibet. True to his promise, Wu got the armistice extended to 31 December but Yuan used the breathing space to prevaricate, holding out against a republic, which he falsely said the powers would not accept. With his troops deserting, Jordan extracted from him the promise to leave the choice of government to the National Assembly, which the British would not influence, but the next day Jordan reported that he was still hedging. On 28 December the Admiralty asked for instructions regarding the cruisers being built for China and was told to delay – for the National Assembly was to meet that day and, according to Jordan, was likely to vote for a republic. The Chinese reforming party had said that it wanted Sun Yat Sen as Provisional President of China and, on the 28th, the National Assembly issued a decree about the proposed form of government: the Provisional President was to be voted in by two thirds of the National Assembly, consisting of three representatives from every province, each provincial government holding its own self-styled elections. The Assembly was to determine the budget, make laws and agree loans and taxes. The meeting ended with a formal request that Sun should be President.

On 29 December Dawson called on Grey again to impress upon him that Sun was the people's choice, that he had been elected President by eighteen of the provinces – the Nanking Government claimed seventeen – and that the Imperial Government had yielded. Yuan, however, had no intention of yielding or finding a peaceful solution and fighting again broke out in Hankow. 'It looks,' said Grey, 'as though the Northern Party is not willing to abide by the decision of the National Assembly.'[6] Suddenly Yuan seemed to lose his nerve, his manner and language changed dramatically and Jordan cabled that he seemed to have lost control of the situation. The scene was volatile and pregnant with the danger of unprecedented violence. On 1 January the diary records press reports of Sun offering the Presidency to Yuan in an effort to avoid bloodshed. On that day, Sun, who had been welcomed by a deputation in Shanghai, entered Nanking and proclaimed an alteration of the Chinese calendar. The diary records a *Daily Mail* report that 'Sun was received in Nanking with rejoicing, 10,000 soldiers acclaimed him and he took an oath to put down the Manchu Government and create a united China with new laws, peace and then retire, so that a new President might be chosen. He got a 21 gun salute and the greatest enthusiasm was manifest.' None of the powers ever acknowledged the strength of Sun's popularity and indeed it never seems to have been communicated by Jordan to Grey. On 5 January the press reported that Sun had completed his Cabinet, including the ablest men in China, of whom two had refused to serve under Yuan; clearly Sun had the flower of youth on his side. On the 6th Sun issued his *Manifesto*, declaring the Government would respect treaties, loans, concessions and the property of foreign nations and would strive to elevate the people, secure peace for Manchus and Chinese alike, remodel the laws, abolish trade restrictions, ensure religious toleration and improve relations with foreign peoples. On 3 January, however, the Germans and Japanese were reported as saying that they opposed a Republic. Yuan, writing courteously to Sun refusing the offer of President of a legally constituted Republic, realised that, with three quarters of the Imperial Guard on his side and the possibility, however inaccurate the reports, of some foreign support, he could afford to wait.

On 7 January the armistice was extended and the Nanking Government in the south cabled to Britain confirming Sun's appointment as President and stating that the new Government would honour all rules governing nations. On Grey's instructions, the telegram was not acknowledged. While Sun was on the ex Viceroy's yacht, inspecting naval ships on the Yangtze, with ships dressed over all and hundreds of people lining the banks, Jordan telegraphed Grey that the Manchus would abdicate peacefully if Yuan was given the Presidency. The weakness of this dual leadership tempted the Russians to recognise Mongolia's independence and the Chinese merchants, seeing the Empire breaking up, persuaded the Manchus to go, first issuing a decree authorising Yuan to rule, pending his election in Peking and Nanking, and offering a compromise seat of government in Tientsin. Yuan tried to secure recognition for his Presidency, but Grey refused to promise anything until the Manchus abdicated, although he did say the British Government was inclined to recognise Yuan as Head of State, pending his formal election as Provisional President, provided the powers agreed. In spite of becoming aware of Sun's popularity as a leader, the powers did not feel he was sufficiently strong to govern China and they would not recognise the Nanking Government, which they claimed was appointed by provincial military governments and not necessarily representative. The Chinese, on the other hand, were deeply suspicious of the Manchus and of Yuan and would not attend the Assembly in Peking, which they said was a sham. There was deadlock. The press reported Sun had taken back the offer of the Presidency to Yuan; fighting broke out; bombs were thrown at Yuan; forty Imperialist generals crossed to the Republic; the Manchus threatened to shoot any princes who left Peking and said they would abdicate in a month. While Morrison and *The Times* reported little or no hope of reconciliation, official sources disclosed that Sun had again promised Yuan the Presidency if he would join the Republicans and submit to election. Jordan felt that if Yuan went there would be no one with sufficient ability to 'cope', but at last Grey seemed to doubt Morrison's judgement, for he commented, 'We know all too little of Chinese forces to be sure of our ground'.[7] While instructing Jordan to deny rumours that the British favoured a constitutional monarchy under the Manchus, he realised at the same time that British recognition of the Nanking Government would not help if the other powers did not follow suit, and in this he was supported by Sir Claude Macdonald in Tokyo, who said the powers wanted whatever government was chosen to remain in Peking.

Suddenly the financial dam broke. Germany and Japan were already lending money to Yuan – the Japanese on the security of the Shanghai Hankow Railway – and the Russians used the alleged threat of revolution in Eastern Manchuria to move troops there to guard their stretch of railway line, which meant that they could do the same. The Merchant Steam Navigation lent on the security of the iron and coal works; the Chinese merchant fleet mortgaged itself to the Hong Kong Shanghai Bank and to Germany and Japan and the Nanking Government promised to mortgage the Salt Tax and started overdrafts with Western banks to be turned to loans. The four powers involved in loan negotiations – America, Britain, France and Germany – now increased their number to include Russia and Japan. Yuan, confident of financial support and with Jordan's personal backing, re-approached Sun, but Sun stuck to his insistence that Yuan's authority must stem from the Assembly and not the Manchus, adding that he would not accept two assemblies, north and south, nor a provisional assembly in Peking because of the turbulence there, but he made no comment on the question of whether he would accept a compromise assembly in Tientsin. If Yuan was prepared to meet these demands he could be elected President of a united China. Yuan's negotiations with Sun did not pass unnoticed by the Manchus, however, who prevaricated again, deciding not to abdicate and summoning Yuan's rival to Peking where they started a reign of terror, forcing titles on Yuan which he was unable to refuse and which would make him yet less acceptable to the Chinese. The British moved troops from Tientsin to Wei Hei Wei, presumably to deal with potential trouble and possibly also to leave Tientsin to accommodate a compromise assembly without fear of foreign pressure. This had the desired effect on the Manchus, who said they would abdicate if they could get good terms, and they issued three edicts in the name of the Imperial Government, the first accepting a Republic and giving Yuan powers to draw up with the Republicans joint schemes for north and south; the second laying down their terms for retirement, and the third securing measures for peace. A new flag was devised and ministers abroad became 'provisional diplomatic representatives'.[8] Sun answered by repeating that Yuan's power must not be derived from the Manchus and by inviting Yuan to Nanking, which produced deadlock.

On 7 February Mr Sheridan Jones called on the Cantlies and asked Cantlie if he would collaborate in writing a book on China to be entitled *Sun Yat Sen and the Awakening of China*. On 9 February a letter arrived from Sun and the diary records that it told how he was 'always busy, much to arrange'. It said that he had accepted the post of President 'while everything was unsettled', and 'expressed constant gratitude for what we had done'. Written on 21 January the letter said: 'I have assumed the Presidency of the Provisional Republican Government in China which I accepted with disinterested fervour in order to render myself an instrumentality to rescue China, with its four hundred million population, from environment of impending perils and dishonour.' It ended by speaking of their kindness 'that I can never nor will forget'. By the 18th, Cantlie was busy writing. Hastily written, the book has a note of urgency. It captures the visionary spirit of the times; of hope, reform, constitutional change, justice, democracy and enlightenment, encouraging a programme of education and economic and scientific training in order to raise living standards. It describes the cruelty and corruption of the Manchus and the part played by the eunuchs; the Manchus' untrustworthiness and determination not to reform, for even Prince Kung – for whose integrity and moderation Sir Nicholas O'Conor had great admiration – did not believe a constitutional monarchy under the Manchus could work. In one chapter Cantlie dealt with the problem of opium smoking, to which the medical missionaries had been drawing attention before the Royal Commission of 1900 had highlighted the dangers. Cantlie had lectured in London on the subject in 1901 and now pointed out here as also in his *Journal of Tropical Medicine* that, although reforms could not come until the Empress had died, now that that event had occurred and the Chinese had begun not only to cut out opium growing and punish offenders but also to enter into an arrangement with the Indian Government to cut down the trade, then there was an urgent need to conform with Chinese wishes. The book speaks of the popularity and esteem which Sun enjoyed based on his personal qualities – patriotism, vision, integrity and humility – the latter of which was to lead him into the greatest mistake of his life, to trust Yuan and hand power over to him. Yuan was a strong, astute politician but, like Li Hung Chang, he had been reared in a corrupt, mandarin administration and had great personal ambition. Li's ambition, however, never led to disloyalty – in a conflict of loyalty, the throne came first – whereas Yuan's ambition was unbalanced, as his declaration of himself as emperor was to show. The book tells of how the Cantlies repeatedly pointed out to Sun the advantages of constitutional monarchies and the drawbacks of revolution. The problem with revolutions is that they so disrupt the fabric of society and the economy that either other nations are tempted to take advantage of national weakness or a dictator arises, leaving the country in either case with less liberty than before.

On 12 February a rising took place at Ili, where the Russians had sixty-five Cossacks stationed, and the High Commisioner and a Tartar general were murdered. The Russians advised the British Consul in Kashgar to send troops from India and thirty men went from Gilgit. Meanwhile the Russians moved troops from Port Arthur, taken from the Chinese by treaty twenty years before, out into the Shantung Peninsula, which had been defined a neutral zone at the time. This alarmed the Japanese, who gave them a five-day ultimatum which meant the threat of war. As if this was not trouble enough, a Manchu prince went to Manchuria to persuade the Viceroy to hold out for the Imperial cause. Seeing the danger of war, Sun again put the unity of China first and offered Yuan the Provisional Presidency, saying he must be elected by the assemblies in Nanking and Peking and by the Bannermen and Mongols. Sun set out five points to be followed in sequence: first, the abdication of the Manchus; then Yuan must swear an oath of allegiance to the Republic; he, Sun would then resign, and

Yuan would be elected President, swearing an oath to support constitutional law. This last point deeply troubled Sun, for the oath was the only protection the reformers had that the rule of law would be obeyed. It was, as Sun feared, not enough, but it seemed the only alternative to the threatened break up of the Empire. Sun wanted, above all, a united China, for he knew that without unity China would drift back into the hands of war lords. The racial solidarity of which he spoke is uniquely Chinese, a mystic identification with the past, present and future, a spirit Sun was trying to recapture in visiting the Ming Tombs in 1911. In deciding to hand over the Presidency to Yuan he was faced with the alternative of splitting his country or compromising. He decided on a compromise: Yuan accepted, and the terms of the agreement were carried out on one day. Grey, pressurised by the powers and advised by Jordan, now agreed to lend money to Yuan, and the press commented that the amalgamated Cabinet which would now govern China was a great advance on previous ones.

The Cabinet now assembled in Nanking for the hand-over of power and then set up a provisional Government in Peking, where it proclaimed the constitution. There was to be 'liberty of speech, press, assembly, association and creed' for all Chinese and Manchus . . . Person and property were to be inviolate under the law. There was to be liberty to live and move as citizens pleased and a right to vote and be voted for in accordance with franchise laws. The President and Vice President were to be elected by two thirds of the provincial representatives. The President was to govern and allocate duties of the executive, but he needed consent of the National Assembly to organise the administration and appoint high officers of state. The Assembly, composed of three representatives from each province, was to deal with all financial matters and consider new laws. Courts of justice were to be public and judges not to be removed without committing some fault under the law. Once these arrangements had been made the powers felt free to negotiate the terms of a loan to Yuan. In the nineteenth century and before, Britain had enjoyed a unique friendship and trading position in China; the banks and trading companies were responsible for loans and trading agreements and the Chinese looked to the British Government for disinterested advice. Policies of European governments towards loans varied; some granted an area monopoly to one bank, others insisted on all loans being government sponsored. The British banks pointed out to Grey that if he only sanctioned loans agreed with other countries Britain would have abrogated her previous unique position, but, in spite of Jordan's judgement, Grey may have had doubts of Yuan's integrity, for only agreement among the powers could prevent them backing different sides in any dispute and thus dragging China into the conflict which thinking people now feared Europe and the world was soon to face.

On 10 March Dr Ho Kai, one of Sun's earliest friends and sometimes known as the Grey Eminence of the Republican movement, was knighted. The British press, with characteristic fairness now that Sun was the loser, began to find complimentary things to say about him. For

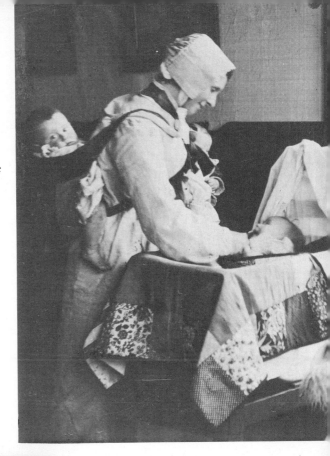

Schools for Mothers, Mabel Cantlie carrying babies Chinese style.

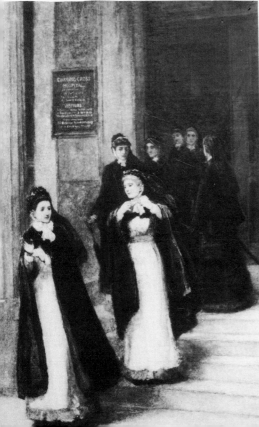

Charing Cross Hospital nurses leaving for the Boer War. (*Charing Cross Hospital*)

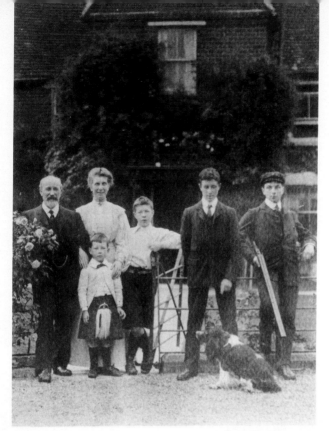

Family Gathering, Sir James an
Lady Cantlie with their four bo
(boys from left to right, Kennet
Neil, Colin, Keith).

Colonel George Cantlie, who,
with his brothers and sister, was a
frequent visitor at Cottered and
Harley Street.

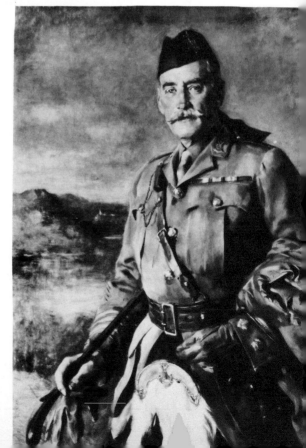

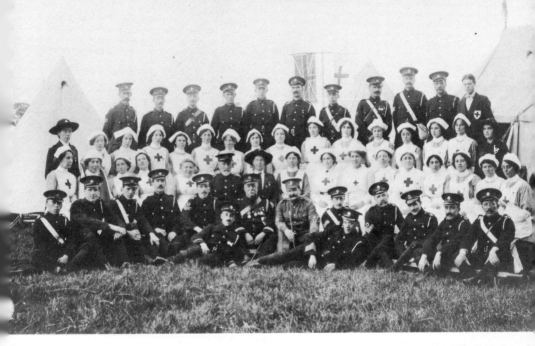

The first Voluntary Aid Detachments, Nos 1 and 2, the Cantlies as their Commandants in the centre.

The White City Exhibition. London Branch Voluntary Aid Detachments in uniform for the first time. (*British Red Cross Society*)

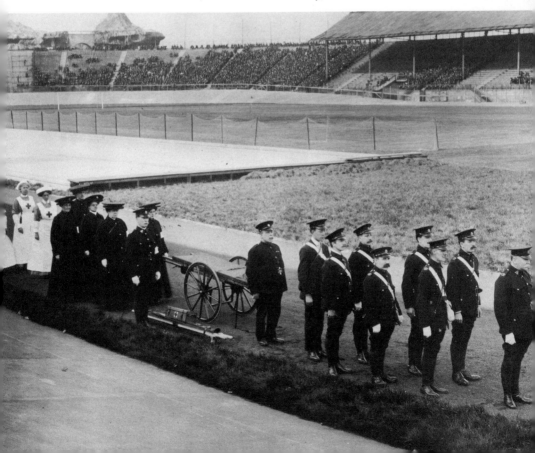

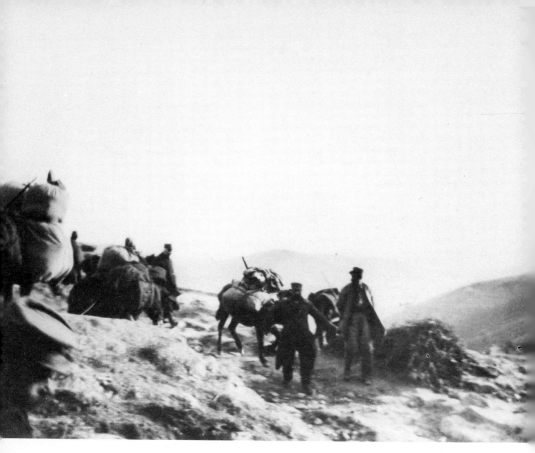

The Balkan War. The Red Cross in action.

Eastcote Camp, Mabel Cantlie on the left.

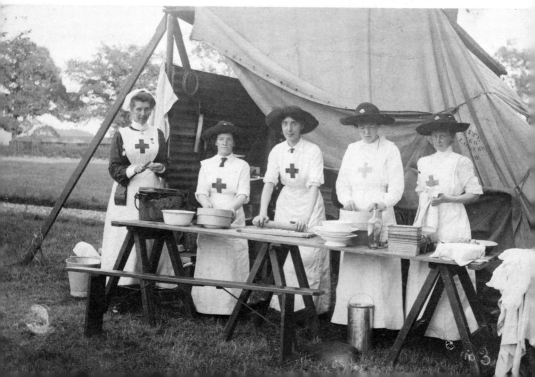

this Christian Saverwin of *Le Matin*, with a seat at *The Times*, was partly responsible. He called on the Cantlies, recounting how Sun had said casually to him in November 1911, 'I am going out to be President of China'. 'I never dreamt,' said Saverwin, 'that it was true.' Having relinquished the Presidency, Sun accepted the post of Director of Railways. He had seen in the revolution the economic, political and military significance of railways; not only to be used positively, as in Canada, to unite an awakening continent, but also negatively by rapacious powers. His map of China, showing existing and proposed railways, demonstrated once more his vision and capacity for detail. Morrison, already Yuan's unofficial adviser, who was sending reports direct to Grey, also realised their significance for he inked in his nominee against the printed name of the suggested Minister of Communications. Throughout 1912 Sun travelled the country, speaking to large audiences and receiving tumultuous welcome. His speeches portrayed his blend of Christianity and Confucianism: 'The Republic cannot endure unless there is that virtue, the righteousness for which the Chinese religion stands, at the centre of the nation's life.'[9] The tragedy was that the revolution had been delayed for so long, for the font at which he had drawn his inspiration, Western and particularly British justice, was losing some of its Christian fervour.

If the choice of Yuan as a leader for China was an example of a new cynicism and lack of confident purpose, many Europeans were nevertheless shaken when Yuan invited two revolutionary generals to Peking and executed them. Characteristically unmindful of his safety and heedless of his friends' entreaties, Sun set out for Peking to condemn Yuan for the atrocities. Following press reports, Mabel Cantlie commented in her diary, 'patriotic and noble, but a dangerous mission'. Sun's reception in Peking was, however, so warm – the crowds turning out in thousands to greet him – that Yuan dared not harm him. In spite of these events, the powers still saw Yuan as the strong man who would pull the country together and encourage trade, and pressed on with their promise of lending him money. Advisers were to be sent to administer the loan with powers over certain government departments. The French proposed a Commission of Control but Mr Bertie, British Minister in Paris, who had been in the Foreign Office in London at the time of Sun's kidnapping, persuaded them that the Chinese would never accept this indignity. The French and Russians then adopted blocking tactics, the French saying nothing could be done until the Balkan War ended. Britain wanted four neutral advisers and the Italians and Danes were suggested. Yuan, however, had already agreed to accept six, which meant that they could be nationals of the countries lending, and this pleased the Germans who wanted to be represented. Protracted discussion and delay meant that money was lost by old loan stock holders and the German far eastern cotton trade expanded at the cost of that in Manchester. In February the French backed the scheme for nationals and claimed a post, leaving the British to abandon their arguments for neutrals. On 19 February the Germans claimed a second post, although the USA was putting up half the

money and Britain a third. The final agreed list was: two audit deputy
directors who were to be French and Russian; a bureau of debt to be
held by the Germans and a chief inspector of the Salt Tax, who was
to be British, with a German deputy chief inspector. The Chinese
Government, unable to see why the Germans should have two posts
while the USA and Japan had none, objected, but the Germans, un-
abashed, claimed a third – that of chief engineer, Tientsin–Pukow
Railways. Grey, however, had had enough and replied 'two or nothing',
blaming the Germans for any future breakdown in negotiations.
Meanwhile the USA, believing the terms too onerous, withdrew. The
Salt Tax – important because the Chinese thought improperly cured
fish caused leprosy – was to be placed, as the Maritime Customs already
were, under foreign control, and the Americans felt that the conditions
of the whole loan touched on the independence of China. Further and
more serious eruptions in China now again brought matters to a
temporary standstill. Sung Chiao-Jen, leader of Sun's party, the
Kuomintang, a future candidate for Premier, was murdered at a railway station. The murderer and witnesses hid in the French settlement
in Shanghai, but were handed over in return for the promise of a fair
trial. On 21 April official sources stated that 'the implication of the
Prime Minister seems pretty clear',[10] and Sir E. Fraser, the British
Consul, reported that papers in code in the house of an accomplice had
been sent by his Private Secretary to whom news of the murder had
been communicated. Yuan's complicity in the plot seemed difficult to
disbelieve and again there was threatened rupture between north and
south.

The first full Parliament had meanwhile met in Peking on 8 April
and Jordan reported that attempts would be made to reduce Yuan's
powers to the minimum, although he would probably still be elected
Provisional President provided Sun did not stand. Now, with the like-
lihood of Yuan's complicity in Sung's murder Jordan commented,
'men like Sun who extol constitutional methods have really nothing in
common with Yuan and older class officials',[11] while other British
spokesmen added 'The Kuomintang stands for party Government and
provincial rights and has little in common with the outlook of Yuan'.
The murder and protracted loan negotiations were again causing
apathy among the Chinese, who felt corruption to be too deep rooted
to eradicate. The Hong Kong Shanghai Bank reported distrust of
Peking so strong that the provinces would probably release no money
to central Government. With characteristic foresight the French now
decided to back both sides and allowed the Banque Industrielle, of
which one of the founders, Berthelot, was brother of the Minister of
Foreign Affairs, to lend £2 million – later increased to £6 million – to
Honan Province. Meanwhile the Germans penetrated deeper into
China, opening schools, appointing an education adviser to the German Legation in Peking and winning new contracts, including one for
electrical work in the British Embassy, about which a question was
asked in Parliament by Mr Touche. Morrison, at last feeling the
anxieties of responsibility as Yuan's official adviser, rightly warned that

if the traditional American and British 'open door' policy of free trade with China was to be abandoned, and Britain's share of the loan cut to a sixth, the far eastern trading companies would scramble to win control over the little left. The situation was critical and fraught with danger, for Parliament had become a pandemonium and Yuan was ruling without it. The Secretary of the Rockefeller Foundation, which had opened missions and hospitals in China, called on the Cantlies to discuss Chinese affairs with them. Sun now decided to approach Jordan to ask for his help to mediate between north and south. He knew his country needed immediate foreign capital to survive, and he saw great dangers in the confused situation, not least of which was war with Russia if she would not withdraw from Mongolia. His request to Jordan was that Yuan should be made to govern constitutionally; that the Presidency be cut to a term of years and defined by law; that offices be apportioned between parties; that Sung's case be dealt with by the courts and that then and only then would Parliament agree to the loans. O'Conor might have been able to mediate, Jordan could not, and meanwhile time was fast running out. The Japanese, while denying Government involvement, were secretly allowing finance houses to send arms to China. On 26 April, having made no attempt to agree with Sun's request to make Yuan govern constitutionally, the powers signed the loan agreement with the Chinese Government on the premises of the Hong Kong Shanghai Bank in Peking. Two days later, both Houses of the Chinese Parliament declared the signing unconstitutional, being a personal loan to Yuan in his capacity as President and not under proper Parliamentary control.

On 30 April a telegram arrived from Mrs Chang which puzzled the Cantlies. It asked them to order newspaper cuttings on Chinese affairs and to send them out daily 'via Siberia'. Possibly she meant via the Siberian Railway, but the wording disturbed the Cantlies who started 'thinking deeply' that evening. The same wording had troubled Grey in connection with a query from a party of missionaries proposing to leave for China. Mabel Cantlie in the morning took the telegram to Mr Whitehead of the Chartered Bank, but his only comment was that Sun was a poor thing, a remark which she felt deeply. On 2 May this telegram was followed by one from Sun, setting out in staccato sentences the full facts of the situation in China. The Cantlies did as they were bid, passed the telegram on to a journalist friend for circulation;

> Submit on my behalf the following appeal to British Government, Parliament, Governments of Europe, and give the same widest publicity in all press. To Governments and peoples of foreign powers. As a result of careful investigation by officials appointed by Government to inquire into recent murder of Nationalist Leader Sung Chiao-Jen in Shanghai, the fact is clearly established that Peking Government is seriously implicated in the crime. Consequently the people are extremely indignant, and situation has become so serious that nation is on verge of most acute and dangerous crisis yet experienced. Government conscious of its guilt and

enormity of its offence and realising strength of wave of indignation sweeping over nation as direct result of its criminal deeds and wicked betrayal of trust reposed in it, and perceiving that it is likely to lead to its downfall, suddenly and unconstitutionally concluded loan for pounds 25,000,000 sterling with quintuple group despite vigorous protests of representatives of nation now assembled in Peking. This high-handed and unconstitutional action of Government instantly accentuated intense indignation which had been caused by foul murder of Sung Chiao-Jen, so that at present time fury of people is worked up to white heat and terrible convulsion appears almost inevitable. Indeed, so acute has crisis become that widespread smouldering embers may burst forth in devastating conflagration at any moment. From date of birth of Republic I have striven for unity, peace, concord and prosperity. I recommended Yuan Shik-Kai for Pesidency, because there appeared reasons for believing that by doing so unification of nation and dawn of era of peace and prosperity would thereby be hastened. Ever since than I have done all I could to evolve peace, order and government out of chaos created by revolution. I earnestly desire to preserve peace throughout republic, but my efforts will be rendered ineffective if financiers will supply Peking Government with money that would and probably will be used in waging war against people. If country is plunged into war at this juncture it will inevitably inflict terrible misery and suffering upon people who are just beginning to recover from dislocation of trade and losses of various kinds caused by revolution. For establishment of Republic they have sacrificed much and are now determined to preserve it at all costs. If people are now forced into life-and-death struggle for preservation of Republic not only will it entail terrible suffering to masses but inevitably also adversely affect all foreign interests in China. If Peking Government is kept without funds there is prospect of compromise between it and people affected, while immediate effect of liberal supply of money will probably be precipitation of terrible and disastrous conflict. In name and for sake of Humanity which civilisation holds sacred I therefore appeal to you to exert your influence with view to preventing bankers from providing Peking Government with funds which at this juncture will assuredly be utilised as sinews of war. I appeal to all who have lasting welfare of mankind at heart to extend to me in this hour of need their moral assistance in averting unnecessary bloodshed and in shielding my countrymen from hard fate which they have done absolutely nothing to deserve.[12]

Unfortunately Sun's plea fell on deaf ears. During the next few weeks there were conflicting reports in the British press, first that the loan was going through, then that Sun's party had stopped it in Parliament. The Chinese needed money, but the terms of the loan were too onerous and without Parliamentary authorisation would be spent without Parliamentary supervision. The British Government, liberal at home but prepared to be illiberal abroad, seemed unaware of the consequences of its actions; the south was again rebellious and Yuan, fearing war, sacked the Tutu in Kiangsi Province, which declared its independence, followed by Kwantung and Fukien. On 2 July Sun, in a telegram, called on Yuan to resign: 'Formerly you were invited to the Presidential Office . . . and now you should leave it in order to save the country being involved in trouble'.[13] The telegram, which set out the principles of the two leaders and the problems facing them, did not appear in the British press until Mabel Cantlie copied it from the Republican *Advocate* and sent it to *The Times*, which published it the next day, 14 August. In it Sun promised the south would stop fighting if Yuan would resign, for Sun had by this time given up all hope of Yuan governing constitutionally. Meanwhile, not only was British public opinion turning against Yuan, but in July the German press reported Jordan as being 'variable and unreliable' – since Yuan's power had grown and the south had to obey his will, so the British, particularly diplomats and press, had drawn away from him 'in a remarkable manner difficult to understand'. What the Germans wanted was 'a strengthening of authority and the maintenance of law and order'.[14] On 26 July Mr F. H. May, former captain superintendent of police, who had apparently not been troubled by the presence of his men at Chinese executions and who was now Governor of Hong Kong, asked Grey if he could deport members of the Kuomintang. Grey refused, although agreeing that they could be asked to move on after finding a place of safety. 'Yuan is unscrupulous, arrogant and intolerant,' said Conyingham Greene, quoting Baron Kato in Tokyo, 'Sun is sincere, impetuous and incompetent';[15] but, while liking Sun better, Kato said he would put his money on Yuan. This is what the powers had done and, after sacking Sun, who left for Canton, Yuan sent his army, well paid and equipped, to rout the army of the south. Sun, Huang Hsing and Chiang Ki Shek fled, accompanied by Charlie Soong, who had been working with Sun on railway projects, and his two daughters. Suspecting that the Chinese navy and merchant navy were loyal to Sun, Yuan tried to arrange for them both to have British protection and financial guarantee payments. Sun now started his second exile, having learnt that all revolutions do is exchange one tyrant for another. Jordan said he was an 'unpractical visionary who wants to bridge a river'. The bridge Sun wished to build was that between government and the will of the people; it was a vision which, for the moment, failed.

Fighting continued. On 7 October Yuan packed the Senate and was declared President, so that the world had to acknowledge him. The Cantlies attended a Legation Reception in Yuan's honour and another for Chinese students, where their British hosts spoke of Sun in glowing terms. Sun wrote from Tokyo, saying he had no fears for the future, 'knowing that his party was stronger than Yuan's'. Reports from Nanking spoke of Yuan's disgraceful reign of terror and the cruelty of his troops. First he sacked the 250 Kuomintang members from the Assembly, and then Mr Alston, Chairman of the Loan Committee, cabled to Grey that all opposition parties had left Peking and Yuan could not get a quorum for Parliament. The Japanese warned that he was creating his imperial court. In spite of this the Germans and French appointed military advisers and the British sent officers to train the navy. On 5 December the diary records a letter from Dr Sun, 'he says he is in excellent spirits. Yuan's behaviour will be his undoing, as people will see what sort of man he is and how cruel and despotic are his ways'. A week later he wrote again, warning the Cantlies of people who might call themselves his friends. Who did he mean? In January Yuan dissolved the rump of the Assembly and ruled on his own. In February the Chinese Minister called and stayed a long time, 'I wonder if Sun is coming back into power again'. Then Mr Whitehead of the Chartered Bank called to ask how much help Sun was getting from Japan. In May Yuan assumed the powers of dictator. In spite of this, however, Morrison, his political adviser, eulogised in his favour in dispatches to *The Times*. On 5 July Sun wired Chinese friends in London, asking them to go to Paris and ask the French to stop handing over Republicans to be butchered by the Chinese Government. The French agreed. The following month the Germans were within 30 miles of Paris and by the end of the First World War China had endured great suffering. If the powers in 1911 had with courage, integrity and unselfish wisdom put Chinese interests before their own financial gain and internal rivalry, how different the history of China at the time might have been. After the second exile Sun lost much of his faith and was not the same man again. Some writers say that the only thing that saved his reason was the companionship and later second marriage to Soong's daughter, Chingli. They claim that she not only gave him love and companionship but provided him with another philosophy to replace the one he had lost. Certainly she was politically much further to the left than Sun. The Great War which followed shook the faith of the whole Chinese people: 'They had been gazing on a new kind of civilisation, with all sorts of glittering merits unknown in ancient China and now, as they gazed, the whole structure was shaken by slaughter, organised on a scale which made insignificant the utmost barbarities of the Orient.'[16]

CHAPTER FOURTEEN

War

'At the beginning of the twentieth century the peoples of Europe, save for a savage patch in the Balkans, had reached an unprecedented level of comfort and civilisation.'[1] Europe was alive to the hardships of poorer members of society and had the ability, drive and zeal to reform their conditions. But dark and sinister forces were stalking the earth; they ran through the literature of the period and threatened the stability of states. In August 1914 Europe went to war. Serbia had emerged too strong from the Balkan Wars for the security of Austria, who felt that her Empire was in danger of breaking up. When the Archduke Franz Ferdinand, heir to the throne, on whom she had centred all her hopes, was murdered, rumour spread that it was the work of the Serbian Black Hand, with Russian-connections. Austrian fears now bordered on irrationality and were encouraged by the Kaiser and his generals with whose backing she ordered partial mobilisation. Russia, although her southern border was flanked by a German prince in Albania and German military advisers in Turkey, nevertheless persuaded Serbia to meet seven out of the ten demands of the Austrian ultimatum, but when these were not accepted she began to mobilise. Germany, the key to stability in Europe because of her overwhelming military strength and geographical position, still had time to draw both Austria and herself back from the brink of war. In vain did Sir Edward Grey strive for peace. The German Ambassador was sent for and told yet again that any invasion of the Low Countries by the Germans in an attack on France, ally of Russia, would be regarded as an act of war. The Germans, confident in the might of their war machine, were undeterred.

In August 1914 the Kiel Canal was opened, and with this opening, according to Major-General Evatt, came a change in German manners and attitude. Their fleet could now sail the seas with access to and from German ports and the Schlieffen Plan, conceived in 1908, of sweeping through Belgium and Luxembourg, outflanking the French, pinning them against their own line of defence and annexing their fleet to defeat the British Navy, became a viable objective. Britain was a force to be reckoned with at sea, but the Germans would, in the Kaiser's words, 'exterminate that contemptible little army'. The reason the plan failed was because of the heroic stand of the Belgians which slowed the German advance; the courage and accurate rapid fire of the British infantry at Mons and Le Cateau, which gave the French time to retreat to the Marne; the genius of General Joffre and the courage of the

French, who, in retreat, turned at the Marne and defeated the Germans before Paris, and the quick thinking of Sir John French who, anticipating the German race to the sea, got there before them, fighting off attempts to break through his line at Ypres, while the Belgians held the river Yser. Four years of trench warfare were to follow with trenches in which men could walk uninterrupted from Switzerland to the sea; a soldiers' war, fighting backwards and forwards over ground riddled with disease, while the list of casualties grew and grew. No one could have seen, when the Archduke fell to an assassin's hand, that the world would suffer a catastrophe of such magnitude or that a whole civilisation would pass away, carrying with it man's innocent hope in perpetual progress and putting out the lights of faith and inspiration which in Sir Edward Grey's words have not been 'lit again in our lifetime'.

'If there is one dangerous job it is to pick up the wounded of a retreating Army': so said Dr Hector Monroe of the Motor Ambulance Volunteer Corps in Belgium, known as the Flying Ambulance. He was with the Belgians during the days of retreat, when heavy medical equipment had to be abandoned. As bridges were blown and city after city – Bruges, Ghent, and, on 10 October, Antwerp – were abandoned in flames, the Germans ignored the rights of non-combatants, tearing up conventions which they had signed, acting 'not as undisciplined hooligans', but in what official reports afterwards described as a 'policy of disciplined terrorism'. 'No Government,' said Mr Souttar, a London hospital surgeon who was with the British Field Hospital for Belgium, 'could have been prepared to anticipate these methods at which a Zulu might blush.'[2] Doctors and nurses returned to Britain with scenes of horror and pathos burnt into the brain such as no human being could describe – dying and wounded lying together on straw, closely packed, with wounds most deadly, never surgically clean and many so foul that it was almost impossible to tolerate the stench. While the English covered the withdrawal of the Belgian Army from Antwerp, the British Field Ambulance, with their wounded constantly on the move, became separated and met again at Furnes. Meanwhile two units of BRCS personnel, doctors, surgeons and trained nurses, left from London under the command of Mr J. Wyatt of St Thomas's Hospital; they went to Brussels, where they were joined by eighty-five surgeons, doctors and trained nurses of St John Ambulance. Both the parties fell into enemy hands shortly after arrival. Although well treated they were detained and nursed German wounded for three months before being repatriated.

Immediately after the outbreak of war Sir Alfred Keogh, late DGAMS and now Chief Commissioner, Red Cross, crossed to Belgium and then went on to Paris and Rouen. In France he found the roads and railways crowded with wounded, whose sufferings in truck trains without brakes, lying on dirty straw, jerked and jostled through long days and nights so moved him that, according to Cantlie in the magazine *First Aid*, he cried himself to sleep for two nights. As the Germans neared Paris and the French Government left for Bordeaux the decision about what to do with the wounded became crucial. The French wounded were taken to the Military Hospital in Paris, the Val du Grace, the peace of its cloisters dating from early convent days, while the British were taken to the Hertford Hospital or to one of its emergency annexes. On 13 September Paris was saved by the Battle of the Marne. On the 30th Sir Alfred returned to London from where he had ordered unlimited medical supplies, motor ambulances – of which fifty had already arrived – and hospital trains to augment those already lent by the French. By the beginning of October a party of nearly 200 British surgeons, doctors, nurses, dressers and orderlies had arrived in Paris, the number of British hospitals had swelled to eight and the Scots, mindful of the 'auld alliance', had sent a hospital of their own. The French had opened scores of auxiliary hospitals in the city. Meanwhile into the ancient cathedral city of Rouen poured wounded from British, French and Belgian regiments, the lorries and ambulances clattering ceaselessly over its cobbled streets until it became a key depot and hospital centre with easy accessibility both to Paris and the sea coast.

What of Britain on 4 August 1914, the day she knew that she was at war? The diaries speak of the heartbreak and the disappointment – 'Oh God, what will become of us?' An American, in an article in *The Times*, wrote in tribute to 'The Silent Briton', and spoke of the self-possession of London, for 'Britain is as London is' – a self-possession and outward calm that hid a great anxiety.

> What may humanity not expect from a land capable of such calm and poise in the most dread hour of her history? . . . Let foemen beware of a nation whose women do not weep and whose men do not cheer at the call to arms . . . I stood in the throng before Buckingham Palace, when the King's Proclamation was read to the people . . . When Their Majesties appeared all heads were uncovered. 'God save the King,' sobbed through the night as though cathedral arches spread about us, and the notes were those of an anthem . . . And when all were gone and the scarlet tunicked sentries alone remained before the Palace, a strangely white moon seemed to sail straight to the centre of the vast space and its light fell as in augury upon the austere head of the old Queen sitting guard over her royal capital . . . As was London that night, so is London this morning . . . The Strand maintains its accustomed appearance. It seems to say to the passer-by, 'Steady my friend . . . All things are episodes to my vast experience. For a thousand years I have borne the tread of regiments and always the tomorrows of London are greater than her yesterdays . . . Take example from me and attend to your allotted tasks as I now proceed with mine.

All day long, in a never-ending stream, people called at the War Office, the Admiralty, the BRCS and St John Ambulance, offering their services to the wounded. The War Office and the Admiralty informed them that the nursing services were adequate for all demands. 'We are always ready, our military hospitals and staff are in full working order.' In addition to the reserve medical services the BRCS had 55,000 trained volunteers and St John Ambulance 71,000; but the deep dread in the hearts of the British people could only be calmed by volunteering. Cantlie's lecture rooms at the Polytechnic were thronged all day with hundreds of people wanting training in first aid and nursing. 'Two days after war was declared,' its magazine reported in August 1914,

> arrangements were made for obtaining instruction in First Aid, Stretcher Drill and Sick Nursing. No sooner had the announcement been made than the Entrance Hall was literally besieged by hundreds who were anxious to avail themselves of the provision made. Every available hall and room in the Institute was requisitioned and from morning until 10 o'clock in the evening lectures in First Aid or practising classes in bandaging were held. Over fifteen hundred students enrolled during the first week and there was a waiting list of five hundred hoping to join. [Trained nurses were given priority and those who spoke a foreign language.] The accommodation of the Polytechnic soon proved insufficient and some of the classes met in the Queen's Hall. A staff of doctors worked under the super-intendence of Dr. Cantlie and the V.A.D.s rendered spontaneous help.

The Polytechnic gave up its third floor to the BRCS and Cantlie used the Great Portland Street Hall for drilling but even this was insufficient. Cantlie's students provided the answer. On 9 September at the end of a lecture they gave him £130 as a 'testimonial' in gratitiude for his well-nigh forty years of Ambulance work, in order that he could start a College of Ambulance, where space could be found for war-time teaching and which they hoped would continue for many years afterwards. Political help was forthcoming. Mr Boyton, the Member of Parliament for Marylebone, offered Nos 3 and 4 Vere Street rent free for a year, and within a month the College was opened a few hundred yards from the Polytechnic. It was to become a centre for teaching and examining ambulance students in advanced diplomas as well as BRCS and St John Ambulance certificates. There was to be a museum, show-ing the history of first aid and containing objects necessary for instruc-tion, a library, lecture halls and club facilities. An editorial in St John's magazine *First Aid* deplored how infrequently certificates were re-newed the necessary three times to qualify for a medallion, and spoke with enthusiasm of the 'object of raising ambulance work to a higher platform and of teaching it in a scientific and technical method'.[3] The aim of the College was also to bring together the members of all voluntary aid societies, including the BRCS, St John's and St Andrew's Ambulance. Mabel Cantlie feared the strain which the new venture might place on her husband, for he was now 63 years of age, but the scheme was the climax of his work and hopes and the demands of war transcended personal arguments. Originally a St John's instructor and holding two of the Order's official posts, Cantlie was also a member of the BRCS Council and Executive Committee as well as chairing one committee and being a member of four, while his love of his native land led to a close association between the College and BRCS Scottish Branch. He was not alone in his aim to bring the voluntary aid societies together; the previous year Sir Frederick Treves had called for a common policy towards the grant of certificates and a redefining of spheres of action to prevent overlapping – although his suggestion of St John aiding the regular army and the Red Cross the volunteers would never have been acceptable. Cantlie believed the roles of the two societies were complementary, St John being primarily responsible for the teaching and training of first aid and home nursing and the BRCS first in the organisation of international relief. As in the Boer War, when the Central Committee had co-ordinated relief, on 24 October 1914 a Joint War Committee was formed to co-ordinate voluntary work in time of war, which happily remained in existence during peace time as a liaison group between the two societies.

'Mr. and Mrs. Cantlie,' reported the press, 'the latter is also a keen ambulance worker, want to see a complete union on the subject of ambulance and humanitarian work in general.' Having brought the College thus into existence, Cantlie went on to outline his plans for a Humanitarian Corps. 'It was,' said the magazine *First Aid*, 'to assuage and relieve distress, not by giving money, but by providing immediate wants.'[4] The editorial hoped it would be put in order as quickly as possible to relieve the suffering during the crisis, for all over Belgium and northern France refugees in thousands were fleeing from the Germans, abandoning homes and packing possessions on carts, bicycles or perambulators and flocking south in a way now familiar, but then tragically new. No Geneva Convention covered their plight. They carried with them risk of infection caused by carriers of disease and lack of sanitary facilities; they were cold, tired and starving. Later, as battles swayed this way and that destroying with shrapnel and shell whole villages between the lines, teams of doctors, including women, came to the aid of homeless inhabitants. The Humanitarian Corps supplied blankets, bedding and clothing and, in its purple uniform, Miss Dormer Maunder left with a small party of trained nurses for Belgium, where she opened a hospital in the casino at Ostend and later escaped with the refugees to Dunkirk, bringing many over to England. Here BRCS, St John and other volunteers met, fed, comforted and opened hospitals for them either in London or elsewhere in the country. West of the River Yser the Belgians were left with a tiny strip of country, fifteen miles by forty. Near the battlefield of Ypres lay the village of Westoutre, later to be adopted and supplied with aid by the Humanitarian Corps. Belgium's plight and heroism was summed up in the famous cartoon representing the Kaiser taunting the King of the Belgians, 'You have lost everything', and the courageous and truthful answer, 'No, not my soul'.

The plight of these refugees brought the Humanitarian Corps into existence, but Cantlie wanted it to survive after the crisis had passed and to have a member in every village in peace as well as war. 'In the village I live in,' he said, 'there is no telephone, the doctor is three miles off, the district nurse has three parishes to attend to and there is no one to render First Aid when an accident occurs. I would place in every village a box of First Aid appliances under the charge of the Humanitarian Corps, whose duty it would be to equip it.' As well as being trained in first aid and nursing, members would give help to anyone requiring shelter or material aid, even if only a loaf of bread. 'Giving,' he continued, 'widens the outlook of the giver and brings joy to brethren in distress.' The magazine *The Queen* called it a splendid idea,

> like looking down an ever widening vista instead of one which narrows to a point . . . for there is absolutely no limit to its possibilities for the betterment of the human race. Here is true culture, for the man or woman who finds an interest in doing kindness to a neighbour will easily discover the best of all that is beautiful in the world can be learned by a wide and deep study of God's most marvellous creation, the human being.[5]

Today, with a proliferation of non-religious societies for human welfare, there might not be need to comment in such eulogistic terms, but then there were only few, of which the Prince of Teck's League of Mercy was one of the first.

A committee was appointed to draw up a constitution for the College of Ambulance. There were to be governors and a council which would award fellowships. Sir Rickman Godlee, Honorary Surgeon to the London and University Hospitals, was appointed President, Mr Boyton, MP, Chairman. A further committee for the Humanitarian Corps included Lady Cromer as President, Mrs Beaumont (Lady Mayoress of Marylebone), a member of the committee, and Mabel Cantlie, Treasurer. There was to be a seven-hour teaching day, which meant that Cantlie, although he had a team of seven doctors to help him, had to find time early or late to see patients and do other first aid teaching. The College never shut before 9.00, and usually 10.00 p.m. There was a weekly attendance of 900 students, and in the first three years approximately 30,000 students were trained. The Council offered Cantlie a fee, but characteristically he turned it down and, although he accepted their other offer of 30 per cent of the profits, the fees were set too low to provide them. Vere Street, with its spacious and elegant rooms, was a splendid background for the displays of models and visual aids used for instruction. In order to explain how to arrest haemorrhage Cantlie attached cotton and string to a skeleton to show veins and arteries, and later had a model made of the human body with pipes running with coloured fluid which stopped when a pressure point was touched. There were splints, stretchers and tent shelters which he had demonstrated during exhibitions; also the Scott-Cantlie sling which enabled the weight of a normally-carried stretcher to be taken by the shoulder, and slings for conveying wounded men on to hospital ships with or without stretchers. Running the length of the hall was a model battlefield, made by Kenneth, showing first aid posts, advanced dressing stations with puffs of cotton wool showing the heaviest fighting, clearing hospitals and lines of communication, with trains running back to base hospital. Standing in the hall was a farm cart driven from Cottered for practising loading and unloading stretchers (carts were still being used to convey wounded from the front), and soon the Great Western Railway offered a railway wagon at Paddington, where students could practise loading and unloading stretchers on and off trains. Cantlie's ingenuity also devised a miniature wooden ambulance railway wagon among his display of models, showing how and where the stretchers were fitted. The longer the lines of communication running back to base hospital the more changes there were from one stretcher to another; between the battlefields in France and a base hospital in England it was calculated there would be no fewer than ten changes from one method of transport to another. In spite of pressure from Cantlie and other ambulance experts, it was not until the middle of the war that regulation canvas stretchers enabled patients to be moved without changing the stretcher also – the method employed of moving a wounded man was the same as is taught today, a tightly rolled blanket. The only way to reduce the pain and shock of the patient was to perfect stretcher drill, for it meant not only courage and discipline under fire, but tender care in lifting the wounded man off the battlefield, carrying him over rough ground without jerking, with the bearers able to turn or climb or halt in unison with the minimum of effort to themselves and the least discomfort to their patient. (The diagrams in Cantlie's *Training Manual* look like the positions in Highland dancing, such was the infinite precision of pace and step in which he trained his bearers to minimise the pain on the journey.)

The lay-out of the miniature College battlefield was the same as that of the Brooklands Demonstration, but then invasion was the fear, whereas now the British Army, with its Allies, was defending Flanders, and with long lines of communication running through France and across the sea the question of where to site base hospitals was crucial. On 29 August Sir Frederick Treves, former chairman of the BRCS, now Vice-Chairman and member of many committees, wrote in *The Red Cross* that the wounded would come home to be nursed and that Netley, where the Red Cross had opened an annexe of 500 beds, was the ideal base hospital. Everything, therefore, would depend on swift, efficient transport by sea and land which would weigh the balance between life and death. The same view was expressed in the RAMC *Journal* which spoke of motor transport revolutionising the treatment of the wounded. 'There is only one place where the wounded can be treated and that is in a general hospital.'[6] The view was not unanimous, one speaker in the discussion preferring the French suggestion of keeping the seriously injured within the battle area by immobilising one in three of the field ambulance hospitals and carrying out major operations there. Mr Souttar of the Belgian Field Ambulance drew the same conclusions, laying great stress on tented hospitals where major operations could be carried out swiftly. Sir Frederick himself had described these tented hospitals in his book *The Tale of a Field Hospital*, envisaging sixty tents, ten marquees, twelve doctors and 200 nurses and orderlies, a picture akin to the tented field hospital which Cantlie described in his *Training Manual*, giving instructions for erection and improvisation.

On 30 September, however, Sir Alfred Keogh returned from France committed to the idea of swift motor transport bringing the wounded quickly as far as possible from the dust, debris and turmoil of the fighting line. On the 9th Mr E. A. Ridsdale had resigned as Chairman of the BRCS Executive Committee and been replaced by Mr Arthur Stanley, Lord Derby's brother, ex-diplomat and MP, who was also Chairman of the Royal Automobile Club. Severely crippled, Stanley had a life-long interest in motoring, and his contacts with touring organisations helped to bring into the Red Cross car owners, drivers and mechanics, and touring cars with long chassis that would support improvised ambulance bodies holding two or four stretchers. As well as the RAC 19,000 Automobile Association members offered their cars and within three weeks repair shops and garages had been set up in London (and later in Boulogne), where sheds rang with the noise of hammering, while these cars were tranformed almost overnight into a fleet of ambulances in one of the fastest uses of a labour force ever known. Within a week of appealing for funds, *The Times* had 520 vehicles subscribed for and by the end of the year 650 ambulances were on the road. 'Day after day, night after night, along roads broken up by shells, often under a rain of shrapnel and rifle fire the ambulances moved to their work steadily, constantly and devotedly, evacuating the sick and the wounded.'[7] With the lights dimmed to escape detection, a man would wade through deep mud with a torch which the leading vehicles could follow.

Just as important as the supply of ambulances was the provision of trains. In September the French generously provided rolling stock for eleven truck hospital trains which the British fitted with improvised steel stretchers. Although make-shift when compared with the magnificent hospital train presented to the Society by Princess Christian in February 1917, those who travelled in them were deeply grateful. Early in September, the fifth hospital train left for the front under the command of Colonel G. A. Moore, Deputy Chief Commissioner of St John Ambulance Brigade, and ran into heavy fighting as the Germans fell back from the Marne to the Aisne. Three medical officers and six orderlies were confronted with 150 badly wounded stretcher cases as well as many walking wounded. Suddenly out of the blue appeared 250 London Scottish, who had just arrived, and hearing of their difficulties offered their services. By evening the worst 150 cases had been removed to shelter and fed and their wounds were just about to be attended to when, relates Colonel Moore, 'as if by magic out of the ranks of the London Scottish stepped four Sergeants, and privates, all qualified doctors, also some medical students and with them their regimental surgeon'.[8] Minutes later three women doctors appeared as if from nowhere. How pleased Cantlie would have been had he known. He was so proud of his association with the Regiment, of which he had been Volunteer Surgeon for so many years. In a family book of press cuttings is the report of this first Volunteer Regiment in action and of their heroism in the line on 4 November. But of this story of quiet devotion, as with that of the first women doctors, many of whom Cantlie had also trained in his early teaching days, there is no mention; it passed unnoticed until afterwards, as did many thousands of other stories during that tragic time.

The other vital factor in sustaining the wounded was the establishment of rest stations along the rail route where they could be fed and their wounds dressed. Fifteen of these were set up by 9 September. During the German race to the coast, following the Battle of the Marne, Boulogne was evacuated and the wounded sent down to Le Havre. To the east, Sir John French was hurrying to Ypres to cut off the German advance, while to the north British Marines and a naval contingent covered the withdrawal of the Belgian Army from Antwerp. Meanwhile the 7th Division, of whose field ambulance Neil Cantlie was a member, landed at Zeebrugge and advanced to Ghent where it met the remains of the Marines, the naval contingent and the Belgian Army. While the Belgians held the line of the Yser, the 7th Division met Sir John French at Ypres, where one of the bloodiest battles of the War was fought and the Allied line secured. As the wounded poured down into Boulogne at the rate of 2,000 a day, hospitals had to be improvised, equipment furnished, stores, drugs and instruments supplied and staff found. 'The Red Cross, the R.A.M.C., and St. John,' said Sir Arthur Lawley in a speech at the Mansion House, 'stood side by side in aiding the wounded, unloading trains and conveying the wounded to hospital.'[9] On 14 October two London Voluntary Aid Detachments, under Mrs Furse of Paddington, were sent to Boulogne to organise a rest station. Joined by the RAMC from Le Havre, they met trains crowded with wounded, unloaded stretcher cases, fed, nursed and dressed their wounds, converting rolling stock and sheds into wards, dispensaries, kitchens and workshops. In all these rest stations the VADs made one of their greatest contributions of the war, which Sir Frederick envisaged in his books and Cantlie had demonstrated at Brooklands. Sir Frederick, in *The Red Cross* journal, described the trains as 'filthy', with the wounded 'just picked off the battlefield, two dead, two shot through the chest, one arm amputated, the sitting up cases dirty but good natured and cheerful'.[10] He spoke of the care required during the long journey, for, after being temporarily patched up in a field hospital in order to travel, the trial of the wounded soldier could be lightened and his sufferings eased by VADs accompanying the train of wounded, feeding, filling hot water bottles, administering stimulants, changing dressings. VADs also set up and staffed the stationary hospitals – wards attached to certain rest stations – so that wounded too ill to continue the journey could be lifted from the train. A member of the RAMC described one such station: 'there was very little light, the platforms were crowded with refugees, shells falling in the town. The work of entraining began, with the method by which we have trained our personnel, using the seats as beds.'[11] Once the line was established at Ypres Boulogne became, with Paris, Vichy and Rouen, one of the vital bases for the rest of the war, a truly hospital city, while along the coast other British and Belgian hospitals opened at Dunkirk, La Panne, Le Touquet, Calais, Le Havre, the French generously providing their allies with the best sites.

Once in the Channel ports, those fit to travel were conveyed to hospital ship and started arriving in London early in September. The first hospital ships were yachts given by private owners. 'A fortnight ago,' ran a press report, 'the social world of England was on the way to Cowes. Those very yachts are now being fitted out as hospital ships.' Soon these private owners were joined by corporations and by the British Red Cross Society, including Scottish Branch, and by other organisations, and again, as with the conversion of cars, the speed with which transformation was effected was miraculous. As with the trains, these ships were rough conversions compared with the splendid ones which followed, including two donated by Queen Alexandra and Princess Christian. Hospital barges, which played an important role in French and Belgian plans, were not as practicable for the British, although the Quakers opened one barge hospital in the Isle of Wight. Cantlie's No. 1 VAD met the first returned prisoners of war early in September, 'many of them,' commented the diary, 'in a pitiful condition'. On the 16th the first party of wounded arrived, 'Hamish's men among the B.R.C.S. stretcher bearers'. 'The returned heroes,' wrote one of his bearers, 'were really the happiest of those gathered on the platform in spite of their terrible wounds.' Just to be home was all they asked and their gratitude was touching. Marylebone Red Cross District helped to meet the wounded with its fleet of fifty cars and two ambulances, one of which was donated by Debenhams, which, with other stores, gave blankets, bedding and accommodation to both wounded and refugees. Men from the Polytechnic and College of Ambulance formed bearer transport sections on duty from 9.00 a.m. to 10.00 p.m. at the Polytechnic on Saturday and the College of Ambulance on Sunday, taking calls from the railway stations, meeting and transporting the wounded. Because of their stretcher drill experience No. 1 VAD was asked to move the special spinal cot cases, many of whom were shortly to go to the new Star and Garter Hospital for paralysed men at Richmond, started with a generous cheque from Queen Alexandra, and to the Queen Mary Hospital for limbless men in Roehampton. Although No. 1 VAD did air raid duties at the Polytechnic and the College, Zeppelin raids were sporadic and duties were given up until the end of 1915, when casualties during night raids became so frequent that they were asked by the police to resume their duties, making the Polytechnic their main centre because of its shelter facilities. For this they were given additional transport by the Women's Reserve Ambulance, which Mabel Cantlie was one of those active in starting, and a member of Cantlie's Detachment described one of these women drivers arriving within minutes of a call in evening dress and satin slippers, with a uniform coat thrown on to give protection on a freezing cold night.

One of Cantlie's first tasks was to train a team of Indian doctors, medical, business and law students, among whom was Mahatma Gandhi. These men offered their services to the War Office to help the RAMC but, being untrained, the War Office turned them down and sent on their application to the India Office, who asked Cantlie to train them with a view to their acting as the Ambulance Unit to the Indian troops shortly to arrive in France. Cantlie enrolled his son Kenneth among the class so that it should be of mixed race, and this example helped to break down barriers – English nurses were soon nursing Indian soldiers in their hospital in Brockenhurst and at Netley. Cantlie was delighted to have doctors among the team for, as with the medical students in the VMSC, he believed first aid to be a specialised branch of surgery which should be learnt by doctors and nurses as well as by laymen (the *BMJ* had quoted him as giving this as one of the aims of the College of Ambulance). The Indian students attended the College daily, took part in demonstrations, recruiting drives, an inspection in Regents Park where they were addressed by Mr Boyton and the Hon. Evelyn Cecil, both MPs, and trained under canvas. By the end of a month on 14 September they were ready to go to France as an Ambulance Corps, where they were attached to the Sikhs and Gurkhas. In appreciation and gratitude they made a presentation to Cantlie at the Imperial Institute where Mr Gandhi said how pleased he was that Cantlie was taking up India now instead of only China. At their last evening at the Polytechnic, the Aga Khan addressed the meeting, saying how much India wished to share the responsibilities as well as privileges of Empire. He said India was well aware of the Kaiser's attempts at peaceful penetration into Asia Minor and his readiness to offer himself as the protector of Islam. 'God forbid that Islam should have such a protector.' The loyalty to England, he said, would never be broken. The Ambulance Corps then left for France where it acquitted itself honourably.

The Indians were not the only people from overseas wishing to learn first aid. A group of Frenchwomen, taking advantage of Dr Sambon's classes in French, asked if they might train and start a Detachment of their own. Meanwhile twenty-five men from Cantlie's No. 1 VAD joined the Red Cross in France, ten of whom went to Rouen, while sixteen more left to join the RAMC as stretcher bearers. They were replaced by recruits requiring to be trained. Realising the urgent need for more men and women, Cantlie staged a Red Cross Demonstration at Wormwood Scrubs and funded another in the Botanic Gardens where he appealed for a million volunteers. On 17 October, with the Channel ports threatened, the order had come through to the College that no more personnel were to go abroad and for the moment there was a standstill. Mr Taylor, Assistant Commandant of No. 1 VAD, commented, 'The V.A.D.s were intended for home service and service overseas was not immediately within the bounds of practical politics'.[12] Nevertheless by the end of the war men from No. 1 VAD had served in

France, Belgium, Egypt, Russia, Serbia, Rumania, Mesopotamia, India and E. Africa. After the first party of nurses had fallen into German hands in Belgium the problems about sending out women VADs were greater, since male chivalry did not want to see women near the battlefield. The women, however, wished to suffer the hardships and dangers of the men. 'It is our turn to be last now', said the nursing sisters to the wounded on a hospital ship torpedoed in the Channel. Mabel Cantlie's Detachment No. 110 included a number of trained nurses and these were among the first to go abroad. Detachment numbers were not intended to exceed those laid down in regulations, but Mabel Cantlie's Detachment fluctuated to between twenty to twenty-five times that number; never far below 350 it rose to 600 by the end of the war, which was nearly a hundredth of the VAD strength of England and Wales. Like her husband, she had a gift of getting people to work together and preventing them quarrelling. It was done in the same way as all the Cantlies' work was done, with kindness and sense of purpose. No wonder the papers commented that like her husband she was always greeted with great applause whenever she spoke in public. Mabel Cantlie had, by September, a number of her Detachment abroad; on 23 August three went to Vichy, followed by six more to nurse typhoid, three to Dieppe, two to Le Havre and one to Paris.

At the College of Ambulance much of the responsibility for the organisation of personnel and supplies fell on Mabel Cantlie's shoulders. An Ostend committee of the Humanitarian Corps was formed and all through September Miss Maunder, from Ostend, was requesting bedding, medical supplies, trained nurses and VADs. On 13 October came a flood of Belgian refugees into Britain and the diary records 110 Detachment members meeting them at main line stations. 'Thousands of refugees pouring into this country, it is so hard to know what to do with them. Poor souls. Everyone trying to help. None of us can work hard enough.' On the 14th nurses arrived in the College from Antwerp describing motor buses crammed with wounded leaving a hospital surrounded by exploding shells and heading for Ostend. On the 23rd came a diary entry concerning a story recounted by Mr Bates,

> He was ordered by the War Office to go over to Ostend at 10 o'clock this morning in a steamer, and when they got there our ships were bombarding the Germans approaching. There were, on the quay, 500 of our poor men on stretchers ready to be embarked. They had been five days with R.A.M.C. Territorial men to look after them. In pouring rain the poor fellows were got into the ships and started for home, operating all the time in spite of rough weather. It was an awful journey.

Women nursing volunteers in Belgium were few. Because the first party of BRCS and St John nurses had fallen into enemy hands the authorities were cautious about sanctioning the dispatch of further volunteers. Among those who had had their offers of help refused by the War Office were the FANYs (First Aid and Nursing Yeomanry).

Raised in 1907 and trained in first aid and nursing and equipped with horse drawn ambulances, the FANYs then offered their services to Queen Elizabeth of the Belgians, with the result that they were now helping to staff hospitals near Calais and running dressing stations behind the Belgian lines. In France volunteers were in greater supply but reports described the suffering of the wounded on the trains and the need for more rest stations and hospitals. In view of this, Mabel Cantlie decided to go to Red Cross Headquarters and ask for permission to continue sending VADs abroad, and on the 22nd the authorities relaxed their restrictions, although they were re-imposed in November because of the gravity of the Allied position in France.

Mabel Cantlie's ability as an organiser was equally important on the distaff side. Sir Alfred Keogh wired for medical supplies, bedding and clothing which had, as it were, to be conjured out of the air. She set up work rooms and advertised for volunteers. Helpers from the Balkan War came forward again, and she soon had more people than she could cope with, moving in August from the Town Hall to the third floor of the Polytechnic and on 10 September to the College of Ambulance. The *Polytechnic Magazine* of September (printed before the move to the College of Ambulance) said:

> Mrs. Cantlie has done splendid service in organizing work for the Red Cross Society at the Polytechnic. We cannot do better than assist her in every way possible. We propose that our Ambulance Classes, which are phenomenal, over 2,000 students within the past month, should be especially associated with this work to provide funds and help in preparing the articles required by the Red Cross. Dr. Cantlie, the unrivalled instructor of our Ambulance Classes, will be in thorough sympathy.

Patterns were cut out, clothes made and bandages rolled. The *Morning Post* described how, on entering the work-rooms in Mabel Cantlie's charge, one found the garment one wanted to sew pinned on a board. Women volunteers were being given lessons in cutting out, others took patterns away to sew and in addition unemployed women were sewing at home for payment. Economy had been pressed upon the Cantlies by their dedication to voluntary work and refusal to accept money. ('There can be few leaders of the Red Cross movement in this country,' said *The Red Cross* journal, 'whose name is known to a larger number of workers than Dr. Cantlie. The sale of Red Cross books now exceeds 274,000 books'[13]; yet Cantlie refused to accept a penny of payment.) Thus, in order to provide for her family, Mabel Cantlie had developed a flair for cutting out shirts and pyjamas requiring the least possible sewing that could be finished in an evening. This aptitude was now at a premium and two days after the declaration of war, Lady Lawley, Lady-in-Waiting to Queen Mary, came to ask Mabel Cantlie to send her patterns to the Queen. She got these ready and dispatched them to Buckingham Palace, where Lady Ampthill received them kindly. It was a great compliment and the press commented, 'The Queen has given a splendid lead in the work of co-operation with other Societies which understand the needs of the sick and wounded in the matter of clothing . . . Since then Devonshire House has a complete set of paper patterns and directions on how to use them.' On 1 September Mabel Cantlie attended St James's Palace at the request of Queen Alexandra and, with Lady Lawley, Lady Northcliffe, and five military and civil hospital matrons, chose the most practical garments to be made by the working parties. By the end of September the Polytechnic party had completed 6,000 articles swelling the total of 53,000 completed by the Red Cross a month later. Meanwhile, in spite of War Office complacency, Lord Kitchener advertised for 300,000 knitted belts and socks and other garments for the Volunteers and Mabel Cantlie installed a knitting machine and sold garments to them at low prices to finance the work party's purchase of material for garments for the wounded. The finished articles were collected by Queen Mary's Needlework Guild, the BRCS and St John.

On 10 October Mr and Mrs Baker of the Society of Friends came to the College of Ambulance asking for help to get a party of Quakers to the front to help the wounded. Through a Quaker forebear on Mabel Cantlie's side, they had already made peace-time contact with each other. The Quakers had a training camp under canvas at Jordans, Buckinghamshire, and they asked Cantlie if he would deliver a course of lectures and teach them stretcher drill. This he did once a week for the next three years, rising at 4.30 a.m., and the Society recorded the debt of gratitude they owed him for his instruction. The Friends also decided to send thirty of their number to London where they attended the College of Ambulance daily on a collegiate basis. By the end of October they had attained such a high standard that they were accepted by the BRCS as an Anglo-Belgian Ambulance Unit, leaving for the front 100-strong on 28 October with equipment and stores provided by the Humanitarian Corps. On their way they assisted in the rescue of the *Hermes* survivors, torpedoed in the Channel, and on arrival tended 3,500 wounded in Dunkirk after the Battle of Ypres. (This unit was later known as the Friends Ambulance Unit, among whose number was Geoffrey Winthrop Young, the celebrated mountaineer.) On 5 November the second party left and a third in January, by which time the units had a Registered Office at the College of Ambulance. Almost immediately they set up an advanced dressing station just behind the British firing line which dressed wounds of soldiers and civilians alike, and on 1 December they opened a hospital for the wounded at Ypres and another at Abbeville. Their work among the civilian population centred on arresting the typhoid outbreak which had decimated armies and civilians in previous wars and was now ravaging Serbia. As Cantlie pointed out in his *Journal*, a retreating army spreads disease since it has no time for sanitation. They disinfected houses, purified water, using chlorine and the gravel and filter technique laid down by Cantlie for camp sites and, above all, inoculated against the disease with the serum discovered by Sir Almroth Wright and tested by Sir William Leishman. They also opened the Queen

Alexandra typhoid hospital outside Dunkirk and the Hospital Elizabeth at Poperinghe in Belgium, from which serious cases were brought to the Isle of Wight. When the Unit returned to England in November the diary records the packing of blankets and clothes and the buying of 48 packets of Quaker Oats, 100 lb of jam, 40 lb of sugar and 40 lb of tea which the Quakers used to start a motor kitchen for refugees, giving special attention to children orphaned by the war. Lady Newman, wife of the Chairman of the Friends, was always active in the College. By the beginning of 1915 the work of the Friends had been extended to helping the French wounded as well. From small beginnings a network of aid had been established.

For months everybody had been working round the clock to organise this aid, finding some solace in shared activity to counteract the horror at the growing toll of dead. 'Late home every night – ten p.m. There is a list of killed and wounded. Oh so long.' In the *Polytechnic Magazine* the roll of students killed continued for four and a half pages in double column in the first month and a large number of helpers had already lost their sons. They shared each other's suffering in compassionate silence. 'It is very sad and makes one wonder how soon may come the dread news,' Colin was in his submarine somewhere in the Atlantic, Neil, who had telegraphed from Aldershot for his sword and his saddle, was at Ypres. George Cantlie with his wife and children was in London, waiting for his regiment to arrive from Canada. The Des Voeux were among those whose sons had been killed: 'We dare not weep because we feel that we too may suffer. God alone knows. Neil only asks for chocolate, I sent him that and another pair of socks.' Dry socks, made of fresh wool, kept out the damp and so warded off trench foot. All through the war, once or twice a week, no matter how tired or ill, Mabel Cantlie never forgot those parcels of socks, cakes and chocolate for Neil and medical supplies for the wounded in his care. In his submarine Colin's needs were different; he wrote and said it would sink if she sent him any more woollies; he was always cheerful and kept other thoughts to himself. Mabel Cantlie was by now in considerable pain, sometimes taking to her bed for half a day in order to keep going the next. Occasionally the Cantlies went to Cottered for a weekend: 'I walked out from the station, and, as I had a heavy basket, it was a bit of a strain. I felt my pains very acutely all evening. Autumn is come and the place looks very sad, but we had a lovely sunset and exquisite colouring.' The words caught the country's mood, determination to keep going, unbelievable sadness, and yet still a capacity for joy at the beauty of the 'warm earth', springing from centuries of Christian conviction. At last two letters came from Neil; one telling how he had not slept in the same place twice since he left nor had his clothes off for three weeks; the second, delivered by the divisional interpreter, describing the landing in Belgium, the advance to Ghent and then a hurried march, before the German lines closed in on them, to Ypres, where there had been twenty-eight days' continuous fighting. Twice he had been blown out of his tent, one horse was killed under him, once he had his tunic shot through. 'But saved. We cannot thank God enough.

Mr. Lloyd, the interpreter, says he is so conscientious, never thinks it a trouble to turn out at any time.' Meanwhile Keith, planning to leave Assam to join a Mahratta Battalion, was sending money home to his parents for the College of Ambulance. At that early stage the generosity of the public was sufficient for the needs of the wounded, but as the war went on and people became poorer, the £1,000 his parents had banked for him had been dipped into for the College. It was what he had intended; all his life he put his hand freely into his pocket to help anyone in need. Kenneth, attending tutors in London, spent much time assisting in the activities of the College.

There was an heroic acceptance of shared sacrifice, set particularly by those who, like Rupert Brooke, had defended Belgium from the savage onslaught of the German army, a spirit typified by his poem 'The Soldier', a feeling that life is transitory – 'there shall be in that rich earth, a richer dust concealed' – a feeling that found expression in the description of the courage of men retiring after Le Cateau, 'not like a retreating army, but more like men returning from a cricket match',[14] chatting and smoking pipes, a brand of heroism that is for others sometimes a little difficult to understand, but which is uniquely British. A great and lasting sadness for all connected with the Polytechnic was the death of the second son of the founder Colonel Ian Hogg, DSO, who died from wounds after safeguarding the withdrawal of his men: 'he would not come back until certain all his men were back and the third shot got him in the lungs'. How many readers of the *Polytechnic Magazine*, when hearing this news, may have remembered the almost prophetic poem of a few years previously, with the note at its head, 'Authorship unknown, Mrs. Hogg requests the insertion of the following lines'?

> If I were told that I must die tomorrow,
> > That the next sun
> Which sinks should bear me past all fear and sorrow
> All the fight fought, all the short journey through.
> > What should I do?
> I do not think that I should shrink or falter
> > But just go on
> Doing my work, nor change nor seek to alter
> > Aught that is gone.
> But rise and move and love and smile and play
> > For one more day;
> And lying down at night for a last sleeping
> > Say in that ear,
> Which hearkens ever, 'Lord within thy keeping
> > How shall I fear?'
> It is his day.

Ian Hogg had quite simply done just that – he had laid down his life for his friends.

CHAPTER FIFTEEN

Wounds and their Treatment: the King Albert I Hospital

Before the first Battle of Ypres the war was one of movement and preparation. After it the armies were bogged down in muddy trenches, fighting over ground which in Cantlie's words was 'strewn with the graves of men and horses'. Little wonder that medical and veterinary men forecast numerous deaths from tetanus, gas gangrene and other bacilli. The story of the next four years is that of mounting lists of casualties and the struggles of the Army Medical Services, aided by the voluntary aid societies, to deal with the fatality of infection. The very nature of the wounds presented the doctors with a hideous dilemma. At the start of the war tetanus took a heavy toll until the inoculation pioneered by Sir Almroth Wright and scientifically tested by Sir David Bruce became routine for all wounds. But other infections such as the deadly bacilli of gas gangrene, carried in soil and dung, caused wounds to putrefy in a way that Mr Souttar in Belgium had described as 'most foul' and contributed to a higher mortality rate than that of the Crimea. The need for immediate operation to open and drain the seat of infection gave the doctors the stark choice: was it better for the patient to travel pre- or post-operation? 'The shells tear such holes in the men,' wrote Neil to his parents, 'that it is a wonder any of them live.' Not only did bullets require to be located (there were reports that some were soft nosed in the early months of the war), but high explosives blew fragments of shell, clothing and debris deep into the body, so that wounds had to be excavated as well as drained. Nor was it easy to find these buried foreign bodies, in spite of one of the great inventions of the war – a mobile X-ray with generator mounted on an ambulance – for this could not always take the minutely accurate pictures of its larger fixed counterpart. Sir James MacKenzie Davidson, one of Cantlie's oldest friends, experimented with a probe attached to a telephone which clicked when contact was made with metal. In view of all these factors the question had to be asked, was it not better to take the patient back to base before opening the wound rather than trying to bring sophisticated equipment to hospitals near the front line. Another factor in the argument was that the Germans paid scant respect to the Red Cross and bombarded hospitals pitilessly, so that operations behind the lines were subject to interruptions, black-outs and evacuations, while the large number of wounded made unforeseen demands on facilities and meant hurrying patients down communication lines to allow more to be received at clearing stations. At the Battle of the Aisne in March 1915, with 11,000 casualties daily, three tented dressing stations were so heavily under fire that two were ordered forward to cope with demands for first aid and one was sent back to comparative safety at Villiers to perform emergency operations.

A field ambulance, as Cantlie described in his *Training Manual*, usually consists of three sections each capable of acting independently, with tents, transport and bearers.

> As soon as an engagement develops, a Field Ambulance halts 2000 yards behind the firing line and sends forward as many officers, bearers and wagons as may be required. After advancing, say 1000 yards, the officer in command forms a Dressing Station, and then breaks up the force into smaller bodies, each with a Medical Officer. The separate bodies advance to within a few hundred yards of the firing line and each establishes an Advanced Dressing Station marked by a Red Cross flag. The wounded are conveyed by road in wagons to the Clearing Hospital, where as near an approach as possible to a fully equipped hospital of 200 beds is set up . . . From the Clearing Hospital to Base is the work of the V.A.D.s.

The men fell in no man's land and often could not be rescued for hours or days under cover of darkness. One of the most poignant suggestions to allay infection was that put forward by Sir Watson Cheyne, who said gas gangrene might be avoided by soldiers carrying antiseptic paste to smear on their wounds, for a wounded soldier moving in no man's land was shot dead. To facilitate immediate rescue Cantlie invented and demonstrated in the Albert Hall in 1915 a bullet-proof stretcher, like a miniature tank, for two bearers, but the idea was not taken up. The wounded were brought into the first aid posts, shocked, hungry and collapsed from loss of blood. Here, often in dugouts, the first dressings were applied. The men were covered in mud – their clothes were impregnated with it – many had lice. It was not easy to decide how much cleansing and antiseptic treatment could be applied at this stage; was it not better, many doctors felt, to stop bleeding or splint a leg and then get the men back quickly to the advanced dressing stations and there cleanse and repair sufficiently to pass them on down the line to the clearing hospitals, where fractures could be set, blood vessels ligatured and emergency operations performed. Even then the question was how extensive could these operations be, for the high risk of infection had not been foreseen, nor the need to cleanse wounds by irrigation, which might continue for days or weeks. If, in view of all these factors, the patient was to be returned quickly to base, then everything had to be done to speed the journey and combat fatigue with food, warmth, stimulants and, if necessary, morphia. Bandages had to be loosened; tourniquets, if used – as Cantlie stressed in his book, this should only be in extreme emergency – had to be slackened every ten minutes. The Japanese attached a red thread to patients wearing tourniquets and the Germans recommended single elastic braces which could be used as emergency tourniquets because they stretched. In the Second World War the problems of succouring the wounded were in some respects different: in most cases the Germans respected the Red Cross emblem for combatant troops in the West, much of the early fighting was in the desert, the discovery of penicillin later in the war meant that wounds could heal and infection be allayed simultaneously, while a well organised blood transfusion service meant that loss through bleeding did not impose so great a threat to life.

According to the RAMC *Journal* ten different organisms were isolated and shown to contribute to gas gangrene, although Welch had first isolated the bacillus in 1892. Antiseptics did not kill spore bearers and had little effect. The ground over which the armies fought was not only arable and rich in manure but had been fought over repeatedly and blasted into fragments, filling the air with particles of dust and debris, so that both ground and air were alive with germs caused by wounds and death. The scenes facing doctors and surgeons were among the most heart-rending in history, for the escalation of war in the twentieth century has been accompanied by an escalation in fiendish devices of destruction. 'To the doctor,' wrote Cantlie, 'engaged in the wearing task of treating the sick, wounded and dying, day after day, week after week, the situation is one demanding a fortitude which few men are called on to endure.'[1] Too often doctors had to watch patients die knowing that medical science had little hope of combating the deadly infection of gas gangrene which set in at the moment or within hours of injury. Lister's revolution of antiseptic and aseptic surgery had transformed operating theatres of civil hospitals, but had made surgeons over-hopeful about its effects in war. Thus it was thought that by operating in aseptic conditions, applying antiseptic lotions (carbolic, mercury, iodine – the list was long enough to give choice – Cantlie was one who recommended carbolic tow), and by excluding air and preventing entry of further germs the wound would heal clean. Not so, as surgeons in Belgium and France discovered, for in the case of gas gangrene the germs were doing their work deep down at the base of the wound. To combat them it was necessary to cut away dead and contused tissue and to drain and irrigate the wound by means of a saline drip, to which was sometimes added $2\frac{1}{2}$ per cent of carbolic or hydrochloric acid, while other doctors recommended as well a glucose solution to stimulate the lymph glands and produce cleansing larva. Mr Alexander Fleming of St Mary's, a temporary RAMC lieutenant, whose early thoughts led to his later discovery of penicillin, believed there were three stages in the disease, that oxygen was vital in the second, while by the third a streptococci infection had set in, with which the patient should be inoculated. Later in the war streptococcal infection, to which was added iodine vaccination, was experimented with with some success, particularly in the French army, and later still antitoxins were prepared from horse antiserum to neutralise the toxins produced by the bacteria. The observation that oxygen was necessary in the second stage was responsible for experiments in the use of hydrogen peroxide, both as a dressing and an injection above the infected part, and also for healing in fresh air, already tried by Souttar in Belgium and now, together with electrically blown warm air, encouraged by Cantlie at the King Albert I Hospital at Rouen.

In November 1914 the Humanitarian Corps became responsible for the running of this remarkable hospital which was started by Miss Dormer Maunder at the request of the Belgian Medical Military Services. A member of Mabel Cantlie's No. 110 Detachment, Miss Maunder was a woman of courage, ability and powers of organisation who set a high standard of work for herself and others. Returning to Britain with Belgian refugees, she was offered a hospital in Paris which she refused and went instead to Rouen, where she opened the King Albert I Hospital for wounded Belgians, under the auspices of the Humanitarian Corps aided by Marylebone Division, BRCS. On 26 November 1914, the diary records, 'Miss Maunder is taking a hospital in Rouen and wants me to send V.A.D.s. She wants 300 blankets, 400 sheets, 400 pillow cases and a gross of towels.' In December, Mabel Cantlie interviewed nurses for the hospital, aiming at six trained nurses with VADs as probationers under them. She also later sent out a Secretary/Treasurer to provide male support for Miss Maunder (she had never forgotten that night in Hong Kong when, during the typhoon, she was in sole charge of a stricken hospital), but, within a short time, she realised that he was placing himself in charge of Miss Maunder and commented, 'We do not want that'. The Rouen Hospital Committee of the Humanitarian Corps was headed by Lady Cromer as President, and included Lady Godlee, wife of the President of the College of Ambulance, Lady Newman, wife of the Chairman of the Friends Ambulance Unit, Lady MacKenzie Davidson, Lady Samuelson, Miss Barber and Baron Goffinet who, together with Mme Depage, was a leading member of the Anglo-Belgian Red Cross Committee. (The names of Baron Goffinet and Mme Depage have been written into Belgian medical history with admiration and affection – only too soon Mme Depage was to lose her life on the *Lusitania* when she gave her life jacket to another passenger while returning from America on a fund-raising mission for refugees.) The first King Albert I Hospital was in the cobbled Rue Saint Lo and contained sixty beds, increased to 200, with an annexe opened later with 275 beds at Orival near Bellencourt and a second annexe with 235 beds at St Aubin Elbeuf. Throughout the winter and spring the Humanitarian Corps bought and sent clothes, bedding, medical supplies and stores to the Hospital, but it was clear by February that a public appeal must be sent out and this was confirmed by the Committee on the 5th. 'May God help us with the new Hospital,' wrote Mabel Cantlie in her diary, 'and may our new Corps bring hope and help to many a one in distress.' Financial help came also from New Zealand, Australia House and the Governor of Ceylon, where Cantlie had given his help to found a College of Agriculture.

Cantlie, who, because of the demands of his teaching, only made two visits to France during the war, was kept informed of conditions at the front by his son Neil. With his experience as a surgeon in the field of injuries and of first aid – he had written articles and made a study of ligature of the arteries, the circulatory system and head wounds – he was able to give his backing for experiments and innovations undertaken by the doctors in the hospital with dramatically successful results. The magazine *The Queen*, after explaining that inquiries about the hospital should be made to the College of Ambulance or the Humanitarian Corps, reported

A striking example of what pure humanitarian work may lead to is given by the work which has been accomplished in the last few months by Miss Dormer Maunder, one of the members of the Red Cross No. 110 of which Mrs. Cantlie is Commandant. She was asked by the General commanding the Belgian forces to become Commandant of a hospital for Belgian wounded in Rouen. She was given a beautiful building, which had been a public school and 200 beds were put in it. It is called the King Albert I Hospital and it received the first batch of patients on Christmas Day. It was publicly opened on December 26th by General de Selliers de Moranville, Inspector of the Belgian Army and Baron de Broqueville, Minister of War for Belgium. Miss Maunder has a staff of fully trained nurses and several Red Cross members who act as probationers and the results are eminently satisfactory, for this hospital is acknowledged to be one of the best managed of the great number which now exist in France.[2]

The King Albert I Hospital was a clearing hospital which took patients suffering from wounds of bone or nerve who required a second operation or physiotherapy treatment. This official definition seems a contradiction in terms, but having an untrained woman in charge the Cantlies preferred the hospital to be listed as 'convalescent' although technically 'clearing' as well.[3] They appeared to do this initially with all the hospitals they ran and then had them transferred to the military authorities afterwards. The hospital also took wounded who could not completely recover, and who were given professional re-education, either manual or intellectual, to equip them for another profession. Dr Deltentre, the senior doctor, liked to get patients to the hospital before their wounds were healed if there was risk of infection, and photographs show them healing wounds in the fresh air and sunlight. There were installations of physiotherapy, thermal therapy (treatment by heat including the blowing of hot air), medical hydrotherapy (douching with water – photographs show patients being hosed, a treatment popular in China), and immersing their limbs in water, radiology and electrotherapy and medical gymnastics. Cantlie had once not been enthusiastic about the Swedish methods used at the hospital in massage and physical education. Just before the war Mabel Cantlie had attended demonstrations of massage done by the blind because it was believed that sensitivity of touch, developed with blindness, was helpful to those with bad injuries unable to stand further pain; but, by 1918, Cantlie had been won over and used the Swedish methods later in his exercises for middle-aged and elderly people. The electrical installations at the King Albert I Hospital were made by the patients themselves under the guidance of Dr Deltentre, and so important a factor was this felt to be in their recovery that he made it the subject of a paper given at La Panne before Queen Elizabeth of the Belgians. The men also learnt wood, basket and foundry work in the hospital and manufactured their own wooden limbs and those of other limbless patients in a workroom manned by eighty wounded soldiers who were too incapacitated to fight any more. Before the war Belgium got her false limbs from Germany so that some change of plan in supply was essential, but the idea of the soldiers manufacturing their own limbs was a novel one which attracted much attention. In 1917 Dr Hendrix wrote a book on the manufacture of false limbs in the factory of the King Albert I Hospital and the Americans thought so well of the work that they asked for a loan of the limbs and spent much money trying to improve them.

Rouen was a depot city crowded with hospitals, far enough away from the front to give security, sufficiently close to study wounds in all their complexities, and almost immediately after the opening of the King Albert I Hospital, the Rouen Medical Society started under the Chairmanship of Colonel Skinner. This followed the pattern of the Hong Kong Medical Society and the Society of Tropical Medicine, giving opportunities for papers to be read by eminent medical men with consequent discussion, observation on clinical experience, remedies and cures. Monthly meetings were attended by army doctors and civilian medical men acting as consultants to the RAMC and reports were sent back to the *Journal of RAMC* for publication. Senior civilian doctors and surgeons see a wider range of injuries and illnesses than their army counterparts and the widest sharing of ideas leads to the best chances of breakthrough in research. Sir Watson Cheyne spoke on bullet wounds and Sir Almroth Wright pointed out at the fourth meeting that almost every wound was infected, and these were not ordinary infective processes but far worse. Tetanus and gas gangrene, which Sir Almroth thought was caused by 'B perfringens', were resistant to antiseptics. He described how the germs adhered to the walls of the wound and advocated injections of saline. (Cantlie had used salt in enemas in sprue because of its healing and aseptic qualities.) At a later meeting the subject discussed was sanitation in order to avoid typhoid and related diseases, and the methods suggested for killing flies were spraying with paraffin and making fly traps with sugar and water. In June 1915 the Society ceased to hold meetings. On the same date Miss Maunder resigned as Matron of the King Albert I Hospital, and the Rouen Committee of the Humanitarian Corps resigned shortly after. Fortunately the hospital was able to continue, for arrangements were made for the Humanitarian Corps to hand over its organisation to the British Ambulance Committee which had always taken a friendly interest in its progress and in November the Rouen Medical Society was revived under the same chairman.

The reason for Miss Maunder's resignation was because, although a VAD, she was not a trained nurse. No one criticised her for not running the hospital well, clearly it was an outstanding institution and, to prove this, Miss Maunder was given the Order of Leopold in March by the King of the Belgians, Mabel Cantlie being given the Order of Elizabeth at a later date. But the attitude of the nursing papers to this hospital was ambivalent. On 2 January 1915 the *Nursing Times* had reported, 'On inquiry at the College of Ambulance we are told that Miss Dormer Maunder is in Rouen, arranging to open a Hospital to be called the King Albert I Hospital. We are told there is to be a Matron and six fully trained nurses, with assistants, for whom preference will be given for V.A.D.s with 4 to 5 years' experience. It is under the French and Belgian authorities.' In a different section it said, 'A hospital in Rouen is to have as Matron of the Nursing Staff an untrained lady and this hospital is run by a Voluntary Aid Detachment'. Again, on the 9th, the paper reported that Miss Maunder was not a trained nurse, although it conceded that she had trained nurses working under her. In another column it carried a report on Schools of Medical Electricity, for which type of treatment the King Albert I Hospital was becoming well known, and suggested training of nurses in treatment by electricity with subsequent examinations. By the 23rd the paper was becoming aware of the possible damage it might have done to Miss Maunder, to the VADs and to the hospital, so it now devoted some space to describe 'its excellent work'. It explained that, as soon as the operating theatre was ready, the hospital was aiming at 400 or 500 patients. 'Certain features make this a specially attractive hospital. Wide gates enable an ambulance presented by Lord Combermere to bring wounded right under cover to the doors of the hall. There are spacious rooms where patients can be undressed, examined and bathed before being taken up the wide convenient stairs.' The report spoke of the large, well lighted wards, many bathrooms, sterilisation of garments, necessary because of the spreading of disease by vermin (Cantlie was convinced that lice played an important part in transmission of infection), and of the beautiful room at the top of the house which was converted into a chapel. Trained at Charing Cross, Cantlie believed that much of the life of a hospital centred round the chapel. Certainly this was praise indeed, but it is always easier to start than to stop criticism, and the Cantlies were also trapped by their own success, for if the hospital was 'convalescent', why was it admitting wounded straight from the trenches, whose garments needed sterilisation, and, if it was 'clearing', then what about the ratio of trained nurses to VADs?

The attitude of the nursing profession towards VADs has passed into First World War history. The reasons for it were complex and mostly centred round the need for state registration, which alone would have given the nurses professional security. In spite of Lord Ampthill presenting a State Registration Bill to Parliament each year since 1908, which was passed by the Lords but not the Commons, the nurses still had no official recognition or centralised examinations. Cantlie's demonstration operating theatre in the College may have made them wonder at what standard he was aiming for VADs, but, as with nurses today in first-year training, they were expected to be present at operations in hospitals in France. The trouble was that many at home were unable to picture the carnage taking place in Flanders, the shortage of medical personnel and the conditions under which doctors, nurses and VADs were working. Dr Monro of the Belgian Field Hospital had one trained nurse in four; the work of the other three, he said, could be done by orderlies or probationers, or, as the *Nursing Times* said, 'by anyone with initiative going ahead in hopeless surroundings'. Civil professional nursing qualifications were impor- tant for anyone running a hospital in such conditions, but almost as important was a training in improvisation and the character qualities of discipline, courage, powers of administration and the ability to keep a cool head (all of which were encouraged by VAD training), provided a person with these qualities had trained nurses working under her. Such a person was Lady Paget, who took a unit of trained nurses and VADs to Serbia – among them men from Cantlie's Detachment – which was faced with a raging epidemic of typhus, small pox, scarlet fever and appalling wounds. About one patient with no eyes or legs Lady Paget said, 'All we can do is to make them as comfortable as possible to the end and to try and do it with a good heart; the one bright spot is their gratitude'. This remarkable woman refused to leave her patients in Skopje when her husband, Sir Ralph Paget, Minister in the Foreign Office, arrived to fetch her three hours before the Bulgars arrived. The Serbs left 200 Austrian prisoners to act as her bodyguards, but this was unnecessary for the Bulgars' admiration for her was no less than that of the Serbs and Austrians and they allowed her to work unmo- lested and later repatriated her and her nursing staff. As Cantlie repeatedly stressed, civil hospital training alone was not necessarily relevant to meet such horrors and dangers.

The trained nurses were also understandably concerned about the effect that the volunteers might have upon payment of salaries, and Miss Maunder's request that her trained nurses should not be paid was not wise. Mabel Cantlie commented in her diary, 'This is not what we wanted'. Again, it is easy to see both sides: professional people, dependent for their livelihood on paid work, see the unpaid volunteer as a threat, but these controversies were out of place when volunteers were desperately needed and the men at the front were sacrificing lives and health for the sake of their country and in defence of their loved ones. The *Nursing Times* hoped that 'Britain would emerge from the war saner and more wholesome, for otherwise human history is an inexplicable riddle and man the sport of an ironic fate which would smite humanity with an incurable paralysis'. It seemed to need a series of appalling crises to make men and women pull together for the sake of their fellow men. On 28 January 1915 the Cantlies reacted to this sniping in their usual way. If the nursing papers said they would respect VADs who could bandage limbs or scrub floors and there were not enough limbs to bandage in Britain and there were difficulties about going abroad, they would get their members to follow up their other training laid down by the War Office and become cooks. Mabel Cantlie wrote in her diary that she inquired at the National School of Cookery about her Detachment training there. This jerked the authorities into reality, for there was an acute shortage of all grades of nurses and the Cantlies' VADs, who totalled around 500, were either trained nurses or efficient probationers. If the country lost the services of such willing nursing volunteers there might be a dispersal that it would be difficult to stop. Two days later, the diary records, 'Sudden demand for our members to go to Boulogne and nurse typhoid. We spent the day hunting up the ones available and having them inoculated.' Two days later the War Office issued a directive asking VADs to become probationers in established military hospitals to release trained nurses to start new auxiliary ones. In February, Charing Cross Hospital spearheaded a movement to train VADs as probationers for three months, an example followed by St Mary's, the London Hospital and others and on the 13th the *Nursing Times* reported that a BRCS VAD Women's Committee had been set up with Lady Ampthill, Mrs Furse, Mrs Ethel Becher (later Dame Ethel), Matron-in-Chief QAIMNS, and Miss Swift (later Dame Sarah), formerly Matron at Guys and now Matron-in-Chief BRCS.

Meanwhile another controversial issue was coming to a head, the question of feeding men returning from or to the front. In Boulogne trains which carried the wounded in, carried combatant troops out and Mrs Furse, who with her Detachment was doing splendid work at the station, would have found it well nigh impossible to issue orders that fit men should be denied food. Nevertheless it was technically in contravention of the Geneva Convention, though the French Croix Rouge, then made up of three societies, the Association of French Ladies (1879), the Union of French Women (1881) and the Society of Relief for Military Wounded from Armies on Ground and Sea (1870), was not unified into a single Red Cross Society until August 1940 and was, therefore, free to give cups of tea to combatant troops if it so wished. The French knew the Germans were waging total war, giving scant recognition to the Conventions, and the Belgian Red Cross, now only recognised by the Germans in contravention of the same Convention as a civilian organisation within a conquered country, also felt free to make its own choice. From the start of the war Detachment 110 and other Detachments had been running a buffet at Victoria Station for refugees, wounded and returned prisoners. The Cantlies had suggested that the Humanitarian Corps should run it, thus freeing it from restrictions and anticipating the work of the Women's Voluntary Service (WVS) and other organisations in the Second World War, but the BRCS would not allow this. On 10 February, however, Colonel Valentine Matthews, RAMC (T), Director, Red Cross, County of London, asked Mabel Cantlie to mobilise her Detachment to run a buffet at Victoria for soldiers and sailors. 'Great publicity has been given to the fact that we are giving food to refugees at stations and the

authorities now want us to give it to soldiers and sailors. They would
not allow that up to now.' Mobilisation meant taking orders from
the War Office and perhaps it was hoped, wrongly, that this would
overcome the difficulties. Letters of help poured in. Queen Alexandra
sent a donation and a letter of good wishes and Sir James Crichton
Browne arranged for Bovril to donate large supplies to the stall. No
sooner had the decision been taken than it was pointed out that the
Geneva Convention was being contravened and the orders came
to close it. The Cantlies refused to discontinue the buffet: 'orders,
counter orders, they are enough to bewilder anyone', and suggested
again that the Humanitarian Corps should run it; 'those in need'
seemed to cover those exhausted young men returning from the
trenches. As usual, a compromise was reached, all Red Cross brassards
and emblems being removed while troops were being fed. A further
coffee stall was opened at Charing Cross and Fenchurch Street, and
others soon followed at main line stations, which were visited by
the King and Queen. When the idea spread to the provinces, Mabel
Cantlie, who had been so closely associated with the work, was asked to
speak in Birmingham and other places in support.

Meanwhile, Cantlie was trying to interest British and Belgian authorities in a hut of his innovation and Mr Pritchard's design which could
be removed and re-erected quickly. It consisted of triangular sections
and long spars of wood, with no walls, the roof tapering to the floor.
Realising that tented hospitals, which had not yet come into their
own, might not be suitable in European winters, Cantlie erected this
alternative on waste ground behind the College of Ambulance and, in
February, demonstrated it to Sir Job and Lady Collins, Admiral
Fremantle, Alfred Sze, the Chinese Minister, and Lord Charles Beresford, who brought General Melis, Inspector General of the Belgian
Army. According to *The Red Cross* journal, 'the hut with its ingenious
fittings can sleep sixteen and be taken to pieces and re-erected in ten
minutes'. The same journal reported that the Belgians had taken up
the idea of a new hospital which was quickly moveable, sponsored by
Lady Bagot, General Melis and the Belgian Minister of War. Hutted
hospitals of both temporary and permanent design were becoming
increasingly popular. The splendid St John Ambulance Association
Hospital at Étaples, situated near the sand dunes, was entirely hutted,
with modern-style covered passageways connecting wards and operating theatres and the King Albert I Hospital in Rouen was later to
move to hutted accommodation in Bon Secours with eighty huts of
wards, laboratory and physiotherapy services.

In 1915, however, the hospital was still on its original site and in
March Mabel Cantlie crossed to France to visit her Detachment in
Boulogne, a French hospital in Dieppe and the King Albert I Hospital
in Rouen. Arriving in Dieppe 'I got a lame man to carry my bag and
take me to some hotel. It was a bit eerie going with him down a narrow
street, and he rang a broken bell and a woman turned up and showed
us a dirty courtyard lined with washing. However, the bed was clean, so
I turned in and dozed a bit until daylight, when I got up.' She found the

King Albert I Hospital in a college in the centre of Rouen with its cobbled streets, spires and quaint old houses. 'The hospital is in excellent order,' wrote Mabel Cantlie, '25 of a staff'. The following day she returned to Boulogne and joined the RAMC and Red Cross at the rest station.

> To the station at 6 a.m. A huge train of poor wounded came in, composed of 20 horse boxes with 18 stretchers each, most pitiable, so bad the men were, but so uncomplaining. We fed them 2 or 3 times with hot milk etc. It took 6 hours to get them to hospital. H would be proud of the bearers for they took such infinite care not to hurt the men when they changed them from one stretcher to the other . . . Trains of wounded came in again last night and several today. There has been an awful fight at Neuve Chapelle. Many men went back in the empty trains and we fed them, they were going to Le Havre and Rouen. Cheery and bright in spite of old wounds. The Rest Station is in old horse boxes painted out, a dispensary, a store, a carpenter's shop, orderlies' bedroom and sitting room for staff.

In April Miss Barber, a member of No. 110 Detachment, asked Mabel Cantlie to return to France to help her in her arrangements to lease a piece of land on which to put up the Tipperary Hut at St John's Hospital at Étaples. While there Mabel Cantlie saw the James Cantlie bed and visited a number of other hospitals in the area before returning to the Boulogne rest station which she was told the authorities wished to close. Within days of her return the reason was clear. The Germans were making another push to the Channel ports from which to launch an invasion of Britain. Again the wounded poured in, this time from the Second Battle of Ypres, and 80,000 wounded were fed. It was feared the British and Belgian lines might not hold for, on 28 April, the diary records: 'Germans using gas. Fearful rush to make masks. Allen and Hanbury's making H's gas masks.' On 1 May the press reported that the War Office had accepted Cantlie's design and the magazine *First Aid* said that the Grenadiers had ordered 2,000. 'Few men have done more for the Ambulance cause than Dr. Cantlie whose name is familiar to all First Aiders. Always on the alert to detect ways and means of alleviating human suffering he has invented a new form of respirator to protect eyes as well as nose and mouth, it is fixed to the cap and unrolled, a strip of mica for the eyes and alkali filter for the mouthpiece.'[4] At the College of Ambulance helpers flooded in to make the mask and the nursing papers carried instructions for designs of various kinds. A description of the first attack appeared in the June edition of the *Journal of RAMC*:

> It was 1.30 a.m. when they reached the Casualty Clearing Station, the gas having been used against them at about 7.30 the previous evening. One man was dead . . . Most of the others were in a choking condition, making agonising efforts to breathe, clutching at their throats and tearing open their clothes. Some were in a condition of

collapse, their faces and hands were of a leaden hue, their heads fallen forward on their chest. The majority of these cases did not rally. 14 died out of 17. The bad cases who lived got severe bronchitis from which they died. Others got bronchitis and lived.

Colonel W. Herringham wrote, 'One battalion with a fairly good pattern of respirator well used stayed in the trenches and hardly suffered at all'. The use of gas in warfare was one step further down the path of what, with the knowledge of modern science, man will do to man. It stiffened the resolve of the Allied armies to resist.

Mabel Cantlie hoped that her March visit to Rouen would help to strengthen Miss Maunder's position, but in June the diary comments, 'I do not think I can save Miss Maunder'. The very success of the hospital may have brought her enemies. She went on to be Red Cross Organiser, under General Melis, to the Belgian Army, for which the Humanitarian Corps continued to send her medical supplies and money. Fortunately Lord Combermere, who visited the hospital just before her resignation, was also a member of the British Ambulance Committee to the Croix Rouge, which now officially took over the hospital, and, although the Rouen Committee of the Humanitarian Corps felt they should resign in loyalty to Miss Maunder, they continued to give their unstinting support to the hospital and Mabel Cantlie supplied all its trained nurses and VADs in 1915. It appears from the diary that it may have been an intervention by Princess Christian, in charge of BRCS convalescent homes, which contributed to the hospital's start and continuance, for when Miss Maunder first went to France the Princess's Physician-in-Ordinary came to the College of Ambulance to find out about Miss Maunder and the importance of the work she was undertaking and to ask Mabel Cantlie how many trained volunteers she could provide – 'what about 500?'. Princess Christian did much kind work of this nature behind the scenes, always ready to hand on a venture to someone else just as credit and thanks were forthcoming. It is impossible to read the minutes of any society on whose committee she served without realising the deep concern she showed for others. She never missed an opportunity to express thanks to those who had done good work, condolence to those who had suffered loss and to promote active steps to help a good cause or those in need. On 28 June, just after Miss Maunder's resignation, the diary records: 'H to Windsor to speak for Red Cross. Princess Christian was in the chair, and spoke so sweetly to H. Lady Spencer Churchill introduced him in the most charming manner as the instigator of all Red Cross work. He much enjoyed his afternoon.'

The British Ambulance Committee, which at the same time as taking over the King Albert I Hospital took over Lady George Murray's Hospital at Le Treport (Lady George was also a keen supporter of the College of Ambulance), had come into being to aid the French, whose sufferings were immense. Their line was six times longer than that of the British, and, as well as the wounded, there were thousands of refugees, women, children and old people whom the Germans had expelled from the land they held. On 10 November 1914 a letter was printed in *The Times* from Lord Knutsford, saying that the arrangements for the British wounded were deserving of great praise, and on the following day came a report in the same newspaper on the British Ambulance Committee, the President of which was the Duke of Portland, the Chairman Lord Charles Beresford, MP, and one of the Vice Presidents Mr Francis Bertie, known to Cantlie from Sun Yat Sen's rescue and now British Ambassador in Paris. *The Times* reprinted a letter from the Committee which had appeared in the *Morning Post*:

> France has used up nearly all the motor cars available for ambulance work, the wounded of our gallant ally are suffering terribly owing to the delay in transport from the front to the nearest hospital. Many have died from blood poisoning . . . Now that the English people have done what was urgent in this matter for our own Army, we venture to ask you to open your columns to this appeal for motor cars for the French Red Cross Society and funds for their upkeep. The Queen has been graciously pleased to say that 'Her Majesty fully sympathises with the objects of the British Ambulance Committee and Queen Alexandra and the Prince of Wales both express sympathetic interest'.

The plea was for drivers and mechanics as well as for funds and cars. There was to be no uniform, just a French Red Cross badge. Soon the Committee was running two convoys of sixty-five ambulances, later increased to 125, and Scotland sent a column of fifty ambulances of her own. As a result of this success Lord Curzon and Sir Lauder Brunton appealed for a French flying surgical field hospital, like that of Dr Munro for Belgium: 'The very soul of France,' said Lord Curzon, 'has put on its armour and gone forth to conquer or to perish', and Lady Linlithgow and Mrs Eleanor Cecil appealed for the French Wounded Emergency Fund. Meanwhile, the American Red Cross was providing fleets of self-contained field ambulance units for the Allied forces, of which the British diverted most of their share to the French. Nevertheless, in May 1915 the press still reported French wounded lying on straw in cattle trucks and at rest stations, although the *Daily Graphic* commented on the devotion of the Croix Rouge workers, who met the wounded with bread, coffee, soup and wine and nursed those too ill to travel further. The article paid tribute to nurses in French hospitals where, with beds almost touching, and a 'sad absence of ventilation' (noted by Mabel Cantlie at Dieppe), their extraordinary courage and devotion saved many lives. Commenting on the qualities of the Croix Rouge nurses *The Queen* magazine wrote: 'the French wounded recover with a percentage that places accident out of the question. Some of the big hospitals have one or two trained nurses, but the majority are run by French women of one of the three societies.'

It was against this background that the British Ambulance Committe, undaunted by the ratio of trained to untrained nurses, took over responsibility for the King Albert I Hospital until it moved to Bon

Secours in 1916, when the Belgian Army Medical Services took it over themselves. Meanwhile, the Duchess of Westminster's hospital at Le Touquet (the third to come under attack in the nursing papers because of her lack of training) increased its trained nurse ratio from fifty to 120 beds. Since Lady Paget's ratio in Serbia remained one to 120 beds it is puzzling why the British should have sought to impose their ratio upon the Belgians in Rouen. With the future of the hospital again assured, Cantlie's home town of Dufftown and the Aberdeenshire village of Tarves, home of Lord Haddo, a Polytechnic council member, joined the list of those who sent money and supplies to the British Ambulance Committee; but the strain of the controversy and uncertainty was demonstrated by the death of Lady Samuelson, nursing at the hospital, just one month after the death of her last son killed in action. On a more helpful note, in January 1916 the *Nursing Times* described the Christmas festivities at the Hospital: 'corridors festooned with ever-greens and mistletoe and Japanese lanterns with messages in English and French; soldiers like excited schoolboys clustered round miniature Christmas trees. Many were on crutches, minus an arm or a leg, but with happy faces.' They might have been describing Christmas in Charing Cross Children's Ward in 1885, when Cantlie and Bruce put on a Punch and Judy show. In all, 23,000 patients went through this hospital during the war, just over 5,000 of these before the move to Bon Secours: 53 per cent went back to fight, 19 per cent joined auxiliary services, 25 per cent had to leave the service, and deaths amounted to 0.5 per cent. This is a puzzling figure because of the missing percentage of 2.5; but even if the deaths had been 3 per cent it is very low, particularly as it includes the deaths from Spanish flu'. The Inspector General of the Belgian Army Medical Services regarded Bon Secours as a unique creation, and so did Queen Mary and Queen Elizabeth of the Belgians, both of whom, with many members of the Allied medical services and aid societies, visited the hospital during the war.

CHAPTER SIXTEEN

College of Ambulance or College of Nursing

Day after day, friends and helpers in the College of Ambulance had lost husbands, sons, nephews; Sir Lauder Brunton, Major Richardson, General Evatt, Lady Strathcona had all lost sons. It seemed it would never end. In April 1915 Italy entered the war, 'The Quakers have gone to Italy', say the diaries, then as fighting flared eastward, 'Colonel Fremantle with 2000 camels goes to Khelat', and in August, 'Warsaw is in German hands . . . Cannot but hope God knows best and hope and hope'. With two sons in the war the Cantlies did not know that Keith, leaving Assam, was temporarily prevented by an ICS ban on volunteering, in spite of a personal letter to the Viceroy. 'God knows when I shall ever see him again.' George Cantlie, now a Colonel, was soon to receive the DSO, 'The Duke of Connaught congratulated him on his men as smart and efficient.' Like all other parents and helpers at the College the Cantlies were anxious and overworked. It was still in its first year and the need to keep up the supply of trained nursing volunteers was paramount. In early VMSC days Hunter and Cantlie had discussed plans in Egypt, away from the distractions; in Tropical School days Manson had taken the Cantlies to Italy to see his successful malarial research. Now everyone was under strain. 'Acute pain today,' say the diaries, 'Sometimes I think it is serious but hope not. Perhaps it is only fatigue. I never get rest. There is so much to do.'

So much to do, and people wanting to do it, but only if someone would organise and encourage them and keep them from quarrelling. That was one of the Cantlies' gifts. Why, Mabel argued, forfeit valuable time recovering from an operation which, if it was cancer, might only alleviate the disease? Was it not better to keep working at a time of national disaster? Thus she hid the truth from her husband almost, it seemed, weighing her life in balance against the lives of her sons. Meanwhile, Cantlie was still rising at four or five a.m.: 'H to a patient at Woking at 4 a.m. I do not sleep much now.' How did either of them keep going at such a pace at their age and state of health with so little rest? Like many others they answered calls made on them, and did not think of themselves. 'Nurse Gordon came in and told of the fighting at Loos and of the advanced dressing stations. Hundreds died in the arms of fifteen women nurses who were with her. Oh God, what scenes.' It was becoming daily more difficult to see life through death or any future at all. Yet five days later the innocent happiness of the King Albert I Christmas party shone through again. 'George Cantlie wrote from France, asking me to get a present for his baby Celia.' In the midst of a nightmare of death there was life. Then in the next entry the horror of seeing Neil off to France: 'My boy. My boy. It shakes one to the root of one's foundations to have to part with them, but one gives them into God's hands.' Knowing how deeply she missed her sons, their friends the Ushers asked the Cantlies to be guardians of their children, Harry and Marjorie, while they were abroad. This meant meeting them at stations, school trunks, having them for the holidays; but their presence was welcome, outweighing extra commitments and at Christmas 'it helped to shut out the saddened thoughts of desolate war hurt homes and hearts'. Only her son Colin, with the same steely self discipline as his mother, was perhaps beginning to wonder if there was not more behind her illness than the fatigue she always pleaded.

As the summer of 1915 ripened into autumn the anxiety of the nation hardened into iron determination. The diary records the report of a Colonel friend back from the front: 'Not enough shells or men. He says there is general grumbling at home and it spoils the spirit of those anxious to make the sacrifices they can to defend their country.' That Germany preparing to invade Serbia was in the grip of a ruthless war machine, bent on subduing Europe, there was no doubt. Lord Kitchener was one of the few who warned that it would be a long war, four years at least, and as German military strength became more apparent so did the weakness of the Asquith Government, which had little grip of the situation and continued its peace-time drift in the face of the worsening situation. Neil told in a letter how the advance parties of soldiers attacked with courage and dash, pushing the enemy back, but went forward too far; and the support party, too late and too small, arrived to find them annihilated. The penetration of the Dardanelles by British submarines was a feat, in the face of dangerous currents and enemy guns, but the disaster of Gallipoli which followed was caused by inefficient organisation and consequent lack of will. The moral of Gallipoli, the failure that was nearly a success, was that only with attention to detail can a crisis in a battle or an illness be surmounted. Although it was not until 1916 that Asquith's lack of leadership in the House of Commons led to the King sending for Bonar Law, and, when he could not form a Coalition Government, for Lloyd George, nevertheless, by the middle of 1915 Asquith's days were numbered and the public knew it, not pulling its punches. Unlike the French and German armies the British Army was still volunteer, and although by October Kitchener had advised conscription from a military point of view, the Government could not face up to the political decision, believing it not in keeping with democracy. Thus, although British casualties were much smaller than those of the French (322,000 dead and 1 million wounded, compared with probably four times that figure) nevertheless the finest young men of the nation, leaders of the future and sons of the experienced, able men who led the country with courage and integrity in the last century, were now laying down their lives as officers and privates in a holocaust where three weeks was the average survival rate for a lieutenant, while others stayed at home. Food was soon to be running short as a result of submarine warfare. Meanwhile, however, the situation in Germany, which had counted on a short war, was worsening and, by the beginning of 1916, reports were coming from the front that their troops were becoming demoralised.

The shortage of nursing staff was critical and in April 1915 Lord Knutsford said that nursing soldiers with only trained nurses must be abandoned. 'Civilians in peace time have never been so nursed. In all hospitals untrained probationers are always to be found working under trained nurses.' Pointing out that the London Hospital had 335 of its 517 nurses not yet certificated, he urged hospitals to increase their strength and get 'some training into more women'. In order to staff military hospitals at home the BRCS now issued new contracts for VADs in Allied hospitals in France, binding them to return if recalled – if not registered they would be counted as part of another organisation. Many of the Cantlies' members were already working in military and the London hospitals and in the auxiliary ones which they had started such as Homeleigh at Harrow, opened in 1914 as a convalescent home and becoming an annexe of Charing Cross Hospital in December. Given by a member of the Schools for Mothers, this hospital was financed by Mr Wellcome and Marylebone Division, Red Cross, until June 1915, when it received a Class A Military Hospital grant and in 1917 became part of the Queen Alexandra Hospital, Millbank, 1,000 patients passing through during the war, of whom none died. Cantlie's No. 1 VAD also provided transport and entertainments for the Queen Mary Hospital for Limbless Men at Roehampton and nursing volunteers to give the male staff Christmas leave. This hospital, financed by Mr J. Pierpoint Morgan among others, was one of the most outstanding of the war and has remained so with passing time. It was started in 1915 with 180 beds to provide convalescent treatment for limbless men, during which they would be fitted with limbs and instructed in their use, to allay the mental and physical shock of amputation. By 1918 there were 900 beds, and Marylebone Division, Red Cross, had provided 600 walking sticks to patients on leaving. Every day now into main line stations poured increasing numbers of wounded needing transport, beds and nursing. Walking cases crawled along the platform 'bowed and listless, moving stiffly from rheumatism', some men 'almost asleep on their feet'. Hospitals to which Nos 1 and 110 sent volunteer nurses or bearers were the Balstrode Street Hospital for shell-shock cases; the Lady Brassey Hospital, with its winding stair, who nicknamed No. 1 the 'Sunbeam Squad' because they were so cheerful; the Endsleigh Palace Hotel Hospital, for which Mabel Cantlie bought beds, made curtains and supplied domestic help from her members, getting mention in the *Nursing Times* for the hospital's airiness, quietness, good upholstery and excellent food; the Livingstone College Military Hospital, where, by 1918, 175 No. 110 VAD members made up the nursing staff on a rota under a trained matron; St Dunstan's where the number of war-blinded called for all voluntary help available; and the Acheson Hospital, opened later, which was run by a House Committee at the College of Ambulance – in connection with which hospital a hostel for VADs nursing in London was opened by Princess Mary in 1918.

By the summer of 1915 the press was trying to make the Government admit the shortage of nurses and decide how to recruit and train more. In France there was also a shortage of ambulance drivers and support staff necessary for the movement of wounded – signallers, motor cycle dispatch riders and messengers. Although the British Ambulance Committee of the Croix Rouge was employing British women ambulance drivers in 1915, the BRCS did not use them abroad until 1916. Formerly the Army Service Corps had supplied personnel for the Bearer Units, but the Maidstone RAMC (T) had been requested, after the Boer War, to spearhead an experiment in making field ambulances independent by using their own staff. Trained bearers were therefore doing jobs which lay personnel could do and, in order to release them, a number of Women's Corps were started and others extended their activities. Mabel Cantlie was associated with the Women's Emergency Corps through the Women's Reserve Ambulance, which provided transport for No. 1 VAD, and in June 1915 she became a member of the Committee and, in July, its Chairman. Meetings were held in Bedford College and the Corps enlisted her help in trying to amalgamate the two movements into one organisation, the Green Cross. A *Lancet* report described the 300 members of the Women's Reserve Ambulance, known as the Green Cross from the early days of war, as meeting trains at all hours of the night, transporting limbless men to Roehampton and supplying workers for the Croix Rouge. Later, the Green Cross and No. 1 VAD coped with the gruesome remains of Zeppelin LZ 31 when it burst into flames over London, killing the crew. In April 1915 the Women's Auxiliary Force (later the British Service Corps) was started as the result of an approach to Mabel Cantlie who was asked to be its first Chairman to organise the opening of the Station Canteen at Waterloo. She then turned her attention to helping to form the Women's Signallers and was instrumental in drawing up their constitution and joining in the suggestion that they be known as the Khaki Cross. The two Corps were officially recognised at the end of 1915, Princess Arthur of Connaught, Duchess of Fife, becoming a patron of the Women's Auxiliary Force, Viscountess French its President and Mrs Parker, a sister of Lord Kitchener, becoming President of the Women's Signallers. In May Australians took over and ran the Buffets at Waterloo, Great Central Street and London Bridge Stations. In August Lady Londonderry started the Women's Legion to provide more women drivers and other support staff.

Meanwhile, in June 1915 the Joint Committee decided to heed Lord Knutsford's warning and accept only a two-year training for staff nurses. *The Times* wrote an article in July praising VADs and implying a lack of liaison between the War Office and reserve forces. It was against this background that Cantlie decided to do all he could to unite the teaching, examining and selection process of the two Voluntary Aid

Societies to promote desired efficiency. (Even in February sixty Quakers had been unable to get to the front because St John would not recognise the Red Cross crash course, insisting on one lecture once a week for three months.) The College of Ambulance was the obvious centre where the societies could attain together a higher standard of first aid training. Sir Claude Macdonald in 1914 had suggested three grades of nurses, fully certificated, certificated and uncertificated, and Cantlie believed that VADs trained by the College could, after serving as hospital probationers, supply the middle grade. During July Mabel Cantlie redecorated the College in preparation for this role and decided, in view of her health, to give up the work party, which should find other accommodation. Its members were, however, determined not to lose her leadership, be dispersed or join the Central Depot in Cavendish Square. The Hon. Mrs Lawson Johnston, whose husband was a Polytechnic council member and who was President of the work party, generously offered her house, 29 Portman Square, with financial help as well. The work party and depot re-opened there in January, still under Mabel Cantlie's direction, with the same committee, including Lady Cromer, Lady Strathcona, Lady Godlee and Mrs Quentin Hogg, 115 voluntary members and a paid needlewoman and two cutters for whom materials had to be bought and supplied.

The College of Ambulance was now able to direct all its attention and space to first aid and in July Mr Stanley, Chairman, BRCS, expressed interest in Cantlie's plan to use it as a centre to teach first aid to the two societies. On 21 July he chaired a meeting of representatives of each society to 'discuss various V.A.D. matters' and on the 28th he moved a resolution at a BRCS War Executive Meeting to set up a Joint VAD Committee, with three Red Cross representatives, including Mr Ridsdale. On 30 July St John nominated three representatives, including Lord Plymouth and Sir Richard Temple, and the first moves were thus made towards a unified programme. Meanwhile, however, the War Office, wanting to release men for the combatant forces and bearer units, was planning to use the VAD's supplementary training and on 1 September issued the General Service Scheme, under which they would be employed as drivers, cooks, dispensers, clerks and other support personnel, joining Voluntary Aid Detachments, but not taking first aid and nursing certificates. Would this two-tier standard in Detachments free those qualified for nursing or dilute standards of emergency training? The new Committee met on 2 September and, on the 7th, the Joint War Committee considered its proposal for a unified selection board, the first step towards a united teaching programme. Then misunderstandings seem to have arisen. According to St John's Ambulance Association correspondence and a report dated 20 September, Sir Richard Temple thought the War Office had agreed to recognise the Joint VAD Committee as it recognised the Joint War Committee and claimed that the War Office, on the 7th, not only refused to give the new Committee direct recognition as it did the BRCS VAD Committee, but did not follow its usual practice of notifying the Joint War Committee, sending the directive only to the BRCS

War Executive, so that St John, unaware of the decision, informed branches and held meetings. On 9 September the diary records, 'H went to see Stanley about the College'. Cantlie proposed that the Joint VAD Committee should build an Extension at the back of the College for administration and that until it was complete the Pritchard Hut could be used for meetings and offices, while the College of Ambulance would be their combined teaching centre. The same day Mr Stanley wrote to Sir Richard Temple: 'We are going ahead with the V.A.D. Extension. I suggested a Joint Selection Board which Lady Perrott refused, but she told me yesterday that she had altered her opinion and would now like it. I am waiting, however, until we have got things a little more definitely established at Devonshire House, as, of course, on her refusal, I went ahead to form the Committee there, and, when that is formed, we can ask St John's to join if they feel inclined.'[1]

A few days later the Joint VAD Committee met in Devonshire House and appointed the Joint VAD Women's Committee. Was this now a venture seeking combined teaching, examining and selection facilities or only to co-ordinate the extension of VAD work under the General Service Scheme? With preparations for the Battle of Loos under way casualties would once more be arriving and all help would be needed. On 11 September Cantlie, seeing no quick decision regarding the College, arranged with Mr Boyton to rent it for £1,200 a year. For a man of 65, dependent on his surgeon's fees in time left over after hours of first aid lecturing, this was a daunting sum, although some of it would be met from the fees of the College and the money that Keith had sent home for the purpose, but which his parents had banked for him. His generosity was not unique at this time. The Grenfell twins had set up the St Pancras Branch of the Invalid Children's Aid Society and funded it themselves before being killed in France. Nevertheless, the Cantlies must have been anxious. On 14 September Mabel Cantlie was invited to discuss with Lady Wolverton, Lady-in-Waiting to Queen Alexandra, the setting up of a permanent BRCS Needlework Society, which would make clothing for the wounded, an idea for which she had been pressing for some time. On 26 September the diary records that Stanley visited the College of Ambulance and 'was delighted with it. The men were all at the College for Sunday duty. He was astonished to see so many fine fellows. Hamish showed Mr. Stanley the piece of ground at the back which would do for a Headquarters, Red Cross Society.' On 4 October Mr Ridsdale, ex Chairman, BRCS, inspected the College and the site, and on the 11th, on which day, according to the diary, Sir Arthur Sloggett, DGAMS, in France, wrote most enthusiastically about the VADs, saying he would like 200 more, the diary also reports: 'Mr. Stanley says he has decided to build a big V.A.D. building at the back of the College and to form a Committee of three St. John and three B.R.C.S. and H as Director. Splendid hope to live up to.' Apparently, therefore, the idea of a joint teaching programme and committee was still in Stanley's mind in early October, and this was borne out when he said at the meeting of the BRCS Voluntary Aid Sub-Committee on 13 October that he wished to form a centre in

London, a headquarters for Voluntary Aid Detachments and 'with it would be connected a large training School'. On 18 October the Cantlies officially complied with the War Office directive to send VADs as General Service Members into military and auxiliary hospitals – they had anyway been using their members in this capacity since February – and the following year a Detachment No. 110 member was chosen Lady Superintendent of General Service Members at Millbank. But on 21 October *The Times*, in a *Red Cross Supplement*, referred to the Joint VAD Committee as having been formed to deal with extra demands of the General Service Scheme: 'In order to cope with this work it was decided to form a Joint Voluntary Aid Committee representing the B.R.C.S. and Order of St. John . . . The Joint V.A.D. Committee is formed to co-ordinate the work of the two bodies, but the control of the B.R.C.S. V.A.D. organisation remains in the hands of its Advisory Committee as hitherto.' Some time, therefore, during October, Cantlie's dream of using the College of Ambulance as a combined teaching college for the two societies had faded.

What was to happen to the College now? In the *Red Cross Supplement The Times* said of VADs: 'Their reward is in the knowledge that in peace time they faced ridicule in order to be ready'. It was this that Cantlie feared, that without the societies having a centralised teaching college it was going to be difficult to supply sufficient certificated nursing volunteers in war and that in peace the Red Cross might give up its training role and the spirit of voluntary service, born of suffering, would die away. *Tantus tabor non sit cassus* – a favourite quotation of Sir Frederick Treves – 'That so much work should not be wasted'. Cantlie cast round in his mind as to what could be done, understanding that a centralised College of Ambulance might well not yet be popular with the trained nurses who had been demanding their own centralised examinations and state registration for twenty years. On 1 November he therefore wrote in the *Journal of Tropical Medicine*, 'In hunting about for a centre for nursing, I would recommend that the B.R.C.S. be selected. In peace the Red Cross becomes a body without a purpose. The National Aid Society did its work from a single room.' He pointed out that the Red Cross Society had no role call of doctors and nurses in peace time and had 'to go into the market in time of war'. Referring to VADs, he said, 'When the war is over this excellent body of willing and well trained workers will melt away.' He realised that a first step towards the permanent establishment of a centralised College of Ambulance for the voluntary aid societies was a centre for the nursing profession, holding examinations and a register of trained nurses. The plan for Red Cross involvement was not novel, for it was the National Aid Society which gave the first grant to initiate army nursing training at Netley. Cantlie had always had great sympathy for the nurses' position and Lady Helen Munro-Ferguson, who first interested him in the movement for state registration, was now wife of the Governor General of Australia, where she had introduced an excellent scheme. In Cantlie's view both were equally important, a centre for nursing and a centre for ambulance.

All through the autumn of 1915 news from the front had been steadily worsening. At the end of October the French Cabinet fell. On 24 October the Germans shot Nurse Cavell, an act of brutality which hardened the resolution of the British – if that was the treatment the Germans meted out to women and a nurse to boot, then it would be a fight to the death. Serbia was being slowly ground down, while in China Yuan was manoeuvring himself into the position of Emperor in the face of British, Russian and Japanese criticism and was expressing pro-German sympathies. As the wounded poured in from the tragic Battle of Loos it was obvious that trained nurses alone could not stem the tide. The figures told the story. There were twenty-three territorial hospitals in Britain with 500 to 3,000 beds and many smaller ones. There were only 20,000 fully-trained nurses, 8,000 for civilians and 12,000 for soldiers and sailors, of which 4,000 were abroad. Staffing in military hospitals was 1 nurse to 16 patients, in civil hospitals 1 to 19, in Poor Law hospitals 1 to 44. The great addition to the supply of nurses in wartime came from VADs and St John Brigade. (The BRCS started the war with just under 60,000 VADs and ended it with 120,000 – that figure allowing for 9,500 St John VADs and General Service Members – while St John Ambulance Brigade started the war with 25,000 trained members and ended it with 65,000.) Those responsible for maintaining the supply of voluntary nurses saw that without hope of time in military hospitals counting towards training, it was going to be difficult, if not impossible, to provide recruits. Volunteer nurses saw probationers, whose work they were often doing, using time towards nursing training, while the medical students also counted their period as orderlies for clinical work requirements. It was understandable, on the other hand, that trained nurses should fear a postwar flood of VADs into hospitals – their very competence made them popular with doctors – and should see in their voluntary status an opportunity to avoid contractual liability which in turn would dilute professionalism.

Cantlie therefore tried, in a series of articles in *The Red Cross* journal in November 1915, to bring the two sides together by helping the volunteer nurses to accept the rules and irksome necessities of hospital life, where split-second reaction and dependability save lives, and explaining to professional nurses that emergency work at the front, for which VADs were specially trained, was far removed from civil hospital life. 'In the railway trains with piles of wounded, dying and dead or in the open air, where everything must be improvised', a particular discipline and training were required, enabling men and women, with courage and compassion, to 'keep going in scenes of horror which either excite or numb the brain'. Differentiating between 'trained' and 'hospital' nurses, he said that this self-control was learnt by repeated stretcher drill, by living up to a code of conduct personified by wearing a uniform and by using non-commissioned officers – vital to any organisation – as a channel of communication to the assistant commandant, for they alone knew 'the strength and weaknesses of individual members'. Then, turning to the role of VADs in hospital, he told them never to lose sight of the objective, the restoration of the patient to health for, with that in mind transcending jealousies and rivalries, 'neither the scoldings of the ward sister are resented, nor do the scathing remarks on VADs affect one's purpose in the least'. (The use of the word 'one's' is typical of the Cantlies' style of leadership, always to identify with those they led.) No work, he said, was then too menial, no order that must not be readily complied with, for 'discipline marches hand in hand with this spirit, one must learn to obey before one is fit to command'. Shakespeare's nurse was still his ideal, 'so kind, so duteous, so diligent, so tender over her occasions, so true, so feat'. Articles in similar vein were written by the Matron of the 3rd London General in the *Nursing Times*, and by the Matron of the 2nd London General, who visited Cantlie's home ground in north-east Scotland and wrote in glowing terms in the *Aberdeen Journal* about the work of the VADs in the area; while another article in the same paper made particular mention of the excellence of Gordon Castle Hospital at Fochabers, with an operating theatre and splendid recreational facilities, including billiards, staffed entirely by VADs under a trained matron. What could be done there, said the correspondent, could be done everywhere.

Providence now put the voluntary ambulance movement to the test in unforeseen circumstances. On 31 October came a dramatic and unexpected call. On that day the diary records, 'H conveyed the King to Buckingham Palace. Ordered by Sir Frederick Treves to have men ready to meet the train. H, Mr. Mitchell, Fulford, Rowe, Taylor and Prescott. They practised all evening together, getting the stretcher in and out of the car. The King had an accident in France, with his horse rearing and falling on him, crushing him.' 1 November: 'Mr. Taylor here to breakfast and then they went to Buckingham Palace to practise on the stairs with a stretcher. Then to Charing Cross Station to practise there. Then to Victoria Station to wait for the train to come in, Sir Frederick Treves being in charge. The removal was made from the bed to the car and from the car to the King's bedroom, and the King said "Magnificent". H took the orders off his uniform.' Sir Frederick measured the platform, so that the bearers knew where the King's bed would be and was only six inches out; the rolled sheet lift was then used. A *Pall Mall Gazette* article said:

> The King was riding a strange horse in France, but an excellent one. The animal, frightened by the cheering crowd, reared up and fell over, pinning him down and causing severe injury and shock but without breaking bones. In the hospital train, although prone and helpless, the King awarded Lance Sergeant Oliver Brookes, 3rd Battalion Coldstream Guards, with the V.C. The Bearer Party was a specially selected party of men belonging to the B.R.C.S. No. 1 London Detachment, the first Voluntary Aid Detachment formed in the country . . . who used the utmost gentleness and care.[2]

The King was attended by English and Canadian nurses from a French hospital barge; a fortuitous thank you for Canadian Red Cross and other war time generosity. On 4 November Sir F. E. G. Ponsonby wrote to Sir Frederick Treves, 'The King hopes you will take an opportunity of conveying to the British Red Cross Stretcher Party employed on Monday last His Majesty's entire satisfaction with the arrangements which were made. Nothing could have been better, the King says, than the quiet and efficient manner in which the stretcher was carried from the railway carriage to the ambulance and from the ambulance into the palace.'

This task of No. 1 gave a real boost to VAD morale, for it acknowledged these men experts in transport of wounded. Thus the Ambulance Column, London District, was re-formed in November and No. 1 VAD joined a composite detachment of County and City of London men, becoming known as Unit 6 of this bearer section of 375 men. They were on twenty-four-hour duty two days a week and also did reserve on-call duty for a further twenty-four hours in case two trains came in together, and one full Sunday in three, making a fifty-six-hour week on top of their own occupations. The London Ambulance Column transported 600,000 wounded during the war, of which Unit 6 transported 55,000 stretcher cases and 42,000 walking cases. At the request of the police No. 1 VAD resumed its air raid duties which had been temporarily given up a month before, and under the new title 'Air Raid Relief Party' the squad covered raids in Marylebone and was also free to help anywhere in London, either using its own newly formed transport section or that of the Women's Reserve Ambulance. Overshadowed by the Blitz twenty-five years later, air attacks over London in the First World War, as indeed the shelling of coastal towns, were far from insignificant, with forty-seven killed in one night and 150 injured. The Polytechnic was used as the squad's duty centre rather than the College because of its underground facilities in which the public could sleep. 'It was a very pathetic sight . . . to see the poor kiddies dazed with sleep, evidently having been pulled hastily from their beds, being carried by their parents, who were in many cases more frightened than their little ones.'[3] In the streets and shattered houses improvisation often had to be the key to rescue – a door placed on a ladder makes an excellent stretcher, as a member of the squad recounted. Although not occurring until later in the war, the direct hit on Odham's Printing Works posed the sort of problems for which the men had been trained.

About six of us went down the narrow stone staircase leading to the scene of the disaster . . . The scene in this room was as weird as could be imagined, the flare of the fire, the steady pour of the water through the ceiling, the woeful figures of the dead and injured with their faces and clothes all smeared with printers' ink. The living victims groaned and cried. Aided by flare lamps, we got quickly to work, and, feeling mostly with our feet, we commenced our search for those still alive, but often had to spend some minutes moving the dead out of the way to get at the living. The dead we carried into the room where the printing machines were, laid them on top of the machines and covered them with blankets. The first victim we

recovered was a woman, but she died soon after. As we found others
they were quickly examined and then sent on an ambulance to the
hospital. In the darkness and water First Aid to any extent was out of
the question. We presently came across a man held down by some
machinery that had fallen across his leg, and for some time we found
it impossible to move it. We had almost decided to amputate the leg
in order to save him from drowning in the rapidly rising water,
when, by the help of a fireman's rope, we managed to get the weight
off and he was saved. We had now been working about fifty minutes,
and had rescued all those who were alive when we started. We turned
our attention next to making a thorough search of all that part of the
room we could get at for any that might have been overlooked in the
darkness and a terrible job it was. We stumbled over bodies and fell
into machine pits full of ink and water, but we stuck it until four
o'clock, when we were sure all who it was possible to get out were out,
and we had sent to hospital some ninety cases. Practically all of these,
as well as the dead, were examined by our doctor, Dr. Hastings, who
stayed down with us all through and cheered and helped us in our
awful task. At 4 a.m. the firemen's chief officer came to the conclusion it was no longer safe to stay in the basement, and we had to
stop work, but we had already cleared the room.[4]

This description shows the need for advanced emergency training in
both war and peace, but times were hard, almost every day there was a
sale of family treasures to give money to the Red Cross and open new
hospitals, so, although on 6 November the diary records, 'The Red
Cross are still considering developing the site at the back of the College', on the 16th it says, 'Mr. Boyton wants £470 for the ground at the
back. Mr. Stanley thinks it too much for the moment if added to the cost
of the hut but he is still interested in building on it.' Undeterred, the
Cantlies continued to prepare the College for advanced classes in first
aid and nursing to be run concurrently with the ordinary certificate
courses. 'In response to a request from the Editor,' said St John's
magazine *First Aid*, 'I visited the College of Ambulance, which, as all the
world knows, is established at No. 3 Vere Street.' Confessing he once
thought the scheme too ambitious, the writer went on, 'to Dr. Cantlie is
due in large measure the present establishment of First Aid as an exact
science, to his credit the R.A.M.C. (T), and to his suggestions and
labour many of the advanced improvements of St. John and Red
Cross'.[5]

During the winter of 1915 the commitments of the voluntary aid
societies steadily increased. In January, Lord Cromer and Lady Sybil
Middleton organised a BRCS unit for Petrograd composed of trained
nurses and VADs and, while Cantlie directed his attention towards
providing an adequate supply of the latter, Mr Stanley turned his mind
towards the establishment of the proposed College of Nursing. On 15
January and 19 February the *British Journal of Nursing* claimed
meetings had taken place at the end of 1915 between the Joint War
Committee and matrons of London hospitals to discuss state regis-

tration and the need for centralised examinations. This was denied, but on 8 January Mrs Bedford Fenwick, President of the National Council for Trained Nurses, replied to Mr Stanley's suggestions concerning the proposed College, that her Committee would consider his letter at their next meeting. Like Miss Nightingale, Mrs Bedford Fenwick was imbued with energy and strong ideas about nursing, wanting a certificated, well trained, intelligent, state registered profession (for which she had started the British Nursing Association), whereas Miss Nightingale thought women of lesser intelligence made good nurses and was not as anxious to see state registration. The BNA was given a Royal Charter and Princess Christian accepted its Presidency, but later Mrs Bedford Fenwick was voted off its Executive and started the Society for State Registration, of which Lord Ampthill became President. On 15 January, in the *British Journal of Nursing*, she criticised St Thomas's Hospital and the Nightingale School for pushing teaching standards rather than state registration and next day, according to the diary, Mr Stanley came to see Cantlie and 'They devised the Nursing College as part of the College of Ambulance. Mr. Stanley is still very keen on the College as a V.A.D. building. They had a long talk on Red Cross work. The difficulty will be when the war is over.' Stanley and Cantlie both realised that without state registration for the nurses the position of VADs, vulnerable as it was in war, would be yet more fragile in peace. Cantlie always went with the current, if it took him in the right general direction, hoping he could paddle himself across into a side stream where he could achieve, together with the main purpose, the original aim with which he had set out. A College of Nursing, promoted by the Chairman of Red Cross and supported by the College of Ambulance, would surely provide the unity sought by all. Had Mr Stanley and Miss Swift, Matron-in-chief, BRCS, not played this vital role in founding the College of Nursing and had the College of Ambulance not given it support and accommodation in the early stages, perhaps the unity of purpose between the nursing profession and Red Cross, which has grown and blossomed ever since, might never have taken root. Although the teaching centre for the voluntary aid societies remained a dream, there were now Joint VAD Committees with Lady Airlie and Lady Ampthill as members, both of whom were life-long friends of the nurses and VADs. Not only this; Devonshire House was soon to open a VAD Club which, funded generously by Lady Cowdray, would move to permanent premises in Cavendish Square. No one could have then foreseen that the College of Ambulance, perishing in the aftermath of the war, would not be revived or that future generations would still have no centralised teaching establishment for instruction in the science of first aid.

It was fortunate for Mr Stanley that his brother, Lord Derby, later Secretary of State for War, set an example of diplomacy and flexibility, for everyone spoke with different voices. The doctors were encouraging and the *Lancet* in January said the College of Nursing promoters were chairmen and governors of leading hospitals and physicians and surgeons who lectured to nurses. The matrons of London hospitals

were mostly in favour, but many nursing societies wanted state registration first. The VADs hoped the College would look kindly upon
them and the Poor Law nurses were pressing for the same pay as the
VAD allowances. On 22 January the *BJN* asked who was behind the
scheme, for, although not allowed to divulge names, it could assure its
readers they were people in administrative positions of importance
'who have the interests of the nursing profession very much at heart' –
nurses would have more confidence if the promoters' names could be
published. The article said the London matrons saw in the idea a
united nursing profession and a way of helping those who 'have
worked so ungrudgingly and loyally as helpers to nurse in military
hospitals' – in other words, the VADs. On 29 January the paper
recommended the Australian scheme started by Lady Helen Munro
Ferguson, with an equal balance of medical men, matrons and nurses
on the council. On 15 February Mr Stanley read a paper on nursing
training to nurses and their representatives who requested further
information before a second meeting, at which he was again
questioned about who was behind the plan. The nurses were convinced
that it was someone in the ambulance movement – 'Was it Lord
Knutsford?' The *Nursing Times*, meanwhile, remained optimistic,
saying the College was finding support among the profession and on 4
March it published a statement of the College aims, 'To promote the
better education and training of nurses by encouraging uniformity of
curriculum'. Certificates would be given for passing centralised
examinations after training and to students trained and examined in
recognised nursing schools. The College would keep a register of
qualified nurses. Two thirds of the first nominated council were to be
matrons and nurses, the other third men and women with medical or
administrative backgrounds, but the government of the College would
ultimately rest with the nurses, since membership would be confined to
those registered and vacancies on the council would be filled by
members' votes. There was to be a consultative board of both doctors
and nurses and an examination board. The College would also concern
itself with relations between nurses and VADs. Mrs Bedford Fenwick,
on hearing this read out, called again for information, 'Who was the
Committee? Who drafted the statement?' But Miss Cox Davies, Matron
of the Royal Free, who, together with Sir Cooper Perry of Guy's, the
Matron of St Thomas's and others had been asked by Mr Stanley to
help in founding the College, suceeded in a plea for unity, for already
the guns of Verdun were rumbling. Yet on 6 March, the Society for
State Registration again told Mr Stanley that they wanted state registration before further facilities for education.

It was a controversial scene, but one in which the seriousness of the
international situation prevented disunity, for meanwhile the breakdown in medical services which everyone had dreaded and prevented
in France and Belgium had taken place in Mesopotamia. Mabel Cantlie
reported in her diary on 16 March: 'There has been a breakdown of
medical services in Mesopotamia. It is a shame when we have plenty of
men and women to go. I wrote to Mrs. Furse two days ago, asking her to

get women out. It is always the same. We are ever late.' The Joint War Committee had, in fact, offered help to the Indian Government, responsible for Mesopotamia, but offers had been refused. Now the Secretary of State for India requested that a Commission, which included Sir Aurelian Ridsdale, former BRCS Chairman, be dispatched to Mesopotamia, where it reported that a serious shortage of medical personnel, ambulances and river transport had been mainly responsible for the suffering of the wounded. Two months later on 13 May *The Times*, commenting on the report of the Vincent Bingley Commission, said that at the Battle of Ctesiphon there was 'no means at all for the treatment of the men actually wounded . . . There was no shelter on the boats where the men were soaked to the skin; hundreds of wounded were sent down under one doctor with no orderlies; wounds were left undressed for days after the application of the first field dressing; many were dying from dysentery and exposure.' The report said no blame attached to the doctors, who were attempting the impossible; there were not enough of them, nor enough of other medical personnel or supplies. 'We cannot afford to sacrifice lives to muddle and inefficiency in organisation.' The need for training, unity and recruits was never more dramatically highlighted, nor the danger of wider outbreaks of tropical and other related diseases. In Serbia people were dying from typhus and typhoid in the streets. In April Charing Cross, in view of these pressures, appointed Cantlie Lecturer in Tropical Diseases.

The tragedy in Mesopotamia united those working for the wounded in a way that nothing else could do. Mr Chapple, MP, a member of the RBNA and the Society for State Registration and a keen critic of the College of Nursing, said he would back Stanley's efforts to found such a centre and at a meeting in Edinburgh chaired by Lady Susan Gilmour, Lady Ampthill's sister, and attended by Sir Joseph Fayrer,[6] a Scottish branch of the College of Nursing was founded. On 27 March the College of Nursing was registered, and on 7 April the first Council met at 83 Pall Mall with Stanley in the chair, when the Minutes report Cantlie present as a member. At his proposal Lady Helen Munro-Ferguson was asked to become a Vice President. Five provincial hospitals were represented on the Council: Bristol, Birmingham, Manchester, Leicester, Ashton-under-Lyne; and, in Scotland, the infirmaries of Edinburgh and Glasgow. The London hospitals represented were the Royal Free, Guy's, St Bartholomew's, St Thomas's, King's College, Whitechapel Infirmary and Chelsea Royal Infirmary. Charing Cross was represented by Cantlie who was appointed to three committees: Education, Establishment and General Purposes, and the Registration Committee, whose task it was to submit to the Council approved nursing training schools which would nominate members to the Consultative Board. The other three London hospitals closely identified with the ambulance movement and the Order of St John, whose history of nursing went back to the Middle Ages, were not represented on the Council – St Mary's, University College and the London – and, this being pointed out, an invitation was extended to

Lord Knutsford, Chairman of the London Hospital, original Vice Chairman, BRCS, and a Knight of Justice of St John. With the College firmly founded it seemed the rocks lay behind, but the critics remained intransigent. The National Union of Trained Nurses saw 'the grant of a licence to the College as premature', and those who feared it might be a back door entry to the profession for VADs interrupted a speech of Stanley's so that he had to alter his description of VAD training in the middle of a sentence. Cantlie again extended the olive branch, offering the College free accommodation in the College of Ambulance. This was not at first taken up because Mr Boyton lent them 6 Vere Street, but nine months later the College of Nursing moved into part of the top floor of the College of Ambulance, where Cantlie gave it free heat and light.

1916 had been a year of few joys and many sorrows. Death was in the air, and the nation was united in a stoic acceptance of suffering. During it Colin had won the DSC, but when his parents congratulated him he made his only request of the war, 'and all he asks for,' says the diary, 'is toothpaste'. Keith, in training now with a mixed nationality Labour Battalion destined for Mesopotamia, wrote home repeatedly for dictionaries and grammars in many languages in order to converse with his men. Neil was in the trenches 'with shot and shell whizzing over his head – and all he asks for is chocolate', and dry fresh socks to avoid trench foot and cakes and sweet things, perhaps to stave off the many forms of nervous collapse which went by the description of shell shock. Mabel Cantlie's own health was deteriorating and money was short. When her husband brought her sole for her digestion she commented, 'I must get well at once, I cannot afford to be ill at that price'. Only in her diary did she confide that by the end of 1916 she wondered if she too 'might have passed the portals of death'. It was the courage of the wounded men and the cheerfulness of the chronically sick and disabled which kept up the spirits of the volunteers. No. 1 VAD had, since the start of the war, taken limbless patients from Roehampton on sight-seeing tours round London and now, at the King's invitation, they went to Windsor Castle. 'Our men will never forget,' wrote Mr Evans of No. 1 VAD, 'the impression which these limbless men created wherever they went.' Concerts for the wounded and disabled had become a feature of voluntary work all over the country. Marylebone Division, Red Cross, gave entertainments at the College of Ambulance and, with St John, at the Regent Street Polytechnic where artistes from the Palladium sang to the soldiers. At a Christmas party for orphans of the war, Cantlie again played his role of Father Christmas. Firms such as Harrods and Whiteleys lent their grounds for functions and gave the 'props' for sports and games. The most moving party of all was at Whiteley's Recreation Ground, Wembley, for the blind, where the men gamely entered into all the competitions: golf, trimming hats, football and blowing soap bubbles. The diary says that at the concert after-wards, 'Mr. Andrews of Roehampton spoke so charmingly of H and all the Red Cross work he had done. It was from the heart and made one shed tears of joy.'

In March the King had again shown his deep concern for the care and transport of the wounded by inspecting the Ambulance Column, London District, at Buckingham Palace and the King and Queen had given great impetus to the entertainment of the disabled and wounded by holding a series of concerts there. On 19 March and again on the 23rd the diary records, 'H to Buckingham Palace to rehearse for a concert for wounded men', and 'H to Buckingham Palace, where the King and Queen entertained 1000 wounded soldiers, our men helped them. Queen Alexandra there. The concert sang Loch Lomond.' Mr Rowe of No. 1 VAD described the occasion: 'It had been announced that the King proposed to entertain 3000 wounded sailors and soldiers, the entertainment to take place on three successive days in March. We were of course delighted to hear that our Detachment had again been selected.' Having attended the rehearsal, after which they were shown the Royal Stables and the King's horse Delhi who, it was explained, would never have caused the accident if he had been taken to France, the Detachment reported at Buckingham Palace to attend the cases from Roehampton during the entertainment.

> I was helping one of my cases to get more comfrotable in his wheeled chair when I heard a voice behind me asking, 'How are you getting on?' It was the King, who had come in absolutely unannounced and was walking between the tables talking to his guests. A minute or two afterwards the Queen arrived at our table and was evidently very desirous that the men should have everything they wanted. Queen Alexandra followed, attended by Sir Dighton Probyn. The latter seemed very anxious that Queen Alexandra should not tire herself, but when he suggested she might rest for a moment, Her Majesty laughingly replied, 'Now, do be quiet, I am quite all right.' Prince Albert was very busy running round with a teapot, and on one occasion when he nearly collided with Lord Charles Beresford, I thought the contents of the teapot would find their way into the Admiral's pocket.

The patients included special spinal cases and many who were up for the first time and had to be wheeled in a wheelchair. At the second of these entertainments one of the wheelchairs assigned to the unit disappeared and reappeared with Queen Alexandra being given a ride by Mr Smith, the pharmacist, telling him to mind the bumps. 'After seeing the patients comfortably fixed up in their various conveyances,' said Mr Rowe, 'I left, feeling absolutely tired out, but having thoroughly enjoyed the most perfectly managed entertainment I ever attended. Even after it was all over, it was impossible to think of one single thing which had been omitted.'[7]

CHAPTER SEVENTEEN
The Tide of Suffering

By now the tentacles of war were speedily drawing in fresh areas of conflict all over the world, and the situation in the Far East was daily becoming more complex and dangerous. Early in 1914 Yuan Shik-Kai had made further moves towards militarist dictatorship and later in the year revived the ceremonies at the altar of heaven. Nevertheless, in May 1915 Britain had supported him in resisting some of the 'Twenty-One Demands' which Japan was forcing on China, for had they all been accepted they would not only have weakened Yuan's position, but would have hopelessly weakened China. On 19 March 1915 Sun Yat Sen had written to the Cantlies warning them of Yuan's pro-German sympathies:

> You can be of great help to me in England by enlightening the public that by helping Yuan Shik-Kai England is indirectly but surely advancing the interests of Germany, for Yuan Shik-Kai is the exact prototype of the Kaiser in his tyrannical attitude and in his greed for power and self-interest. Yuan Shik-Kai is pro German through and through and if Germany comes out victorious in this war, then China will surely become Germany's dependency. England will not only not gain anything by befriending Yuan, but will certainly lose the ground she has already gained in China.[1]

Throughout 1915 Yuan continued to strengthen his own power at the expense of democracy and Parliament and on 1 January 1916 he proclaimed himself Emperor. On 18 January Sun wrote again to the Cantlies, warning them against British support for Yuan:

> The English officials in Hong Kong, Shanghai and Singapore zealously co-operate with Yuan in persecuting our patriots, and act as if they receive orders from Yuan Shik-Kai and not from their Government . . . Such action on the part of English officials here is surely going to bring bad consequences on their Government, for very soon our party, the younger and more progressive elements in China, will get into power. Therefore I beg that you will get those of our friends in the Parliament to bring this subject before the Government as soon as possible, and do so in a forcible and strong way. In the past our people have always looked upon England as a friend and have reciprocated wherever and whenever possible.

Unless such persecutions are stopped and policy changed, henceforth the Chinese peoples cannot help but look upon England in another light. England is doing herself injustice by continuing her persecutions of our patriots and stands as our stumbling block. The English Government should not keep her eyes glued to the present and the temporary, but look farther into the future if she desires friendship and not enmity from the younger generations of China.[2]

By the end of March the revolt against Yuan of which Sun had warned was becoming widespread – Yunnan had taken the lead in declaring its independence and province after province was following in quick succession, so that a rival government was set up in Canton. In June the problem was solved by the death of Yuan and his replacement by the Vice President Li Yuan Hung – also once a Manchu general, who had crossed to the Republicans early in 1911. It was a fortunate change for China and the Allied cause. Cantlie sent Li a telegram of good wishes.

Meanwhile in the West the summer of 1916 was the most crucial of the war. 'The defence of Verdun and the battle of the Somme rank among the greatest achievements of human endurance and the saddest tragedies of human waste.'[3] But although on the face of it little seemed to have changed in ground lost or taken, in reality the balance between the two sides had been tipped in favour of the Allies. When the French held off the attack on Verdun and the outstanding effort of the British on the Somme had died away, 'the old German army, the best trained and most highly skilled body of fighting men which the world had ever seen, was no more'.[4] At the Somme the Germans realised that the British Army was capable in numbers and fire-power not only of standing up to attack but of launching a deadly offensive; and for the first time the British invention, the tank, which played a decisive part in 1918, made a real, if limited, appearance. The diaries record these events. Miss Grenfell, a loyal helper at the College of Ambulance who had lost brothers and cousins, including the poet Julian Grenfell who laid down a gifted life with courage and self sacrifice, heard from a brother at the front that the Germans had lost the initiative and were becoming demoralised. Meanwhile in the heartland of France the toll of human life and destruction of towns and villages was devastating. Describing the aftermath of the battle which had raged round Verdun, the centre of which was a shell, the poet Laurence Binyon wrote in a *Times* article on 14 July, 'Only a strange silence about it presages the hurt within . . . Not a house but is maimed or shattered'. Along the road from Bar-le-Duc to Verdun had roared and rumbled the lorries carrying supplies. 'Today,' said Binyon, 'it was solitary and silent in the windy sunshine. But suddenly, as if from nowhere . . . appeared a single soldier tramping towards Verdun.' The poet described this soldier's spirit of heroism and the gratitude he shared with his fellow *poilus* for the help received from Britain and the Dominions, which strengthened the friendship and liaison between the French and British armies.

That help is inspired by a spirit that has won the heart of the French soldier, because it brings him comradeship and affection beyond and above the material aid. It is the spirit of the volunteer . . . These unpaid Red Cross workers talking to him in his own language have developed an extraordinary respect and love for the simple *poilu*. They have seen him in his time of trial and suffering . . . uncomplaining and cheerful . . . How infinitely France has suffered . . . [her homes and industries broken by] the enemy's devilish will to maim her for an age to come.

Allied medical services were faced with a great variety of shell and bullet wounds of which perhaps the most tragic were the spinal patients, suffering paralysis and threatened with early death. British soldiers went to the Star and Garter Hospital in Richmond where, with a view over the valley, they were given every care. 'He has fought his fight,' said Treves, 'let him feel the loving kindness of the land for which he died is around him when the bugle from afar off summons him to the Last Post.' Gas gangrene remained an intractable enemy, Sir Almroth Wright repeating that the bacillus was carried in 'vegetable and dung' and that 'the presence of foreign bodies is fatal to the speed of infection, even if air is present' – a speed which Sir Anthony Bowlby said could prove fatal in sixteen hours. The need for immediate treatment was emphasised also by a woman doctor serving with the French Army who described how air bubbles and streaks showed up on X-ray, how the proximity of limb to soil increased the danger, that deep-seated shell injuries were six times more prone than bullet wounds and how infected clothing carried the microbes. Cantlie always stressed the importance of keeping free from lice to allay all infection. Trench fever, a form of relapsing fever, was certainly spread by lice and he believed that the infection-by-soil theory in gas gangrene in no way discounted transmission by lice. Trench foot, however, was caused by wet and cold and treatment included experiments with oxygen passing through an ozoniser to increase the supply of blood, kill any germs and form oxyhaemoglobin, while prevention lay in keeping feet dry and warm with fresh socks, rubber boots, oiled silk or other material soaked in linseed oil. Other wounds demanding immediate operation and treatment were those of the abdomen because of the risk of haemorrhage, and these reacted least favourably to the bumping horse ambulances still used on bad roads. Nor were all sicknesses of external origin; adrenalin exhaustion following upon the strains of battle meant that otherwise fit men had to be withdrawn temporarily or permanently from the trenches, the deficiency resulting in lack of vascular tension, with irregular heart function, lack of hearing and other nerve sensory reaction, all loosely called shell shock. Doctors stressed the importance of lessening shock for all desperately wounded and ill patients far from home and friends, frozen, hungry, suffering from loss of blood and thrown temporarily off balance. 'It is,' said one press report, 'a wonderful comment on the backbone of the nation that the patients were all so cheerful . . . The cheapest remedy is hope.' 'The inclination,' said Cantlie in the *Journal of Tropical Medicine*, after his return from France, 'in approaching one of these men is not to speak, but just to sit beside him asking no questions, a sacred silence, for these men have in defence of hearths and homes but recently faced death.'[5] 'It can only be hoped,' he commented elsewhere in the *Journal*, 'that new medical facts will emerge from the horrors of war.' 'In spite of wounds,' said the RAMC *Journal* in July 1916, 'nearly all of them are asleep. There they lie on stretchers with muddy or wet clothes, bandaged limbs or head. Some ask for food. Only a few are excited. Many who are asleep are suffering from profound collapse.' It was essential to keep them warm, persuade them to take hot soup or cocoa or sometimes a little alcohol before they dropped off once more into deep exhausted sleep. 'Sometimes the seemingly pulseless men pulled round, they were so nearly dead that it could be several hours before any attempt could be made to dress their wounds.'

There is nothing more demanding on human nature than the giving of courage and the will to live to those who are suffering, and to give it freely with compassion, care, discipline, and love. Doctors were described as 'patient, indefatigable, tender, encouraging and brave'; Army nurses, who with the Reserve had increased their strength from 2,223 in 1914 to 10,404 in 1918, were complimented on their 'tender care, splendid, marvellous untiring energy and unfailing cheerfulness'. Backing them in all places were members of the Voluntary Aid Societies, 'renowned for their cheeriness, good temper, hard work and desire to give every possible help', while the spirit of the VADs was said to be the 'finest thing on earth'. Their voluntary role, as Binyon said, gave them an aura, but nevertheless it also deprived them of a status. Those in military hospitals under six-monthly contracts were paid a minimum of £20 a year, but if in auxiliary hospitals or working for the Allies they received no payment nor proper expenses. Yet their presence was vital in hospital and on lines of communication, for if trained nurses could not stem the tide in 1915, what was to happen at Passchendaele, Vimy Ridge, Amiens and the Third Battle of Ypres? In April 1916, with the threat of an offensive again imminent, Cantlie staged a Red Cross demonstration at the College of Ambulance showing methods of improvised medical aid at the front, and in June he was asked to repeat it at the Economic Exhibition at the Princes Skating Rink. Cantlie was in bed with influenza, and telephoned Mabel Cantlie at Cottered to bring straw ropes and corner props to make beds. She brought the ropes to London and spent the evening filling biscuit tins with gravel to act as corners for the straw rope mattresses. The following day, the diary records, 'The Queen came round and was quite charming. H showed her all his new ideas.' Meanwhile the College of Nursing, installed at 6 Vere Street, was given publicity by the *Nursing Times*, whose reporter was 'whisked into a passage and shown the waste space at the back. "That is where I see it, [said the Secretary] a great building, storey above storey".'[6] That was where Cantlie had seen his BRCS and St John's office to administer a combined teaching

College of Ambulance, but his generosity in laying aside the idea to help to start a College of Nursing was already paying dividends. 'Are the trained nurses doing enough to help the VADs?' asked the June edition of the *Nursing Times*, reflecting a new spirit of co-operation. 'VADs can be quite good nurses in eighteen months.' And again, 'What is this work going to count for when the state register is drawn up?' If a woman who had nursed, said the paper, could qualify by a central examination, she should be entitled to register. Unfortunately this view was far from universal and trade unions now added their voices to those who argued that volunteers were a threat to the labour force. Yet without grading and promotion under proper supervision, which alone could provide them with the hope of having their time counted as part of professional training, it seemed as if it might be impossible to find enough recruits.

At the end of June, with the Battle of the Somme imminent, Lord Ranfurley and Mr Stanley appealed for volunteers for St John and the BRCS and in July came a rush of wounded. 'H's men were unloading wounded all night,' the diary records. 'One of our men told me they had transported 9991 stretcher cases and 9792 walking cases during July – 362 bearers.' But in the same month she commented, 'V.A.D.s are becoming very difficult to obtain. I had a talk with Mrs. Cave, Devonshire House about my members at Netley. They are being used for scrubbing, when, after 14 months probation, they ought to be nursing. I need more recruits.' According to BRCS records at the Imperial War Museum, the idea of grading VADs had been suggested by the War Office in February 1916, but it had lapsed. On 29 July *The Times* put forward the idea again, 'It is imperative to advance the voluntary workers who have gained experience and so relieve the fully trained.' Instead the War Office, relying on a short war, reacted to the crisis by cutting VAD contracts from six to three months, following the lead of the civil hospitals who were providing three-month courses for probationers, and introduced Special Service Probationers who needed no first aid and nursing certificates at all. This cut across what the College of Ambulance stood for, the supply of qualified, experienced VADs. Understanding their disappointment and fears for the supply of nurses, 'Kind hearts at the College, mostly Quakers, I believe', presented the Cantlies with a motor car, for which Mabel Cantlie had constantly prayed, 'a small one now,' the diary says, 'a larger one to follow'. The Quakers, like the Indian students, had taken every advantage of the specialised training in the College. As well as training at Jordan, where Cantlie also lectured, their students had done a nine-hour day at the College for six weeks and in this way the Society had trained 1,180 volunteers by 1916, many of whom were in France, where the Humanitarian Corps helped to supply them with medical stores and food. Official Red Cross history was warm in its praise: 'Perhaps no class of volunteers did more to strengthen mutual understanding and respect between the Allies than these. In parts of the country devoid of the ordinary medical practitioners, these services could not be appraised too highly and in this particular field the Friends Ambulance Unit was conspicuous and civilians as well as soldiers benefited.'

Support also came from the RAMC. On 12 August Sir Alfred Keogh, DGAMS, wrote to *The Times* inviting reporters to visit London military hospitals and see the debt the public owed to modern surgery and surgeons, of which people had a wholly inadequate idea. On the 17th the RAMC invited Cantlie, Hon. Colonel RAMC(T), to France. He was met by Neil at Boulogne, stayed with him at 2nd Army Headquarters at Hazebrouck, visited a casualty clearing station in a Trappist Monastery, casualty clearing stations at Vimy, field ambulances at Poperinghe and Vlamertinghe; then to Ypres, where he saw field hospitals, rest stations and casualty clearing stations. Then he went on to 1st Army Head-quarters at Hesdin where he stayed, dining with Sir Arthur Sloggett, DGAMS in France, and so returned via St John's Hospital, Étaples, where he visited his bed and saw the chapel donated by Lady Strath-cona, an active member of the College of Ambulance and Humani-tarian Corps, and the harmonium presented by Lady Mountstephen. While Cantlie was away two articles appeared in *The Times*.[7] The first was on British women volunteers in France, including drivers, mes-sengers and workers in canteens, whose Corps Mabel Cantlie had helped to form, singling out in particular the underground canteen in the Gare du Nord, with baths and rest facilities, a luxurious replica of the station canteens for which she had worked so hard. The second article, on Queen Mary's Hospital, Roehampton, with which No. 1 VAD was associated, described the manufacture at the hospital of the patients' limbs with the help of five British and two American firms – an idea practised at the King Albert I Hospital, Rouen, where the soldiers helped to make their own – and the running of an employment bureau. The hospital was, said *The Times*, 'the crowning wonder of the war'.

While much was being done, therefore, to aid the ambulance movement to overcome its difficulties in finding voluntary recruits, Mr Stanley was also running into problems over questions of entitlement of trained nurses to register with the College of Nursing and to elect members to the proposed General Nursing Council, which was delay-ing amalgamation with nursing associations. Not only were specialist nurses – fever, mental and children's (as well as VADs) – posing a problem, but Poor Law Nurses (with 94,000 beds out of a total of 178,000) felt they were under-represented on the Council and in this they were supported by Princess Christian and by Cantlie, who had seen their good work at Kingston Infirmary, where he examined in first aid. In August the College of Nursing published its aims to reassure the profession: to organise and promote the advancement of the nursing profession, state registration and standards of training, with a uniform curriculum, one examination and headquarters in London. Proposed conditions during a period of grace included those of age, good character, a certificate of three-year training from a nurses' training college recognised by the Council, or a certificate of two years' training, followed by two years' bona fide practice as a nurse, or evidence of training to the satisfaction of the Council (before 1899), followed by five years' bona fide practice as a nurse. It was a bridge across a river, too broad for some and too narrow for others. The leaflet did much to publicise nursing, reassure the profession and draw in recruits, but the shortage of VADs was almost more critical and they could draw little hope from this statement. Dame Katherine Furse had 500 places that she could not fill: 'Are the wounded going to remain neglected,' she asked, 'because there is no one to nurse them?'

At the beginning of September the King, who was on a visit to France, focused attention on the need for succouring the sick and wounded, and on the 16th Lloyd George set up a Committee consisting of Mr Bridgeman, MP, Lord Commissioner of the Treasury, Lord Knutsford and Sir Frederick Treves, Captain Boulton, Chairman of the Queen Victoria Jubilee Institute of Nurses (one of the first bodies to press for state registration), and Dame Katherine Furse, Commandant-in-Chief, BRCS, 'to consider the existing system of training nurses for hospitals for sick and wounded soldiers at home and abroad and to make such recommendations as they consider necessary'. 'The services rendered by nurses during the war,' said *The Times* in its editorial of the same day,

has added the lustre to a noble calling. We rejoice therefore that certain difficulties that have arisen are about to be the subject of consideration. A large body of women have become nurses in the last two years and . . . are anxious to remain in the ranks. These new recruits have not yet received the full three years' training which is considered essential by the great hospitals and therefore in some cases friction has arisen between them and the fully certificated nurses. This was inevitable but it has produced a situation of some delicacy and has, to a certain extent, curtailed the supply. A more important matter is the future of these voluntary nurses. Surgeons and doctors who have had V.A.D. members working under them in military hospitals make no secret of their desire to employ them after the war. They are very good material, yet it is clear that most of them will resent having to start on a three years' training after having done a year or more in a military hospital. It is suggested that the civil hospitals should allow probationers who have served in military hospitals to count part of their time in these hospitals towards a general training. This would be a great inducement to women to begin training as war nurses. While the scheme for the College of Nursing advocated by Mr. A. Stanley has opponents there are reasons for believing it is a step in the right direction. There is the further question of registration which would at least prevent the nurses' uniform being used by the unworthy.

On the same day Mabel Cantlie followed this editorial up with a letter to Sir Frederick Treves, asking for some remission from training for VADs who had nursed for three years in military hospitals. And, also on the same day, the Belgians conferred on her the Order of Elizabeth in recognition of the work she had done for their wounded soldiers and refugees, particularly in the King Albert I Hospital, where full use had been made of VADs working under trained nurses. The whole question had now come out into the open, with the ambulance movement, supported by people in prominent medical positions, pointing out that it was impossible to maintain the supply of VADs if they had no grades or proper nursing status and one day might be doing domestic work and another acting as staff nurses in wards of seriously ill patients, as the wounded poured in from the front. *The Red Cross* journal called for an intermediary role for the partially trained, suggesting more frequent transfers from critical to intermediate stages of nursing, rather than the patient passing through only two, hospital and convalescent. (These three stages of nursing, intensive, ordinary and convalescent, have now been accepted, as has also the concept of 'practical' or 'enrolled' nurse.) Underneath its editorial on nursing and VADs *The Times* printed a poignant poem,

> But Thou has done well leaving me with the humble,
> Whose doom it is to suffer and bear the burden of power . . .
> For every throb of their pain
> Has pulsed in the secret depth of Thy night,
> And every insult has been gathered in Thy great silence,
> And the morrow is theirs.

The morrow, however, proved little better, for by the time the College of Nursing Council met on 21 September the trained nurses were up in arms about the choice of Committee members, feeling themselves under-represented. The National Council of Trained Nurses, early into Belgium in 1914, had asked then for the DGAMS to set up such a committee and the regular and reserve naval and army nurses had answered every call made upon them. The Council bowed before the storm and wrote to Lloyd George, saying that it questioned if the appointment of the Committee was opportune: 'The Committee, as announced, is not such as to command the confidence of the nursing profession and the trained nurses look upon its appointment as a slight, while the Matrons have shown a willingness to co-operate with the Army Nursing Board'. Next day a representative of the Army Nursing Board, set up by Royal Charter to advise the Secretary of State, was appointed to the Committee. Cantlie was present at the meeting at which the letter was drafted; he knew it was vital not to alienate the nursing profession, but he disliked controversy and greatly respected both Lord Knutsford and Sir Frederick Treves. In future Cantlie only attended College of Nursing meetings when he had something to report, such as when giving his findings as a representative of the Poor Law Nurses Association. But five months later he gave the College accommodation in the College of Ambulance and on 10 February 1917 the diary reads, 'We have finished the partition for the College of Nursing on the top floor. I expect the Secretary will come on Monday.' Lord Knutsford withdrew at once from the Committee, followed by Sir Frederick. Matrons, nurses and others concerned with nursing were appointed and the brief was changed, 'to ascertain the resources of the country in trained nurses and women partially trained in nursing, so as to suggest the most economical method of utilising their services for civil and military purposes'.[8] The new members included Lady Airlie, Mrs Becher, Matron-in-Chief, QAIMNS, Miss Sidney Browne, Matron-in-Chief, Territorial Forces' Nursing Association, and the matrons of many leading hospitals. While they deliberated, the College of Nursing worked to get agreement with other nursing associations about elections to a General Nursing Council which, in spite of temporary failure, did result in one meeting of the first National Council, of which Sir James Crichton Browne, an old friend of Cantlie who had pressed upon the Select Committee of 1905 the need for state registration, was a member. By the following month trained nurses were almost impossible to obtain and in view of this the College, having failed to get agreement, decided to present its own Bill. Stanley issued a statement, saying that the birth of the College and the achievement of state registration would be a 'worthy memorial to the countless women who have served their country in our hospitals at home and abroad often at the cost of health and too often of life itself'. Cantlie, who was a signatory, saw both these aims as first priorities, after which he hoped to put the College of Ambulance on to a permanent basis and to secure recognition of nursing time for experienced VADs. Thus on 7 December the Minutes of the College of Nursing record that the Registration Committee, of which he was a member, added the following conditions for registration during a period of grace: 'In deciding upon applications of candidates, whose training does not fulfil the above conditions, the Council may have regard to exceptional experience obtained subsequent to qualification or to professional status'. The wording of this was sufficiently vague to cover both VADs and children's nurses, the fever nurses having been recognised in October.

What above all the ambulance movement did not wish to sever was its link with the consultant surgeons, which Sir Alfred Keogh had stressed, nor to abandon the principle that, with training, a high standard of professionalism could be achieved in first aid and nursing by lay volunteers. St John Ambulance Association thus chose this time to sanction war-time demonstrator certificates to lay teachers of its Brigade members and VADs and Sir Alfred Keogh directed each hospital district at the front to have a consulting surgeon to sanction major operations. The ambulance movement believed first aid was a science of its own whose links were with the casualty departments of civilian hospitals and the casualty clearing stations at the front. (It is to the credit of the nurses that whereas first aid is still not included in the curriculum of medical students, it is now part of the training of student nurses.) In the gloomy winter of 1916–17 the gravity of the crisis of how to succour the wounded brought the people of the nation closer together – the RBNA ratified its amalgamation with the College of Nursing and the *Nursing Times* demanded that the newly appointed Nursing Committee should be frank in its assessment of the crisis. 'If we have really come to the end of the supply of trained nurses let the Committee be frank enough to say so.' Then, in January 1917, came a London disaster which brought home to everyone the horror of high explosives and the need, in Lord Knutsford's words, to get 'some' training into more people – the Silvertown munitions works blew up. 'Just after tea,' says the diary,

> we heard a fearful sound of explosion which blew open our hall door. Then we heard about ten o'clock that an ammunition works had blown up at Silvertown. So H and I went down in a hansom cab, no taxi could be got, to the Albert Docks Hospital. Many fearful casualties were brought in there, but they only took the worst. Some were burned. Some were blown up terribly. The poor things were dying in the wards as we stood there. Fires were burning. Houses were wrecked all round.

The disaster highlighted the need for emergency training and skilled volunteers working under professional supervision. A month later Lloyd George's Committee concluded its findings, although the report was not officially published until later in the year. The press welcomed the recommendations on hostels, increments, pensions for nurses, increased allowances for VADs and better arrangements for accommodation, but commented that the only substantially constructive suggestion was that VADs should be graded after thirteen months. There was a feeling that the Committee had identified the problem but not solved it and in order to identify herself with the difficulties faced by her VADs Mabel Cantlie had gone to a hospital where they were employed and washed up with them from 8.00 a.m. to 3.00 p.m. A fortnight later, with letters appearing in *The Times* about the poor conditions under which they were working, the diary records that a visit was to be made by Princess Christian to the College of Ambulance. It acted like a tonic and, strengthened by this support, Mabel Cantlie visited Colonel Bates, Director, County of London BRCS, and told him that her VADs were on night duty for too long hours with too many patients.

All this while the war was becoming increasingly international and entering a yet more dangerous phase, with consequent anxiety about the safety of the wounded. While the Allies had been offering stern resistance in the west the Germans had taken 450,000 Russian prisoners in ten weeks, and, with Rumania coming to Russia's help, had entered Bucharest at the end of 1916, commanding an area rich in corn, oil and natural resourses. The discord the Germans had sown in Russia was now reaping its harvest, and Europe was astounded to read that the Czar had abdicated for himself and his son, and on 17 March there was no news of where the Czar or his family were. Meanwhile in China the situation hung in the balance. On 11 March the diary records, 'China enters the Entente'. Certainly the National Assembly was in favour of so doing, but Sun, appointed High Adviser to Li Yuan Hung, feared the additional strain that war would impose on the fledgling democracy and telegraphed his fears to Lloyd George, while Li demurred and did not sign the papers. Sun was right; German gold, working through the banks, had been doing its work and a military coup came two months later. The dangers in the spring of 1917 were of a weakened Russia, with consequent German increased strength on the Western front, and, although German interference in peaceful shipping with her U-boats and her intrigues in Mexico were soon to provoke an American declaration of war, for the moment the skies were dark indeed. It was against this background that Lord Derby made an appeal in the Albert Hall for ten times the number of VADs and Dame Katherine Furse said in the columns of *The Red Cross*, 'Someone has to do the drudgery, and you, with your experience and training, do it so much better than the raw recruit'. In another column of the same journal, however, came the familiar question, 'What is going to happen to V.A.D.s at the end of the war, are they going to be cast off like old shoes?' On 13 April, while Cantlie was again trying to interest St John's men in the teaching facilities of the College with personally conducted demonstrations, *The Times* was exhorting women to come forward as VADs despite the lack of salary: 'It must be faced . . . the vacancies among the nurses must be made good at once. Our soldiers must be nursed and we know that there are hundreds of women who will come forward willingly and gladly when once the need is known.' But exhortation does not have the same appeal as example. The next day Princess Christian visited the College of Ambulance, and both *The Red Cross* and St John's magazine *First Aid* reported, 'Princess Christian visited the College of Ambulance and witnessed a display of ambulance work given by No. 1 London V.A.D. of the Society. H.R.H., who was received by the President and Principal of the College, Sir Rickman Godlee and Colonel James Cantlie, first inspected a transport section of 50 cars and 4 ambulances and visited the Museum before proceeding to the large hall where the display was given. The display consisted of stretcher drill for men and women.' Following the display, Sir Rickman Godlee asked Princess Christian to accept the first certificate of Honorary Fellowship of the College and the Princess, in turn, made similar awards, on behalf of the College and the Humanitarian Corps, to a number of distinguished men and women, including members of both Voluntary Aid Societies.

Again the ambulance movement took heart. The letters which continued to appear in *The Times* about the VADs, claiming they were being given more to do in a morning than three servants in a day – 'Girls should not be asked to perform these duties in such unnecessarily long hours of work'[9] – culminated in a letter on 30 April from 'Observer' calling for some form of promotion for voluntary nurses. The nursing profession, the writer said, 'has recruited the best and most highly principled of our womanhood and it is losing these recruits for both the duration of the war and for service in years to come by a policy at once short sighted and unconstructive'. The editorial of the same day referred to them as a 'very important reserve of strength' who had received a nursing training extending over a period of years (many had trained for many months in civilian hospitals prior to service) and 'proved their vocation under a searching test, yet official promotion is denied to them'. It suggested that army nurses be recruited from VADs as a means of ending a 'blind alley' occupation, while not jeopardising the position of the professional nurse. The next day Mabel Cantlie wrote an outspoken letter to *The Times*:

> Your leading article today draws my attention to what is proving a detriment to the enthusiasm of women who offer themselves to help in hospitals. It has been a great privilege to deal with many hundreds of women since the commencement of the war who have joined the Voluntary Aid Detachments. At present my own is 500 strong, so I speak with some experience. A great number of our members have become excellently trained and act as staff nurses. I am most anxious that their services should be at present and after the war retained to augment the supply of nurses necessary for the well-being of our nation. The prospect at present of years of devotion to hospital work leads, as your article says, to nothing but a blind alley occupation. Surely the doctors and matrons could meet and devise a scheme whereby the experience these women have gained may be retained and employed in the future.

The Cantlies knew that the proportion of VADs wishing to nurse after the war would not be high, so that, war-time recruiting apart, it was a pity to lose so many nurses from the profession, particularly since after the war the understaffing in the Poor Law hospitals and among the district nurses would be unacceptable. Mabel Cantlie's letter received much support, but it provoked some nurses to anger. She was by now a sick woman, although her remarkable self discipline disguised her sufferings. To take up such a controversial cause was a drain on her reserves of energy, but she saw it as her duty. Two days later, 'I am feeling very weak and have come home quite collapsed'. Then, with no break, 'Painted five baths. 143 wounded to tea in the afternoon in the College. Blind men. Men without legs. How awful it is, but how cheery they are.' It was the courage, hope and cheerfulness of these wounded and disabled men which set an example of resilience to those concerned with their welfare, and the constant thought of their loved ones in danger which inspired them to carry on. On the following day, 'Neil came home to our joy', then 'Turning feather beds into 32 pillows.'

With the Red Cross and St John taking an increased interest again in the College, Cantlie gave a demonstration there to the medical profession on 10 May reported in the journals of both voluntary societies in June:

> Colonel James Cantlie gave an interesting and instructive display of ambulance work before a large audience of medical men and their friends – Sir James Crichton Browne and Sir James Porter. [Porter was actually the young man whom Cantlie had taken a hansom cab to coach before his entrance to the navy.] Cantlie demonstrated the

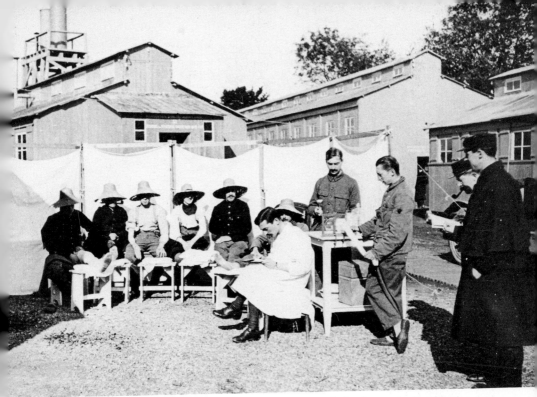

The King Albert I Hospital, Rouen. Healing wounds in the open air. (*Musée Royal de l'Armée et d'Histoire Militaire*)

The King Albert I Hospital, Rouen. Treatment by warm running water. (*Musée Royal de l'Armée et d'Histoire Militaire*)

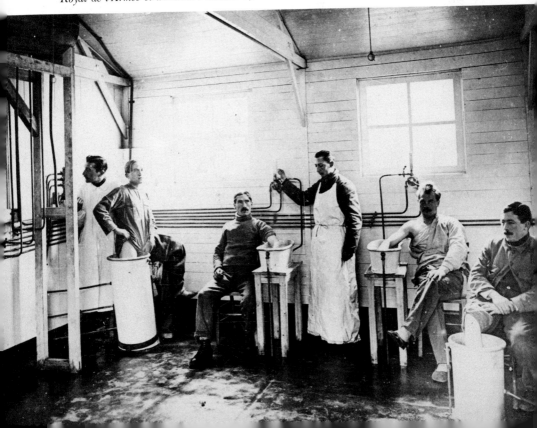

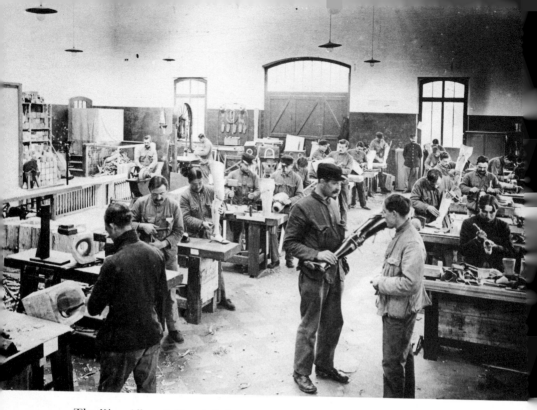

The King Albert I Hospital, Rouen. Patients making their own limbs. (*Musée Royal de l'Armée et d'Histoire Militaire*)

HM Queen Mary visiting a hutted hospital in France, July 1917. In the picture Red Cross and St John nurses and ambulance drivers. The Queen visited British, Commonwealth and Allied Hospitals, including St John Hospital, Étaples, and the King Albert I Hospital, then moved to Bon Secours. (*Imperial War Museum*)

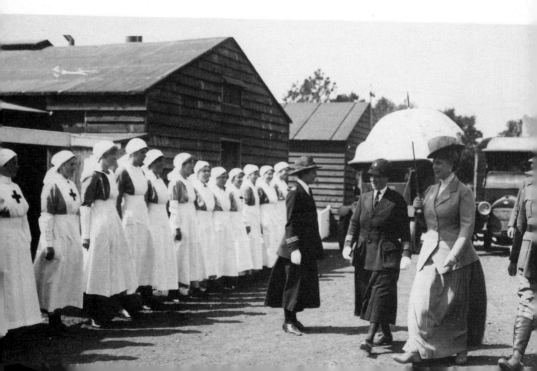

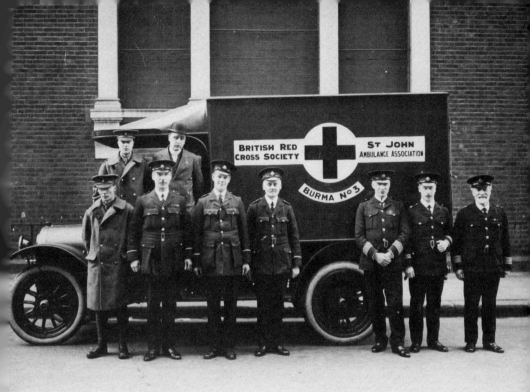

The Ambulance and Stretcher Party which conveyed the King in 1915. James Cantlie on the right. The ambulance was a gift from the Ladies of Burma. (*The Polytechnic of Central London*)

One of the later ambulance trains in action with attending Army Medical Service. A Casualty Clearing Station in France. (*The Imperial War Museum*)

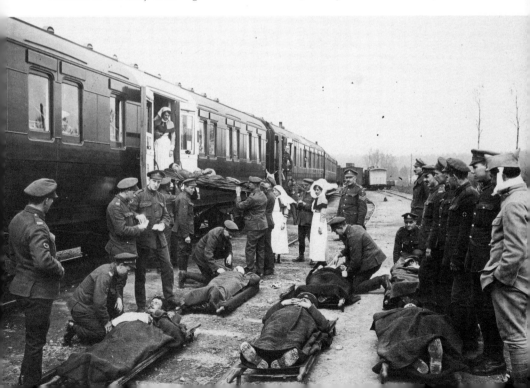

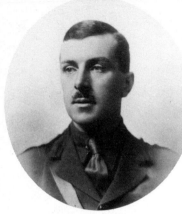

Sir Keith Cantlie.

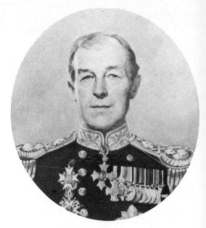

Admiral Sir Colin Cantlie.

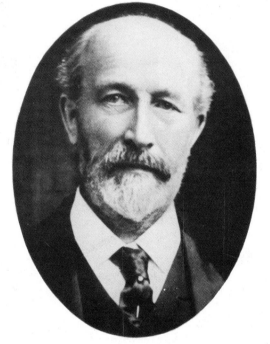

Sir James Cantlie.

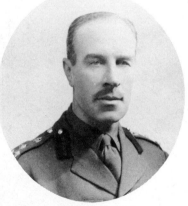

Lt General Sir Neil Cantlie.

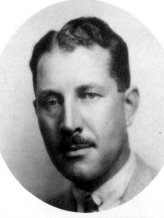

Lt Colonel Kenneth Cantlie.

transport of wounded men from battlefield to hospital ship by means of a magnificent model, occupying the whole length of the museum. V.A.D.s demonstrated loading, unloading stretchers from trains etc.

The Scott Cantlie sling was on display, along with Cantlie's invention of the bullet-proof bearer's shield. Three days later Mr Percy Harris, MP, visited the College and suggested that Cantlie should teach first aid to the Territorial Army as was done in Canada, where nearly a quarter of a million copies of Cantlie's *First Aid Manual* in English and French had been sold, while in the British Army the idea was still experimental. Just as it seemed, however, that the nation was heeding the warning to get some training into more people to stem the tide of suffering, a *Times* letter of 14 May criticised nursing volunteers and landed a snide under-cut at hutted hospitals with which the ambulance movement had been particularly identified. The writer compared VADs 'to the very excellent war huts, temporary structures, most efficient for their specific purpose, but necessarily roughly equipped and inadequately supplied and built on a shallow foundation that can have no permanent stability . . . VADs have scant knowledge of medical diseases . . . They should submit to training and thus maintain the prestige of British nursing and the ideals of Florence Nightingale.' Certainly it was true that VADs in military hospitals had less knowledge of medical than surgical nursing, but fever and children's nurses were equally special-ised, one recognised, the other not. Four days later 'Observer' answered, pointing out that civilian nurses were not ideal at the front, 'some huts have fundamental virtue of construction, which are absent in some buildings of a conventional kind'. Nevertheless the writer saw no peace-time role for VADs, nor any need to allow their service to count towards training, the stumbling block to lack of recruits. On 29 May *The Times* reported that the supply of VADs had gone dry; 'This state of things calls for immediate attention'. The Wednesday before it had published the official report of the Lloyd George Committee, which defined the problems facing the nursing profession and the VADs as the want of increments and pensions for the former and the need to grade, pay expenses and provide better accommodation for the latter, but offered no real solutions of how to fill these areas of need. 'Increase the staff in military hospitals to secure leave.' 'Give recognition for satisfactory service for all nurses nursing wounded.' It was to work out ways for doing this that it had been appointed and *The Red Cross* was outspoken in its comments: 'The wrong tool used for a purpose it was never designed for, three people of common sense could have made them all. It seems a pity that so much heart burning as the appointment of the Committee occasioned and the expenditure of so much energy on the part of able men and women, all or nearly all engaged on other important work, should have resulted in the War Office being told what it could have ascertained by simpler means.'[10] What was more serious, however, was *The Times*'s claim on 29 May that, with the exception of the distinguishing stripe for thirteen months service, none of the Lloyd George Committee recommendations concerning VADs had yet been put into effect. Some were walking ten miles to work, others were paying their own medical expenses and uniform. On 15 June Princess Mary took a decisive and influential step. The Princess started a Voluntary Aid Detachment of twenty-five members in Buckingham Palace, and Cantlie was asked to teach them. *The Times* reported, 'Princess Mary has organised a Voluntary Aid Detachment which has been registered under the War Office. Colonel J. Cantlie is giving a course of lectures on First Aid to the Detachment.' These lectures were twice weekly and the Detachment was registered at the War Office, simply as Princess Mary's Detachment. On 11 July Queen Mary attended the lecture and the diary reports, 'H showed the Queen all his slings for stretchers. She astonished him by remembering she had seen them before at the Economic Exhibition, where the College had a stand. Wonderful memory.' The Queen asked questions about the model of the eye – almost, it seemed, with second sight, for, having already caused minor sporadic trouble, by next year Cantlie's eye was causing severe pain and had to be removed. On 13 July the King and Queen left for France where the Queen visited military and auxiliary hospitals, including Allied, British and Commonwealth hutted hospitals, at Boulogne, St John Étaples, Wimereux, Hesdin and Rouen. 'The Queen entered minutely into methods by which the highest forms of surgical knowledge and appliances were used in the service of the wounded.' The ambulance movement took heart from Royalty's lead and *The Red Cross* reported in July, 'Colonel James Cantlie is giving a course of advanced instruction for V.A.D. Officers and others at the College of Ambulance. There are twelve lectures and practical demonstrations.' Sir George Newman of the Quakers asked him to write a pamphlet on first aid for the munitions industry and St John Ambulance Association spearheaded a movement to bring first aid into factories and schools. With 7,000 trained nurses now registered with the College of Nursing and Surgeon General Sir George Evatt calling in *The Times* of 14 August for the DGAMS to be appointed to the Army Council, it seemed that co-ordination of organisation, recruitment of nurses and volunteers and the dissemination of ambulance training were in the forefront of the public mind.

At last Mabel Cantlie gave in to her ill health and an operation was performed. She was told the trouble was not malignant, which it was. 'The Library a bower of flowers. So many letters.' Earlier in the year she had been at Colin's bedside in Plymouth where he was suffering from typhoid fever, with high temperature and hallucinations, and now, on leave, he was able to be at hers. Neil wrote daily from France, 'I do prize his letters'. Keith, now with his Labour Battalions of Kurds, Persians and Arabs in Mesopotamia, sent telegrams. Because of his wife's health Cantlie thought about giving up lecturing so that he could devote more time to her, and she, worried about his health, wrote, 'I am sure he will kill himself if he does not'. Evatt in another letter to the press had drawn attention to the long hours and the over-worked, under-staffed and under-paid nature of the job of examining recruits, which Cantlie had spent much of his life doing. He had worked too hard at too many things which did not bring him sufficient income to shoulder the enormously increased costs of the College of Ambulance. There is a photograph of Princess Mary coming down a flight of stairs with Cantlie at her side. He looks an old man, 'H so thin with all his hard work', says the diary. But it was impossible for either of them to give up, for these were heartrending months, when the only reality seemed to be death. 'Mrs. B wants to go to a canteen in France,' says the diary, 'poor little lonely woman with no son now to look after and she has a longing to see the grave of her dear lad. Alas! Alas!' The thunder of guns could be heard across the Channel as the British tried to force their way through to Belgium in one of the most costly campaigns of the war. But a spirit of love and unity which has often confounded our enemies was now shining through the suffering and silencing the discord.

Perhaps it was Cantlie's invitation to instruct Princess Mary in ambulance work, perhaps it was the gravity of the national crisis and the will of the public to succour the wounded, with which he had been so much identified, perhaps it was the extent of Mabel Cantlie's illness and her courage in never giving in to it, but suddenly and unexpectedly, as the diary records 'People keep writing and saying why did we not get decorated. It is quite absurd.' Cantlie had never worked or looked for honours. But his friends, particularly Sir James Reid and Surgeon General Sir George Evatt, were very disappointed that he had not been honoured in the August list and said so quite openly. Sir Arthur Stanley courteously 'wrote and apologised and said there had been some mistake and that Voluntary Aid would have been in a bad way without H or I'. The man who never sought awards for himself was now, so his friends thought, being singled out for receiving none. On 17 August, however, came a letter to *The Times* which said VADs were enrolled to give patriotic and voluntary help and not to gain status for themselves. It struck the wrong note. Suddenly a dam broke and there was a rush of gratitude to the Voluntary Aid Societies, the VADs, the College of Ambulance and to the Cantlies for all the work which they had done in the cause of voluntary aid. On 24 August came a moving tribute in *The Times* from the father of a boy, thanking all those in army hospitals in France who tried to save his son's life. He said he was expressing the sentiments of all anxious relations in the BRCS hostel, 'To all of us the perfection of the medical and nursing arrangements and the more than courtesy, the loving care lavished on us was a revelation ... I would especially thank the Red Cross and V.A.D. young ladies who, without fee or thought of reward, conduct the hostels for relations and whose cheerful solicitude lightens the days of nerve racking anxiety.' On the same day the Secretary of State for War appointed Sir Rickman Godlee, President of the College of Ambulance, a member of a committee of inquiry into personnel and administration of the Army Medical Service in France, and, in the following month, *The Red Cross* answered the sentiments expressed in *The Times* letter of 17 August: 'Those who are really worthy of decoration, whether they receive them or not are usually much above giving more than a passing thought to such questions. Their work is, after all, what they will be judged by. Shakespeare would have been no greater had he been Sir William. Indeed perhaps the highest honour of all is to leave behind a name which by common consent it would be affectation even to prefix Mister.'

In October the Bishop of London opened the session at the College of Ambulance and said he would like to start a Parson's Ambulance Corps; this was a great tribute and St John's magazine *First Aid* in reporting the visit described the width of training and number of students who passed through the College. In the same month also came a 'thank you' to the Victoria Station Buffet, 'never closed,' said *The Times*, 'day or night since 1914'. In November Lord Knutsford called for fewer inequalities in the bestowal of honours. It was, however, the inspired pen of Sir Frederick Treves who in *The Times* of 3 October gave to the whole Red Cross movement the tribute to their work for British soldiers that Binyon had given to those working for the French. ' "Where do you come from?" was the question of a dying man to a VAD who held a cup to his lips. "I come from Home," she answered, and, smiling a little, presently the man was dead. She came from Home and all that the Red Cross brings comes from Home and Home is where they must come from for Home is where love is.' Love and mercy and compassion, and all the other human virtues assailed by the terrible carnage and devastating assault which surrounded them – somehow in tears and tribulation the compassion of men and women for each other still shone triumphantly through.

CHAPTER EIGHTEEN

The Armistice

Throughout 1917 the international situation grew daily more serious, everywhere the skies were darker. The Czar and his family were prisoners in the Palace of Petrograd and the Council of Workers and Soldiers Delegates kept this a secret from the people. The Kerensky Government was weak and vacillating in the face of defeat, food shortages and anarchy. The Germans had their eyes on world domination and were planning a Socialist hegemony in Central Europe. In Italy the struggle was hard and unavailing, the taking of Vimy Ridge brought no respite in losses. Although America entered the war in April 1917, it was a year before the main American Army arrived in Europe. In China, *The Times* reported that the German banks were involved in espionage, and on 5 June there was a military *coup d'état* under Ssu Shih-Cheng which drove Sun temporarily out of China, so that he wrote to the Cantlies saying he had written 'another Manifesto and was retiring to private life because it was impossible to get the Chinese to pull together'. On 5 July the German-backed boy Emperor returned to the Forbidden City and Kang Yu-Wei, Sun's rival in reform and revolution, was made Vice President. At that moment *The Times* must have doubted its judgements based on Morrison's dispatches from Peking for, if Kang was pro-German, so had been Yuan. Morrison's deathbed confession of having wrongly judged Sun, which was made to Cantlie whose advice he sought on terminal cancer, was only a dotting of i's and stroking of t's. 'Whether,' said *The Times*, 'a puppet Emperor and a handful of adventurers will improve the internal conditions of China seems doubtful.'[1] The regime only lasted five days, after which Sun returned to Canton. On 14 August, Li Yuan Hung, who had dispatched a Labour Battalion to France earlier in the year before his Presidency was overthrown, made a formal declaration of war on behalf of the Peking Government, followed one month later by a declaration from Canton – for most of the next decade, China was divided into North and South, a division which both China and Britain had sought to avoid. In Britain, by the last year of the war rations were scarce, money short, air-raids frequent and endurance a way of life. Although the fight against the U-boat had been strengthened by the convoy system (the credit for which must go to Lloyd George and to Sir Maurice Hankey, Secretary to the War Cabinet), improved anti-submarine warfare and the deployment of the American Navy, nevertheless supplies crossing the Atlantic were short.

Similarly, although American loans filled Allied empty coffers, borrowed money is no substitute for real wealth and the lack of funds was reflected at national and personal level. November was a month of hard won victories. On the 21st the diary records, 'Great victory. Hindenberg line smashed. Our tanks in action.' In the Middle East Gaza was taken and Beersheba, but in France the taking of Passchendaele Ridge at such heavy cost of life – although it drew fire from the hard-pressed French – did not live up to *The Times* expectations 'that the worst of the work is over'.

As trench warfare developed into more open fighting, so did the difficulties of transporting the wounded at the firing line increase. The main dressing stations moved forward, followed more slowly by the casualty clearing stations, so that the distances between the two were greater. It was now that the tented operating theatres, used increasingly in 1917, began to come into their own and also the mobile ambulances with operating theatres, ice-making equipment, heating, lighting, bathing, laundry and disinfecting plants, with which the American Red Cross had originally led the way. As well as assisting in hospitals and mobile ambulances in support of the medical services, the Joint Committee of St John and BRCS had by now taken over all relief work on lines of communication – at one rest station in a week 30,000 men were fed and 1,500 dressings done. By 1918 trains were fully victualled, but in 1917 wounded soldiers were still fed from platforms, forty minutes allowed for each train, while another train, during the fierce fighting, was queuing up outside the station. All these relief activities demanded an increasing supply of nurses and VADs. The College of Ambulance had received much recent publicity but, since the idea of a combined teaching College for the two Voluntary Aid Societies had been put aside, it was becoming increasingly difficult to see under whose aegis the College could be carried on. Marylebone District, Red Cross, had used it since 1914 as its headquarters and examining centre and the voluntary aid societies and many other organisations and individuals wished it to continue, but both the Cantlies were in failing health and at the College and Harley Street they were facing rent increases, so that Cantlie was forced now to ask the College of Nursing to pay him rent. As she had feared, Mabel Cantlie's health was only marginally better, the diaries recording temperature, weariness and pain. 'Walked home, but oh, so tired, as not feeling quite so well.' Then, when Cantlie was away, inspecting a German prisoner of war camp at Stanley's request, 'Woke up feeling very ill, with pulse going at 120 per minute'. Yet, with that astonishing resilience, she was back at the College in the afternoon.

Meanwhile Sir Arthur Stanley was running into further problems over the amalgamation of the College of Nursing with the RBNA. The College had originally intended to recognise various branches of nursing, and, in September 1917, its minutes record that evidence of nursing training was to include at least twelve months in a general hospital. This sounded like a compromise, and the Privy Council's alteration of the Charter of Amalgamation with the RBNA in which it changed the words 'uniform curriculum' to 'equivalent curricula' was sufficient to arouse the nurses' fears that the College intended to recognise different branches of the profession and that the three-year general training could be avoided. In spite of a cogently worded letter from Stanley, the RBNA withdrew. Cantlie followed these matters only sporadically, when attending the College Council as a representative of the Poor Law Nurses. Perhaps this was fortunate considering his identification with the VAD movement because, realising how strongly the trained nurses felt about their position, the College of Nursing sent a statement to the *Daily Mail*, recorded in their minutes, to set their fears at rest. 'Our endeavour will be to draw a clear line between trained nurses and V.A.D.s and to encourage such of the latter, as are suitable, to obtain a three years' certificate from a general hospital, which will enable them to become members of the College of Nursing.' Although on 15 November an attempt was made to put the matter to all their members and the secretary was asked to write, no action seems to have followed. On the same day Dame Katherine Furse resigned as Commandant-in-Chief to start the WRNS, saying that the arrangements for General Service members were difficult to operate and that she wanted more women on the Joint VAD Committee and more grading for VADs – although, following the recommendations of the Lloyd George Committee, they could now become assistant nurses with one blue stripe. Lady Ampthill took her place and Mabel Cantlie's diary records, 'I went and saw Lady Ampthill and found her quite charming. She congratulated me on my members getting Military Medals for bravery. She is now our C-in-C and I think will prove an excellent one.' Mabel Cantlie chose this moment to ask for a promotion stripe for VADs working for the French and Belgians and to ask that Dominion members could wear the stripes of their country of origin, in which latter request she was successful.

At the end of December, Cantlie was awarded the KBE for his work for Red Cross and voluntary aid. The *Polytechnic Magazine* said, 'It is with the greatest pleasure that we saw that Dr. Cantlie's indefatigable labours for the Red Cross and St. John's Ambulance have been thus honoured. Sir James Cantlie was the originator of the Voluntary Aid Detachments and has for a great number of years been the head of our Ambulance Classes.'[2] Cantlie was in company with others whose work he respected: Lady Ampthill and Lady Dawson, the latter Honorary Secretary of the Queen Mary Needlework Guild which had many branches in the country, including one in Glasgow, were both made Dames Grand Cross; Mrs Locke King who had organised the display at Brooklands in 1914 was made a DBE, while Scotland's contribution to voluntary aid was honoured by its BRCS President, the Duchess of Montrose, being made a Dame Grand Cross. Scottish Branch, BRCS and St Andrews Ambulance had provided ambulances, X-ray ambulances, hospitals and hospital wards in France and Russia and had organised all the transport in the hospital base city of Rouen. A large number of helpers in the College of Ambulance and Humanitarian Corps had also been Scots. Two weeks later came the news that Neil, to his parents' joy, had been awarded the MC. At the end of January Sir Alfred Keogh retired and wrote a letter on 26 January to the Commandant of the Ambulance Column, London District, of which Cantlie's No. 1 VAD formed part of Unit 6:

> I know of no organisation of the kind in the country which deserves so much unstinted praise and commendation as that over which you preside, and that, I think, is saying a great deal, for in all the great centres there are similar organisations doing the most glorious voluntary work for the sake of the wounded, but here in London, the work may be said to have continued without any remission day and night. The centre which they serve is enormous. In all weathers, at all hours, the Ambulance Column has been found at work, making long waits at the Railway Stations and long journeys to the destinations of those whom they carry. When we come to consider that this work is being done without pay, that it has not been advertised, and that every single member of the organisation appears to have abandoned every moment of his spare time, while engaged in his own occupation, in order that the sick and wounded should be cared for, what can be said by way of praise. Those who know, know also that this work would not be well done, if it were not accomplished with kindness and tenderness towards those whom they succour. In this respect, whoever has witnessed the work will recognise the extraordinary devotion to the patients whom they thus voluntarily serve. Many people, no doubt, think that the organisation is an official one in the narrowest sense, and that the workers draw large emoluments and do nothing else. The Column has no desire that people should think otherwise, I know, but I often think the men from the Front and the public generally should know what a splendid and devoted body of men we have in this London organisation and let me say also in all the similar organisations throughout the country. You will perhaps permit me to say this and to ask you to convey to the Officers my own deep appreciation of the splendid partiotism and devotion I take off my hat to every one of them.

This letter was included as a frontispiece in the detailed record of the work of Unit 6, compiled by Mr J. Abrahams, Quartermaster, who was orginally a quartermaster of No. 1 VAD before it became part of Unit 6, and kept a daily list of all the wounded the Unit transported across London, either to other stations or to hospital, loading and unloading the ambulances, and taking the patients to their beds in the wards. They were on duty for twenty-four hours at a stretch, and often trains were still arriving at four in the morning. 'I well remember when the pushes were on in France, we had 26 hours duty right off without a break and spent the whole night on Waterloo Station.'

Throughout these months the diaries had been recording the grave news of the war, the anxiety about the boys, the air raids and the difficulties in getting round London because of the crowded tubes in which people were spending the night. Mabel Cantlie did not go out so much now in the evening to the College of Ambulance because of the state of her health and spent the time instead making clothes for hospitals and for her husband and family to aid their ailing finances. Her son Kenneth said to her of a sermon on loving your neighbour as yourself, 'You do not do that, but give the neighbours all the love'. Work at the College of Ambulance continued steadily and throughout the winter plans were made to put the VAD movement on a firmer footing. In December, Dr Alfred Sze, the Chinese Minister in London, arranged for a party of Chinese ladies to enrol at the College in order to nurse the Chinese Labour Battalion in France (his children, at school in England, were soon to become Cantlie's wards when their parents returned to China). On 9 December the diary records, 'Germans massing on the Western front. I fear a terrible offensive ahead'. In February *The Red Cross* reported the co-ordination of hospital and convalescent treatment to be nearing completion; VADs would be properly utilised and would receive efficiency stripes, entitling them to undertake responsible duties. A club was to be opened for them and then, in the throwaway line, came the statement, 'An agreed length of service as V.A.D.s should entitle nurses to sit a central examination'. This was what the Cantlies had repeatedly requested, but the controversy was unending, like looking down a corridor of mirrors with reflections perpetuating into the distance. The answer, with hindsight, was so simple: VADs with promotion stripes could have had remission for one year's service, as was done by the London Hospital, of which Lord Knutsford was Chairman. The Nightingale School, on the other hand, insisted on a three-year training, but allowed a remission of fees. On 26 January the *Nursing Times* felt free, after the publicity given by his knighthood, to link Cantlie's name for the first time with the start of the College of Nursing, instead of only claiming that it was someone in the ambulance movement. 'Certainly it was an open secret at the time when the College of Nursing began to be mooted that some idea of a great permanent V.A.D. organisation, analogous we imagine to Dr. Cantlie's First Aid College in Vere Street was in the air.' The periodical was casting a fly and insinuating a connection with the inevitable result that, during the same month, the College of Nursing came again under attack from the RBNA and the trade unions. Not only was there a real fear in the minds of the nurses that the VADs would enter the nursing profession without what they considered proper training, but to the unions they represented privilege, being people of financial independence. This may have been understandable, but it was unfortunate at such a moment. All this controversy coupled with anxieties about his wife's illness and fears for the future of the College did nothing to improve Cantlie's health – he was 70 and working harder every year. In February, the diary records, 'H has a bad right eye. He must lie in a darkened room.' Then, returning to the worry about the College for which two months' rent was owed, 'H sees Sir Job Collins, who is very anxious to help him and wants to affiliate the College to London University'. It would have been an ideal solution, but it unfortunately came to nothing. On 16 March the Cantlies decided they must appeal to the public and Mr Boyton agreed to let them keep the College on for another month. Notices appeared in the press and welcome donations immediately came in. It was just in time, for volunteers were again to be needed in large numbers. The next entry in the diary shows the need: 'A bad night with a thumping heart, big offensive at St. Quentin. All this anxiety about the boys prevents me from sleeping.'

By now the Kerensky Government in Russia had fallen and the Germans had taken 435,000 square miles of Russia, driving the people before them like sheep. Only Eastern Russia was not in the hands of the Bolshevists. People were deeply anxious about the weight of men and armaments which the Germans would be able to hurl against the Allies on the Western front. The blow fell on the Fifth Army on 21 March. Immediately the attention of the public turned again to the need for the ambulance movement. On the 22nd came the entry in the diary, 'Reporters over the College. Sir James Crichton Browne came full of sympathy, wanting us to keep it on. H showed Mr. Edwards, Secretary of St. John's over the College.' The next day *The Times* reported that Sir James Reid was to preside at a public meeting of the College of Ambulance in Vere Street as a result of which it was 'hoped that steps will be taken to establish it on a permanent national basis'. At the meeting Sir Malcolm Morris moved a resolution for its incorporation. 'For the last three and a half years,' said the paper, 'the College has been carried on with remarkable success by Colonel Sir James Cantlie. Well over 20,000 persons of both sexes have received instruction in first aid and ambulance work and are now attending to the wounded at home and abroad.' For two days now the guns had been rumbling as the German onslaught forced the British back on to the Somme line. 'The most terrible fighting, since the retreat from Mons,' said *The Times*, 'The Emperor is boasting the battle is won . . . The battle has not been won, the boast is vain and false. The British people are fully aware the situation is grave, and even critical, and they look at the facts with steady eyes. The French are acting in the closest co-operation . . . The men bear themselves with calm and dauntless courage, unsurpassed in the annals of any army . . .'; and then, quoting Tennyson, 'with courage never to submit or yield.' Had the poet foreseen the holocaust when he wrote of the legendary court of King Arthur with its Round Table and Order of Chivalry, and did he fear a bloody war and wrongly forecast the defeat of chivalry? For it was chivalry for which the battle was being fought – chivalry in its widest sense. Again, as the fighting became fiercest, appeals for nurses appeared in the pages of the press. On 16 March had come a letter from 'Mere Man' saying the VADs did not have sufficient leave or time off for dancing. Dancing – with an offensive about to begin! No doubt kindly meant, it was answered by 'Mere Nurse' who said the VADs did not want to dance, so many had lost their loved ones. Responding to these criticisms, Lady Ampthill went to France to see conditions for herself and an ex-army sister sprang to the support of the VADs, showing the co-operation between navy and army sisters and VADs on the field of battle. 'Thank God,' she wrote to *The Times*, 'for the spirit of patriotism that stops these girls from complaining. It is a little of the wonderful mystery of which our men have so much'. She spoke of how she had worked with trained nurses and VADs, eaten frozen eggs, been unable to write with frozen ink and welcomed the fact that, at the same time, the men were snug in bed; likewise in sweltering heat that they were on cool sheets. 'Ours the privilege to spend our love and energy on those who had spent their lives for us, to work by day and night if by so doing we could assuage the suffering of one man.'

'Still terrible fighting,' reports the diary at the end of March, 'for both Arras and Amiens, but the Germans have stopped advancing for the moment. So anxious about Neil . . . Could not sleep all night . . . Post card from Neil. He is safe, thank God.' Then, on 2 April, 'Sir Arthur Stanley came and Sir James Boyton. Sir Arthur wants the two top floors of the College for the College of Nursing . . . Perhaps we might let him have it.' This would have meant a house in Vere Street virtually split in two. It is difficult to see how it could have worked, for the trained nurses would have feared dilution and influence by the VADs, and the ambulance movement, while happy and anxious to promote the cause of the trained nurses, equally did not want to be taken over by them. Sir Arthur may have felt that a centralised examination centre, about which he had made inquiries, could produce a compromise solution. He continually expressed his gratitude to the Cantlies for all they had done for voluntary aid and no doubt he did not wish to lose the teaching and examining facilities available at the College of Ambulance. Meanwhile, in France, although the first German attack had failed, the crisis was quickly reaching a climax. 'The Germans ready to attack again. Colin came in from Dover. He is going to dine with Admiral Colville at Portsmouth tonight, but of course does not tell us why. He said if Amiens did not remain in our hands the whole Army would suffer greatly and it would even perhaps knock us out of France for the present. H heard ships were ready at Boulogne and Calais to evacuate.' But the nation, with characteristic resilience, was holding fast to spiritual values. On 10 April the diary records, 'I went to a service at St. Paul's for the nurses who have fallen in the war. It was a very impressive sight, some 4000–5000 nurses and V.A.D.s being present. It seemed like a dream to see St. John's and the Red Cross come in and to feel that H had been the guiding star to them all. Band of the Grenadier Guards played the Dead March in Saul. Last Post sounded. All very impressive.' On the same day *The Times*, with infinite sensitivity, reported in the midst of one of the bloodiest battles of history the return of the swallows; the joys of nature, sometimes passing unnoticed, are welcome in periods of great stress.

A few days later the diary reports, 'Bad news from the front. God is near us when the darkness is greatest. Germans have Armentières. Seem to be getting on and it takes a bit of courage to make one feel at ease. As the news seemed serious, I went round to the Detachment this evening just to prevent the women getting nervous. Miss Sharpe came in tears. She will have to give up her Nursing Home as she cannot get food . . . Germans creeping on, taking more ground. It is impossible not to give a shudder now and again.' Then, on the 13th, 'Sir Douglas Haig has sent forth a clarion call. No more ground must be given up. Our men must stand by to protect the ports of France. Very grave outlook . . . Anxious Sunday. A sort of agony in the air. So terribly anxious about the Western Front. May God find us worthy of victory. One feels one cannot pray enough.' Sir Douglas Haig's message had been brief and to the point: 'With our backs to the wall and believing in the justice of our cause, we must fight to the end'. On the 16th the diary continues, 'We have lost Baillent to the Germans and Messines Ridge'. As the Germans rolled ever onwards, fears of a German occupation of France and of an attempted invasion increased. In the face of over-whelming odds the British retreated. The Germans were in the sub-urbs of Amiens. Hospitals which had been far back from the line of battle were becoming casualty clearing stations, and the roar of the cannon and the casualties, filthy from the field of battle, left the nurses in no doubt as to the dangers they faced. The public was reminded that the 'untrained' VADs were involved near the battle line in the most terrible war of history. On the same day as Sir Douglas Haig's clarion call the *Nursing Times* came out with the statement that 'most matrons agree there should be time off training for V.A.D.s', and on the 15th *The Times* set out a leave schedule, showing the VADs lagging behind. Leave – at such a moment! Why could people only forget their differ-ences in moments of deadly danger?

On 18 April came the King's letter to the Red Cross and St John on the day the results of their appeal reached £10 million: 'I earnestly trust that the Joint Committee will be enabled until victory is won and the peace of the world assured, to continue without abatement its sacred mission to the wounded, the sick and the prisoners, whose welfare has our unfailing solicitude and our heartfelt sympathy'. The King went on 'The value of the help thus rendered to our sick and wounded cannot be estimated'. On the same day *The Times* leader said, 'The supreme trial is upon us . . . The forces of liberty are locked in a death struggle with those of absolutism.' But the morale of the British Army was high. On the 18th also Mabel Cantlie received a letter from Neil, typical of others from many sons, in which he sought to set her mind at rest: 'He says he is full of beans, their line has been dented and the policy is to wait and see. I feel so thankful to hear from Neil that the world seems brighter'; and, on the 20th, 'Another letter from Neil. He is fit and well. We have fought for Givinchy and have given the Germans a good defeat there.' Then, on the 22nd, 'Colin wrote in his usual quiet way and we wonder what he was doing'. The Royal Navy was in fact preparing for Zeebrugge and, on the 24th, 'Tremendous fight for Zeebrugge. Our men took old cruisers filled with cement which were sunk in the harbour. They did splendidly. A traditional British fight under Admiral Keyes.' However, on 26 April came the thrust for Mount Kemmel and its fall to the Germans. Again the skies were dark in retreat. On the same, day the Queen sent a message to the men of the Royal Navy, the Army and the Air Force.

I send this message to tell every man how much we, the women of the British Empire at home, watch and pray for you during the long hours of these days of retreat and endurance. Our pride in you is immeasurable, our hope unbounded, our trust absolute. You are fighting in the cause of Righteousness and Freedom, fighting to defend the children and women of our land from the horrors that have overtaken other countries, fighting for our very existence as a people, at home and across the seas. You are offering your all, you hold back nothing and day by day you show a love so great that no man can have greater. We, on our part, send forth with full hearts and unfaltering will the lives we hold most dear. We too are striving in all ways possible to make the war victorious. I know that I am expressing what is felt by thousands of wives and mothers when I say that we are determined to help one another in keeping your homes ready against your glad home-coming. In God's name we bless you and by His Help we too will do our best.

On 1 May came the news recorded in the diary, 'Our men gave the Germans a great beating yesterday near Mount Kemmel, it was splendid and we have not let them come on'. *The Times* headline was 'German defeat south of Ypres'. The country and the Commonwealth were resolute and united – their sailors, soldiers and airmen 'deeply sensible of the debt and duty owed' and warmly appreciative and respectful in their thanks for Their Majesties' inspiring messages and for the confidence placed in them. 'The soul in us,' wrote Binyon, 'is found and shall not die'.

The day before the publication of the Queen's message was Princess Mary's birthday and the *Daily Telegraph* re-told the story of the Princess's Voluntary Aid Detachment and of Cantlie's lectures at Buckingham Palace. The Princess, now a qualified VAD, was nursing at the Great Ormond Street Hospital for Sick Children, thus identifying the VADs with their nurses who were also having problems about recognition and time required for general training in order to register. Cantlie was at this time again lecturing to the police in first aid, and the *Nursing Times*, with welcome good humour, commented that the best qualification for a VAD was six months in a children's hospital and six months as a policewoman. Humour was needed, for the dangers of invasion were again real as the German armaments were hurled against the Allied troops defending the Channel ports. It was against this background of crisis that the decision to incorporate the College of Ambulance was confirmed and Sir James Boyton agreed to let No. 3 Vere Street to the College for a further year, offering at the same time No. 8 to the Marylebone Red Cross as their headquarters so that the College could accept the support of other organisations, including St John's Ambulance Association and the Territorials. Cantlie now staged another demonstration to a wide audience at the College, addressed by Sir Havelock Charles, during which, according to the diary, Dr Attwood Thorne 'told H that 18 Field Ambulances are to be raised from Volunteers in London (to meet the threat of invasion), with a

request from each 18 that H would have charge. Splendid testimony.'
The next day, with the Hon. Evelyn Cecil, MP, Vice Chairman, BRCS,
in the chair, Cantlie lectured on the relation of first aid and National
Service, for, in spite of the work and initiative of Colonel Synge Hutch-
ison, VC, first aid teaching in the British Army was still only sporadic.
On 4 May Cantlie went to the House of Commons to discuss with the
Red Cross Director, County of London, a plan to use the College for
all ambulance instruction, civil and military. This had always been
Cantlie's aim and he went also to see Sir Dyce Duckworth who was
appreciative and promised his support.

In early May, as the fierce fighting swayed this way and that
and the fate of the Allies in France hung in the balance, letters continued in *The Times* about the shortage of VADs and the conditions
under which many were working. On 11 May the main body of
American troops arrived in Europe to an enthusiastic reception. On
the 14th the Order of St John 'despatched a solemn communication to
the Order of St. John in Prussia protesting against sinking of hospital
ships, ill treatment of sick and wounded prisoners of war and other
breaches of the Geneva Convention'. On the 16th there was a further
appeal for VADs. On 24 May *The Times* reported the Germans' fourth
inhuman blunder, the bombing of Étaples, as this

> latest exploit in bombing deliberately a well known group of British
> hospitals in France and in sweeping the cots of the wounded men
> and the devoted nursing sisters and attendants with machine gun
> fire . . . After dark on Sunday night two squadrons flew over the
> camp and for two hours dropped heavy bombs on the hospitals and
> swept the hostel tents with machine guns. Throughout the attacks
> the attendants refused to leave the patients. Many paid the price of
> heroism with their lives.

Since Étaples was the site of St John's hospital, as well as of others, and
since this hospital was staffed with Brigade members and VADs, the
role of the volunteer was brought, as never before, into the mind of
the public. On 25 May the *Nursing Times* recommended centralised
examinations for VADs; on 5 June Mr Evans of St John came to the
College to recruit for the Brigade instead of only for VADs and on the
6th Sir Arthur Sloggett, DGAMS, wrote to the BRCS thanking the
Society for its generous assistance during the war. On 27 May came a
further German attack and then at last, on 8 June with Allied air power
beginning to play a significant role, the combined effect of British,
French and American forces halted the German offensive.

As the Allied forces began their advance to recover lost territory they
found houses destroyed, agricultural and industrial equipment gone,
tuberculosis rife and, just as in the Second World War, a vast network
of aid organised by government and charitable institutions. As soon
as conditions made it possible the Humanitarian Corps adopted the
village of Westoutre, near Ypres. Slowly the British nation began to
turn its eyes towards the longed-for peace and the formidable task of

reconstruction. Thus began a new involvement of government in social welfare, which brought drawbacks as well as advantages. In February 1918 Cantlie warned in his *Journal of Tropical Medicine* against doctors taking part in politics – he regarded Sir Watson Cheyne as an exception – 'The healing art was not considered to have anything to do with politics', and also turning doctors into civil servants in a nationalised health service. 'You lose . . . the stimulus of work for work's sake. It will lead to specialisation and mean that "my own doctor" will no longer be a friend. There will be a divorce between laboratory work and clinical practice.' In March 1918 Cantlie spoke at the Medical Society of London, trying again to increase the interest of the medical profession in first aid, which he saw as the finest way of encouraging the public to recognise their duty to each other. 'We want the best appliances, the best teachers and our foremost physicians and surgeons to take the matter in hand.' 'We quite agree with this statement,' said *First Aid* in March,

> for we have always maintained that the medical profession was the backbone of ambulance work, and it is due to them and the S.J.A.A. that the many thousands of workers in all fields of industry have acquired the knowledge, enabling them to render able assistance to a fellow worker in case of accident. The more medical men who impart instruction in ambulance work the greater facilities will the layman have in receiving instruction. Unfortunately the medical and nursing schools do not take the subject in their curriculum and it is only by coincidence that a medical man becomes interested in the subject.

Cantlie pointed out that 'In military work the medical department sent out trained men under its control to bring in the wounded, but in civil life, surgeons and physicians waited for the injured to be brought to the hospitals, but took no responsibility or control for how or in what state the injured were to be brought to them. Universities and medical schools took no part in the training or teaching of first aid bearers or ambulance workers.' In June, following the lead given by St John's in co-operating with the new government legislation regarding first aid in industry, Cantlie staged a demonstration at the College for those employed in agriculture, dressing his members up as agricultural workers and exhibiting remedies for kicks, poisons, tears, bruises and severed limbs. Although this demonstration concerned injuries to agricultural workers, he always emphasised, since Keithmore days, the links between first aid for animals and for humans – Florence Nightingale's first patient was reputed to be a dog with a broken leg – and it is notable that some books written by army veterinary surgeons who had served in France relate animal injuries such as sprains and strains and their remedies to those of humans.

On 31 July the College was officially incorporated and Sir Rickman Godlee asked the College of Nursing to move its office out in order that the whole building could now be used for the teaching of first aid. Under the Chairmanship of Admiral Sir Edmund Fremantle a Council was elected and there was a welcome financial recovery in College funds. But the following month the good news from the front that peace was in sight resulted in the fall-off in numbers in all centres of instruction in first aid and nursing and the College was no exception. The nation was war weary and did not yet realise the vital peace-time and reserve role that the BRCS, St John Ambulance Brigade and Association and the VADs were later to play. In spite of efforts to interest the public in peace-time first aid and its importance in dealing with any accident or emergency, the ambulance movement was for the moment swimming against a tide. Cantlie was so used to overcoming difficulties – 'the greater the obstacles the greater his determination to overcome them' – that he did not realise that the drop in numbers was to last for years, not months. On 6 August Admiral Sir Rosslyn Wemyss opened the Debenham Ward of the West End Hospital, which special-ised in shell shock cases. It was in this hospital that Mabel Cantlie raised the first Women's Detachment, No. 2 VAD, and became its first Woman Commandant as well as the first woman VAD until, in her own words, 'a better one can be found'. The Cantlies had always wanted doctors and trained nurses to join Voluntary Aid Detachments and play their part in training and working alongside lay volunteers, and had this been achieved nation-wide many difficulties would have been avoided. 'The fully trained nurses who are V.A.D.s do not look down on those members who are only half or a quarter trained and realise the valuable work they do.'[3] Mabel Cantlie had therefore handed over her leadership of No. 2 to Dr May Thorne of the West End Hospital (who remained its Commandant until she left for Malta and who, on her return, became, at Cantlie's request, a Vice President of the College of Nursing), while Mabel Cantlie, at the request of Bedford College, started and became the Commandant of Detachment No. 110. As Sir Arthur Keith said of the Cantlies, 'Their unselfishness took different directions, his was to give himself to the service of the community in which he lived; hers was to give herself to the service of her husband' as well as to the service of her country.

'Our 34th Wedding Day,' wrote Mabel Cantlie in July, 'what a privilege to live with H. Only I want to be strong again, so that I can do more to help him.' The problem was that neither of them could be strong again, the war had taken its toll; Cantlie had hardening of the arteries, and the malignancy from which his wife suffered was now to spread to the liver. At last they took a holiday, the first since the war. They went to Scotland, where the Duke of Richmond and Gordon gave them fishing and showed them over the splendid hospital in the castle. They spent a 'golden day' at Glenfiddich and then, going home, the pony cart overturned, injuring Cantlie's eye. He returned to London in intense pain and for two months struggled on while glaucoma developed. At the end of August Keith, who was now an Acting Captain, Labour Directorate, Staff Officer, Persia, was mentioned in dispatches for Gallant Service in Mesopotamia. On 28 September came the last battle of Ypres, a decisive German defeat. Neil, Acting Major, Deputy Assist-ant Director Medical Services, was soon to be advancing with 9th Corps through Belgium. During the summer a further horror struck the nations of Europe – Spanish influenza, which crossed the Channel in early autumn, taking a heavy toll of life among nations under-fed and war weary. 'Many people dying of flu',' says the diary, 'it is like plague.' Cantlie's remedy was whisky, which saved lives because it 'sweated out the flu' ', while providing necessary stimulation for the heart. Also in the autumn the work rooms were saddened by the death of Mrs Quentin Hogg who had 'tired herself out', said the *Polytechnic Magazine*, 'while refusing to give up her beloved duties at the work rooms. She was indeed a gift from God.' At the end of October Cantlie had to succumb to pain and have his eye removed, although he was lecturing five days later, and on 9 November *The Ladies Field* reported, 'Princess Mary, in common with the King and Queen has been distressed by the fact that Sir James Cantlie has had to have his left eye removed as a result of a recent accident, following an earlier trouble with his sight'. The paper spoke of the Princess's instruction at Buckingham Palace. 'The Royal V.A.D.s made particularly rapid progress under the cheery, kindly and most competent surgeon from Banffshire.' Cantlie was so touched that he wrote to Lady Ampthill and a day or two afterwards there is an entry in the diary, 'The Princess sent H flowers and a sweet note'.

At last, on 11 November, came the Armistice and the bells, which might have heralded the invasion, rang again to pronounce the longed-for peace. The diary described the scene at Buckingham Palace, 'The King and Queen came out on the balcony with the Duke of Connaught. There were many thousands of people. The National Anthem, the Old Hundredth Hymn, Auld Lang Syne, Keep the Home Fires Burning, Now thank we all our God were played by the band. It was a very grand scene. The King made a short speech and the Queen looked very happy.' Then, on the 12th, 'Miss Grenfell and I went to St. Pauls to the Thanksgiving Service. The King and Queen were there. The Cathedral had been full since 9 a.m. Many people waiting all night. It was most wonderful to hear the bells again after their silence for so long. God guard our peace.' Tragically it was only twenty-one years before they were silent again. Already in 1919 Cantlie was warning in the *Journal* that the Germans would come again, this time in the name of Socialism.

So many young men of all nations had died. The flower of manhood had perished in the almost unendurable suffering of the mud of Passchendaele and Ypres and the Somme, and it was to the Flanders poppy that the nation – its heartbroken parents and sweethearts – turned as a symbol of remembrance. An article by a VAD in *The Red Cross* captured the deep emotions of 1917, the shared suffering, courageous endurance, faith and fleeting moments of hope and joy: 'In the shadow of a great Cathedral the hostel waits. It waits quietly, with a great courage, if one out of thirty has hope they all have hope. If one mother leaves with her son off the danger list her happiness gathers in all those waiting guests and warms them. There are flowers everywhere, in the cobbled courtyard, along the narrow gallery and in the living room and dining and bed rooms.' At birthdays and anniversaries also came the request from relatives to plant flowers on the graves: 'I thought at first I could not bear to be here. It was such a long journey. Now it is only as if they were going a little way off. Like a crossing from France to England.'[4] On 4 August Mabel Cantlie had taken to church one flower for every person she had known who had been killed in the war and placed them on the altar, just as she had planted violets on the grave of a young man in far away Hong Kong. Five of her Detachment members had laid down their lives, two had been awarded Belgian decorations, one the Military Medal, another the Croix de Guerre and a fifth the Special Service Medal. On 19 December Mabel Cantlie was awarded the OBE and said 'I shall feel shy wearing it'. 'Lady Cantlie,' said *The Red Cross*, 'was the first woman V.A.D., whose unfailing optimism and sympathy have been the inspiration of her detachment.' On the same day *The Times* published a letter from Countess Michel Karolyi, The Government Commission of the Hungarian Red Cross, expressing thanks for the remarkable work of Lady Paget in Serbia. Without a nurse's training herself, with very few trained nurses and dependent on VADs and orderlies, she had done one of the most remarkable jobs in the war, for the suffering in Serbia was such that no regulations or ratio of trained to untrained staff could apply. 'We know she has been but an English lady, the perfect incarnation of her generous race, of its ancient virtue, which is always to assist, never to strike the fallen and helpless. In the name of our heartbroken mothers I bow to this great heart.' The following day *The Times* in its editorial spoke a 'word for the modest, a request for some thank-you to the unpaid; St. Martin, who gave his cloak to the beggar would make a good Patron of the Order'. These words described the spirit of the volunteer during the war, of the British Red Cross Society, St John's Ambulance Association and many others; quietly, modestly, courageously, without mentioning it to anyone: the work of the hospitals and the inspiration given by St Martin's to Charing Cross. As Cantlie said of the VADs in 1918:

As volunteers they assumed a national burden and without anticipating pay or reward they have given of their best and for some five years of their lives they have attended to the sick and wounded in hospitals, in the fields and on the railways and in the ambulance wagons ... Not a few have laid down their lives in the cause of humanity and many more have contracted illness or become permanently disabled in their gallant endeavour to help the sick and wounded. This is known throughout the length and breadth of the land, for from tower and town and hamlet they came to supply Britain's need. Their work will remain a glorious legend in the nation's history and a sacred memory of Christian endeavour.[5]

Epilogue: The Crossing

Perhaps the story, already tinged with sadness, should end there before the people in it begin to make their own crossings and the reader is swung into the changed circumstances of the modern postwar period. The leaves of autumn had left the trees of Cottered before the boys had returned to their parents' joy. Keith was first home. The people of South Sylhet had, before his leaving India, presented him with an address of esteem, thanking him for his good manners, kindness and justice. 'Keith wants one day to be [Deputy] Commissioner with the Naga,' the diary records, 'they are a primitive people in Assam.' There in a life of service, he never altered his gentle style of leadership, which made him much beloved.[1] Colin came next, arriving from Scotland. Submarines had helped to mould his character: self disciplined, efficient, admiring courage, deciding on a course of action and seeing it carried through, while showing concern for the welfare of his men, these qualities enabled him to build up a venture 'almost from scratch to an efficient organisation in a remarkably short space of time'.[2] Neil did not come home until 1919 and the diary for that year is missing. His task had been hard for a boy of 21, to care for the wounded and the dying. Like Keith he inherited much from his father in unselfishness and sensitivity and a beautiful singing voice, and, although partly hidden under the quiet determination commented on by his professors, it was this dedication to duty combined with rare humanity which accounted for his popularity. As DGAMS he did much to continue his father's work of fostering the link between military and civil medicine, which he feared might be weakened by the move from Millbank.[3] It is impossible to read the diaries without being aware of how much his parents owed to Kenneth's unfailing optimism and cheerfulness as well as to his help with transport and demonstrations at the College. Now a qualified engineer he was soon to be back in China serving as technical adviser to the Chinese government on railways. 'When Sir James died,' said Sir Arthur Keith, 'his only fortune was his four sons.' Again, the Commonwealth had proved itself to be a family of nations, and in December George Cantlie passed through London on his way home with his regiment which he commanded, the 42nd Battalion of the Black Watch of Canada. 'There are those who remember Colonel Cantlie,' said the press, 'leading his battalion as it advanced on the enemy position at Feneck Graben in open country in broad daylight, while the shells struck and burst. Those who saw him that day could not believe they would ever see him again ... The things he served and stood for will never die so long as there are those whose values are as sound and straight as they were in him.'[4]

On 11 November a poem appeared in *The Times* over the initials
C.A.A.:

> And us they trusted; we the task inherit.
> The unfinished task for which their lives were spent;
> But leaving us a portion of their spirit,
> They gave their witness and they died content.
> Full well they knew they could not build without us
> That better country, faint and far descried.

Was the nation going to be worthy of the task? Britain had spent herself
fighting for the right to live in justice and freedom under the law,
without fear of oppression, believing in leadership by example and not
by intimidation. The chaos into which the world had been thrown by
the clash of democracy and totalitarianism imposed on young and old a
daunting task. Some opted out, others with hope and optimism set
about the job of reconstruction. On what was it to be founded, on a
sense of duty towards one's fellow men or on self interest? It was
against this background that the Cantlies continued their work, in
hopelessly failing health with the road still winding uphill. The end was
drawing near but, nevertheless, it is perhaps worth recording the most
noteworthy of Cantlie's medical achievements and pronouncements
during the period. Understandably, interest in the ambulance movement had dwindled with the Armistice and was not to revive for more
than a decade. 'If,' as Cantlie said, 'the care of the injured person falls as
it must upon the public, it is imperative that those who undertake
the work should be provided with the means of study,'[5] but, for the
moment, this was to remain a dream and, in the changed circumstances
of the 1920s, it was going to be difficult enough to keep the VAD
movement together.

Cantlie concentrated much of his time and energy after the war on
aids to the disabled, in which the King Albert I Hospital in Rouen had
made a significant contribution. He publicised in particular a table
for an armless man invented by Mr Thompson in Edinburgh, which
enabled the man to feed himself and do simple mechanical work. He
also took over the mobile X-ray, so useful in diagnosis with a patient
difficult to move, and handed it over as a going concern to the voluntary aid societies. His concept of the barefoot doctor bringing first aid
and nursing to those suffering from tropical diseases in the East led to
an invitation to give a course of lectures on the subject to Princess
Mary's Detachment in Buckingham Palace and to the subject consequently becoming part of the curriculum at the London School of
Tropical Medicine. In 1921 he became President of the Society of
Tropical Medicine which became Royal in that year. In 1919 he was
given an LLD at Aberdeen University. During the same year Mabel
Cantlie was busy helping the Quakers who were sending clothes to
English wives starving in Austria; they both crossed to Westoutre to
bring help to the village adopted by the Humanitarian Corps and
Mabel Cantlie retired as Commandant of her Detachment, showered
with gifts and gratitude.

Cantlie's medical pronouncements during the period were, as usual, racy. Aware, no doubt, of his own circulatory troubles, he advocated and participated in exercises to music for the middle-aged. Music he believed eliminated fatigue and Highland dancing and fast walking, 110 steps a minute, helped to create new air passages, combat chalk-like deposits in the arteries, remove bumps on joints and help lumbago. For rheumatism he recommended aired beds and clothes, for longevity the need to keep slim: 'Don't let your husband go to sleep in his chair, it is bad for him.' 'Long walks,' he said, 'cure more illnesses than most medicines . . . Do not be afraid of your heart . . . If your heart palpitates when you go up and down stairs, keep on taking exercise gradually until it stops palpitating . . . Exercise! Exercise! Regularly but in moderation.' He warned against alcohol, tea, coffee and tobacco, particularly inhaled cigarette smoking; 'Tea,' he said, 'is bad for the stomach, coffee for the heart.' 'I'm ninety five, I'm ninety five,' rhymed the press, 'and to keep active I'll contrive, for Cantlie says if I jump and run, I'll probably live to 101.'[6] To the children he said 'Do not eat stodgy puddings . . . Throw away your toothbrushes and massage your gums' (by this he meant hard toothbrushes), 'and do not eat or drink anything too hot'. He claimed that infants' teeth and gums were being ruined by mothers feeding milk to them at 20 degrees beyond blood heat and that the use of comforters produced malformed jaws and nasal obstruction. He worked to secure a shorter working day for children in industry both at home and in Hong Kong and, although he fostered and was president of movements to enable more young people to engage in physical sports, he continued to warn them against swimming in cold water before breakfast because of the strain on the heart and kidneys and bicycling fast in a racing position because of the constriction of the heart. He also warned young people against insufficient clothing, particularly the wearing of the Eton jacket, which gave no protection to the kidneys. Fresh air and milk were the best things for health – 'We can't hope to have good digestions,' he said of London, 'breathing the air we breathe' – but, as Moses instructed, it was important not to drink milk or eat milk puddings after eating meat. The press were delighted, 'Moses, M.D.' they headlined, and 'The Peril of the Pudding'. For the working population he also had advice: 'Trams and trains are playing ducks and drakes with the nation and so are the Trade Unions. They are making the nation lazy.' Measuring energy by foot tons, he said that the average worker was only expending half the energy he once did and that physical work consumed less energy than mental work. 'The labourer is doing nothing compared with the man at the head of affairs and if this state of things goes on the working man will disappear and then the nation may look to itself.' The press said his platform style was unique, suggesting John Knox in a frock coat with a touch of Harry Lauder and just a dash of Plato. Carrying on his work for first aid in prisons – he had demonstrated at Wormwood Scrubs all through the war – he did a course of lectures on health and first aid in prisons in company with other doctors. On a lighter note he still enjoyed his role as Father Christmas at the Seamen's, Charing Cross and the West End Hospitals and was yearly host at a Claridges party given for Dr Barnardo's Homes. He was also much in demand as a preacher on Hospital Sunday, when his favourite theme was the Good Samaritan, in whose name (the Good Samaritans) he sent out his last Christmas card. But the Cantlies' work was over. No amount of forcing and disciplining themselves to continue could keep either of them going much longer. His wife's illness dominated his thoughts at this time. She was living on will power and determination to stay at his side. Dinners were cut short, receptions not attended unless she could be with him. She continued with her work as long as possible, but by late summer she was at Cottered and then in August the diaries cease.

Mabel Cantlie died on Christmas Eve 1921. The funeral was at St Peter's, Vere Street, on 30 December. The coffin, draped with the Red Cross flag, was borne into the Church by VAD officers, lady nurses acting as pall bearers. Three representatives of the Serbian Red Cross attended, a fitting thank you for the work she had done for them during the Balkan and Great Wars. 'The world', said an obituary, 'will be much poorer at the loss of such a generous and hard working lady. Her whole life has been devoted to the relief of the suffering.' But perhaps Sir Arthur Keith's words are the best tribute, 'That Cantlie was able to pursue such altruistic objectives was made possible for him by the unselfishness of his partner in life'. With that must be set her own words in her diary, 'I would be nothing if I was not H's wife'. She was indeed his guardian angel, her choice of fancy dress in Hong Kong, and it was as that that she would want to be remembered. Her gratitude to him for his love and kindness to her was what she wanted him to know to the end. 'Thank you for what you have done,' were her last words, 'not only now, but always, always.' So much of him died with her, it was impossible for him to imagine life without her; as he turned away from the grave he said, 'Where's Mab?' Of his work and writings after her death there are few records, although the press reported him from time to time. But the spirit that made him write and speak and teach was broken by her illness and death and by his own failing powers. 'The war had cost Cantlie dear. His almost superhuman efforts for the relief of suffering had taken toll of even his immense reserves of bodily and mental energy . . . and his wife's death had dealt him a blow which time could never heal.'[7] They were all in all to each other, and without her and in failing health, his inspiration had gone, his concern for her suffering shining through his writing of the time. It was his kindness for which she loved him, his generosity of spirit, his refusal to take a hurt without giving some gift or kindness in return, his generosity in never sparing himself in the service of others, without any desire to receive reward in return, his unfailing optimism, coupled with that Celtic sensitivity that moved him on occasions to tears. Now, however, his mind as well as his hand was failing. What was it the Admiralty had said of his teaching in those early days? 'Mr. J. Cantlie's mode of instruction appears to be as nearly approaching perfection as it is possible to imagine.' These powers were gone.

So great was Cantlie's devotion to his work that it was not, however, until 1925, after a severe illness, that he could be persuaded to give up the last of his teaching, that for the BRCS. Sir Arthur Stanley replied to him in the kindest terms:

It is difficult to find words in which to thank you for all that you have done for the British Red Cross Society in this connection during many years past. It is no exaggeration to say that the excellent work by the V.A.D.s during the war was largely due to the very efficient manner in which they had been taught by yourself, and on behalf of the Society, I beg to offer you our most grateful thanks for all that you have done for the Society in this and many other directions. I will place your letter before the Executive Committee at its next meeting, but I know they will wish me to ask you to remain on the British Red Cross Council and Executive Committee and also to retain your post as Examiner in Ambulance work. I should like to take this opportunity of thanking you most gratefully for the loyal assistance and support you have given to me on all occasions.[8]

In September 1925, Cantlie left for Scotland by sea, bent, aged, his work over, financially as poor as when he arrived. He went to his sister's in Fochabers where it was hoped he would recuperate, close to Keithmore and the scenes and memories of his youth, and be able to write his memoirs. The music of the mountains had been part of his inspiration, the strains of Marshall's Strathspeys echoing through the house; the healing quality of music, which soothes the sad heart and aching wounds and makes men think and feel. 'Suddenly,' wrote a poet, after one of the fiercest battles of the war, 'a shepherd's pipes broke the stillness of horror.' Likewise, the haunting strains of a violin, taken to war by a young orderly in the RAMC, echoed down many a darkening hospital ward. Can men not learn to share without that terrible suffering? Was that the lesson which the war had tried to teach.

One of the Christmas cards that Cantlie received that last December was from the Princess Royal, Commandant, VADs and the following year Commandant-in-Chief, BRCS. It was of a church with a light in the windows and a couple approaching it along level ground. The road wound uphill no longer. Instead, there was a light for all who came, a candle in the window making a welcome. In January a serious haemorrhage necessitated his removal to Aberdeen and thence to his old nursing home in 30 Dorset Square, where under the care of his former matron, Miss Sharpe, he passed peacefully away on 28 May 1926. The Memorial Service was at St Peter's, Vere Street, on 1 June, when a guard of honour was formed by the British Red Cross Society. He was buried with his wife at Cottered Cemetery, where three of his four sons now lie buried with him.

His great heart and warm nature could flourish only in a community which shaped life towards happiness rather than riches . . . To spend and be spent for others was his guiding principle, for, greater than his great achievements were the purity of the motives and sincerity of the purpose that inspired them. It was for these that he was loved and it is for these that he will be remembered. He was a knight errant in the fields in which he fought for the alleviation of human suffering, believing with a simple faith in his fellow men of every race and serving them with a rare humility.[9]

On his tomb is carved in Chinese characters a verse from the New Testament taken from a presentation given by a friend of Sun Yat Sen's. The same verse is inscribed on the memorial to him in Cottered Church erected by his dear friend Dr Sao-Ke Alfred Sze. It reads:

Blessed are the merciful for they shall obtain mercy.

Notes and References

1 Early Days

1 Macduff, Thane of Fife, was created Earl in 1057. In 1389 the title reverted to the Crown, there being no heir, and was revived in 1759.
2 Adam Duff was given a grant of lands at Keithmore in or around 1650.
3 N. Cantlie and G. Seaver, *Sir James Cantlie* (London, 1939).
4 ibid. (Introduction).
5 J. Mackinnon, *The Constitutional History of Scotland* (London, 1924).
6 I. Brown, *Summer in Scotland* (London, 1952).
7 Cantlie and Seaver, *Sir James Cantlie*.
8 ibid.
9 ibid.

2 Charing Cross Hospital and the Start of First Aid

1 W. Hunter, *Account of Charing Cross Hospital and Medical School* (London, 1914).
2 'Lines spoken on the occasion of the Jubilee of the Medical School' (MS Cantlie Papers, 1884), and *Charing Cross Gazette*.
3 *3rd Statistical Account of Banffshire* (Glasgow, 1961).
4 J. Cantlie, chapter on 'The influence of exercise on health' in M. Morris (ed.), *The Book of Health* (London, 1883).
5 J. Cantlie, chapter on 'Accidental injuries – their relief and immediate treatment' in *The International Health Exhibition Handbook* (London, 1884).
6 ibid.
7 St John's Annual Report, 1887.

3 The Volunteer Medical Staff Corps

1 Account of raising VMSC in *Charing Cross Hospital Gazette* (July 1900–January 1901).
2 Cantlie and Seaver, *Sir James Cantlie*.
3 By 1893 the VMSC totalled 1,433 men and Glasgow and Norwich had also started Companies.

4 Hong Kong and the College of Medicine for the Chinese

1 Newspaper cuttings, 31 January and *c*. 1885. Cantlie Papers (see Bibliography). Also J. Cantlie, 'Degeneracy amongst Londoners' (1885).
2 ibid.
3 Newspaper cuttings, 28 October 1885. Cantlie Papers (see Bibliography). Also J. Cantlie, 'Life in London hygienically considered' (1885).
4 Newspaper cuttings, Cantlie Papers. Also Cantlie and Seaver, *Sir James Cantlie*.
5 J. Cantlie and S. Jones, *Sun Yat Sen and the Awakening of China* (London, 1912).
6 Lo Hsiang Lin, *Sun Yat Sen and his European and American Friends* (Taipei, 1951).

5 Hong Kong Surgeon

1 *China Mail*, 16 August 1888.
2 Trans. of C. A. Pekelharing and C. Winkler, *Beri Beri — Researches Concerning its Nature and Cause and Means of Arrest* (Edinburgh, 1893).

3   Report on the conditions under which leprosy occurs in China, Indo China, Malaya, the Archipelago and Oceania (London, 1897).

6 Medicine in China – the Bubonic Plague

1   *China Mail*, 23 July 1892.
2   *China Mail*, 25 July 1892.
3   Cantlie and Jones, *Sun Yat Sen and the Awakening of China*.
4   ibid.
5   L. Ride and Jen Yu Wen, *Sun Yat Sen: Two essays* (Hong Kong, 1970).
6   Sun Yat Sen, *Kidnapped in London* (London, 1969).
7   *China Mail*, 20 February 1923.
8   On 15 March 1849 a Scottish MP proposed a resolution to set up a Select Committee to inquire into the best means of establishing libraries freely open to the public. The first of these was opened in 1850.
9   J. Lowson, 'Medical report on bubonic plague to the Hong Kong Government.' (*Hong Kong Government Gazette*, 13 April 1895).
10   Lecture on 'The spread of plague' (*British Medical Journal*, January 1897).
11   W. J. Simpson, *Report on the Causes and Continuance of Plague in Hong Kong and Suggestions as to Remedial Measures* (London, Colonial Office, 1903).
12   Article on plague, *BMJ*, 25 August 1894.
13   Introduction to D. Masters, *The Conquest of Disease* (London, 1925).
14   Undated press cuttings, Cantlie Papers.

7 Turmoil and Tribute

1   Foreign Office 17/1234, No. 141, 16 April 1895.
2   FO 17/1239, No. 403, 23 October 1895.
3   ibid.
4   FO 17/1239, No. 414, 30 October 1895.
5   FO 17/1239, No. 421, 31 October 1895.
6   Hong Kong Sessional Papers, 1896.

8 Kidnapped in London

1   Cantlie and Jones, *Sun Yat Sen and the Awakening of China*.
2   Sun Yat Sen, *Kidnapped in London*.
3   FO 17/1718, No. 113, 12 November 1896.

9 Tropical Medicine

1   *BMJ*, 9 January 1897.
2   *Lancet*, 13 February 1897 and 'Medical report on bubonic plague to the Hong Kong Government' by James A. Lowson (*Hong Kong Government Gazette*, 13 April 1895).
3   Edinburgh was the first university to accept students from the College of Medicine for the Chinese for MB ChB after its incorporation in 1907.
4   Dr A. Davidson was the author of *Hygiene and Diseases of Warm Climates* (Edinburgh, Pentland, 1893).
5   W. Byam and R. G. Archibald (joint eds) *The Practice of Medicine in the Tropics* (London, H. Frowde and Hodder & Stoughton, 1921–3).
6   Cantlie and Seaver, *Sir James Cantlie*, Appendix.
7   Chamberlain to SHS, 2 February 1898, Minutes SHS.
8   *BMJ*, 5 March 1898.
9   *The Organisation of the Colonial Medical Service of the Empire* (priv. print.).
10   *Lancet*, 26 March 1898.

10 The End of an Era

1 Cantlie and Seaver, *Sir James Cantlie*.
2 Regent Street Polytechnic, 1901–2, Prospectus.
3 The Army Medical Services. Paper read by J. Cantlie before the Charing Cross Medical Society, 25 November 1897, entitled 'The relations of civil and army medical men in Britain'. Cantlie Papers.
4 H. A. L. Fisher, *History of Europe* (London, 1936).
5 Letter, *Polytechnic Magazine*, 9 May 1900.
6 B. Oliver, *The British Red Cross in Action* (London, 1966).
7 Two articles in the *BMJ*, 18 and 25 August 1894. Lecture to the Epidemiological Society, December 1896, published in the *BMJ*, 9 January 1897. Two articles in the *Practitioner*, November 1899, October 1900. Also printed privately, Cantlie Papers.
8 *Journal of Tropical Medicine*, January 1901.
9 ibid.
10 *Journal of Tropical Medicine*, February 1901.

11 Family and Friends: Hands across the Sea

1 *Journal of Tropical Medicine*, 15 July 1901.
2 K. C. Wong and L. T. Wu, *History of Chinese Medicine* (China, 1932).
3 *Journal of Tropical Medicine*, 16 July 1906.
4 ibid.
5 Appeal to China Association for funds dated 5 April 1909 and made by Cantlie on behalf of Hong Kong College of Medicine Committee formed by him in London in 1907. Cantlie Papers.
6 Cantlie and Seaver, *Sir James Cantlie*.
7 Letter from James to Mabel Cantlie 3 April 1910. (If separated they wrote or telegraphed to each other daily.)
8 William Marshall, *Scottish Airs, Melodies, Strathspeys and Reels* (Edinburgh, 1822).
9 *The Immortal Memory* (priv. print. by Elgin Northern Scottish Office, 1912). Also undated press reports, Cantlie Papers.

12 The Threat of War

1 'Lecture on the art of healing', *Polytechnic Magazine*, October 1906.
2 'Report on the founding of the Voluntary Aid Detachments', County of London, BRCS Annual Reports.
3 *Polytechnic Magazine*, April 1912.
4 St John's Magazine, *First Aid*, February 1914.
5 Letter from Sir Frederick Treves to Cantlie, 20 June 1912, in Cantlie and Seaver, *Sir James Cantlie*.
6 Letter from Mrs Locke King to Cantlie, 20 June 1912, Cantlie Papers.
7 *The Red Cross*, August 1914.
8 S. Unwin (ed.), *The Work of V.A.D. London 1 during the War* (London, 1920).
9 ibid.

13 Sun Yat Sen: First President of China

1 FO 371/1093, p. 237, 14 October 1911.
2 Fisher, *History of Europe*.
3 FO 371/1094, p. 207, 4 November 1911.
4 FO 371/1095, p. 166, 14 November 1911.
5 FO 371/1096, p. 558, 8 December 1911.
6 FO 371/1310, p. 120, 2 January 1912.
7 FO 371/1311, p. 374 *et seq.*, January 1912.
8 FO 371/1312, p. 520, March 1912.

9   FO 371/1315, p. 521, 25 March 1912.
10   FO 371/1623, p. 207, 21 April 1912.
11   FO 371/1624, p. 30, 19 May 1912.
12   Original telegram, Cantlie Papers.
13   B. Martin, *Strange Vigour: A Biography of Sun Yat Sen* (London, 1944).
14   FO 371/1624 (Glanville in Berlin to Grey), 15 July 1912.
15   FO 371/1624, p. 288, 17 June 1912.
16   H. Hodgkin, *China and the Family of Nations* (London, 1928).

14   War

1   Fisher, *History of Europe*.
2   H. S. Souttar, *A Surgeon in Belgium* (London, 1915).
3   *First Aid*, November 1914.
4   ibid.
5   *The Queen*, 6 February 1915.
6   *Journal of RAMC*, July 1914.
7   *The Times Red Cross Supplement*, 21 October 1915.
8   G. A. Moore, *Birth and Early Days of our Ambulance Trains in France* (London, 1922).
9   *Times Red Cross Supplement*, 21 October 1915.
10   *The Red Cross*, November 1915.
11   ibid.
12   S. Unwin, *The Work of V.A.D. London 1*.
13   *The Red Cross*, December 1914.
14   J. Terraine, *Mons: The Retreat to Victory* (London, 1960).
15   *Polytechnic Magazine*, April 1903.

15   Wounds and their Treatment: the King Albert I Hospital

1   Obituary to Surgeon General Sir Joseph Fayrer, *Journal of Tropical Medicine*, 1 June 1907.
2   *The Queen*, 6 February 1915.
3   It was referred to as both in *The Times Red Cross Supplement*, 21 October 1915.
4   *First Aid*, July 1915.

16   College of Ambulance or College of Nursing?

1   Report by Sir Richard Temple dated 20 September 1915, St John Ambulance Association Papers.
2   *Pall Mall Gazette*, 2 November 1915.
3   S. Unwin, *The Work of V.A.D. London 1*.
4   ibid.
5   *First Aid*, December 1915.
6   Son of Surgeon General Sir Joseph Fayrer.
7   S. Unwin, *The Work of V.A.D. London 1*.

17   The Tide of Suffering

1   Cantlie Papers.
2   ibid.
3   H. A. L. Fisher, *History of Europe*.
4   ibid.
5   *Journal of Tropical Medicine*, 1 September 1916.
6   *Nursing Times*, July 1916.
7   16 and 18 August 1916.
8   *The Times*, 4 October 1916.

9 ibid, 25 April 1917.
10 *The Red Cross*, May 1917.

18 The Armistice

1 *The Times*, 5 July 1917.
2 *Polytechnic Magazine*, January 1918.
3 T. Bowser, *The Story of a V.A.D.* (London, 1917).
4 *The Red Cross*, November 1918.
5 Cantlie and Seaver, *Sir James Cantlie*.

Epilogue

1 In the Second World War Keith led a Khasi Porter Corps behind the Japanese lines which took supplies to our troops during the siege of Kohima and carried back wounded. In recognition of his services he was knighted in 1944.
2 Admiral Superintendent, Rosyth Dockyard, 1939–44. In 1944 Colin followed another submariner as Director General, Indian Dockyards.
3 During the Second World War Neil served in North Africa and India and on his retirement was appointed Governor of Osborne.
4 *Montreal Star*, 19 April 1955. On the occasion of a special parade to honour his 70 years' unbroken service as a Volunteer, the press described him as 'a gallant old figure, bearing himself erect, every inch an officer and a gentleman'. The Black Watch of Canada was the only regiment to send three battalions to France in 1914–18.
5 Cantlie and Seaver, *Sir James Cantlie*.
6 *Sunday Pictorial*, 26 June 1921.
7 Cantlie and Seaver, *Sir James Cantlie*.
8 ibid.
9 ibid.

Bibliography

1 The Works of James Cantlie

1878   *Handbook. Aids for Cases of Injuries or Sudden Illness* (London, Order of St John). Until 1885 *The Handbook* was published under the name of Peter Shepherd, with an anonymous reference in the Introduction to Cantlie who had enlarged and edited it. From 1885 to 1901 it was 'Edited and rewritten' by Robert Bruce of the Royal College of Surgeons. From 1901 it was rewritten and appeared under the name of James Cantlie until 1928, after that under the name of 'the late James Cantlie' until 1937 when it was rewritten.

1883   With D. Colquhoun, *William Meade's Manual for Students Preparing for Medical Examination* (London, Renshaw).
      M. Morris (ed.), *The Book of Health* (London, Cassell), chapter on 'The influence of exercise on health'.

1884   *The Health Exhibition Literature* (London, Clowes), chapter on 'Accidental injuries, their relief and immediate treatment'.

1885   'Degeneracy amongst Londoners', lecture at the Parkes Museum, London (priv. print.).
      'Life in London hygienically considered', lecture at the YMCA, Exeter Hall, Strand (priv. print.).
      'The effects of certain anatomical relations', lecture to the Medical Society of Charing Cross Hospital (London, priv. print.).

1886   *A Text Book of Naked Eye Anatomy* (London, Bailliere Tindall).
      Trans. of C. J. Witkowski, *Bones and Muscles of the Hand* (London, Bailliere Tindall).
      C. Heath (ed.), *Dictionary of Practical Surgery by Various British Hospital Surgeons* (London, Smith Elder), articles on 'Ligature of the arteries', 'Nerves of the cranium', 'Management of the sick room'.

1888   R. Quain (ed.), *A Dictionary of Medicine, Including General Pathology, General Therapeutics, Hygiene and the Diseases Peculiar to Women and Children by Various Writers* (London, Longman), article on veins with S. Boyd.

1890   *Leprosy in Hong Kong* (Shanghai, Yokohama, Singapore, Kelly and Walsh).

1893   Trans. of C. A. Pekelharing and C. Winkler, *Beri Beri – Researches Concerning its Nature and Cause and Means of Arrest* (Edinburgh and London, Young Pentland).

1894   *British Medical Journal* (18 and 25 August) two articles on plague.

1897   *Report on the Conditions under which Leprosy Occurs in China, Indo China, Malaya, the Archipelago and Oceania, Compiled Chiefly during 1894* (London, Macmillan; reprint. 1898, Bedford Press).
      'The relations of the civil and army medical men in Britain', paper on the Army Medical Services read to Charing Cross Medical Society (priv. print.).
      'The spread of plague', lecture to the Epidemiological Society, 18 December 1896 (priv. reprint. from articles in *The Lancet*, January 1897).

1898   'The organisation of the colonial medical service of the Empire' speech
of 2 March at the Imperial Institute (priv. print.).
'The treatment of the tropical invalid in Great Britain' (priv. reprint.
from *Treatment*, August 1898).
'On a new arrangement of the right and left lobes of the liver' (priv.
print. from speech to the Anatomical Society in Ireland in 1897).

1899   'The plague' (priv. reprint. from article in the *Practitioner*, November).
S. Thomson (ed.), *Dictionary of Domestic Medicine* (London, Griffin),
article on 'Guide to the maintenance of health and management of
disease in warm climates'.
P. J. Anderson (ed.)., *Aurora Borealis Academica, Aberdeen University
Appreciations, 1860—1889* (Aberdeen University), chapter on William
Pirie.

1900   *The Plague: How to Recognise, Prevent and Treat Plague* (London, Cassell).
'History of Raising the VMSC' (*Charing Cross Gazette*).

1902   'Suprahepatic liver abscess' (reprint. from *International Clinic*, Phil.,
Lippincot).
'The health of the people' (priv. reprint. from the *Practitioner*, March).
Tropical Life as it Affects Life Assurance (London, Gray).

1903   'Liver abscess and its treatment' (priv. print.).
B. Scheube (ed.), *The Diseases of Warm Countries – a Handbook for Medical
Men* (London, Bale), addendum on yellow fever.
Article on sprue, pub. in the *Practitioner*.
MS speech on 'Need for systematic teaching of tropical medicine'.

1906   *Physical Efficiency* (London, Putnam). Preface by Sir Lauder Brunton;
foreword by Sir James Crichton Browne.
'Subhepatic liver abscess', in *Journal of Tropical Medicine* (January) (priv.
reprint.).

1907   'Tropical hepatic ailments', in *Journal of the Polyclinic* (London, the
Medical Graduates College).

1909   Ed. three numbers of the Medico Chirulurgical Series (London, Bale).

1911   'Plague and its spread' in *Journal of the Royal Society of Arts*.
British Red Cross Society Training Manual (London, Cassell).

1912   *British Red Cross Society Nursing Manual* (London, Cassell).
British Red Cross Society First Aid Manual (London, Cassell). (Cassells
printed eight editions of Cantlie's *First Aid Manual*. His basic text was
used until after the Second World War. During both wars it was trans-
lated into French and used by some Commonwealth countries. After the
Second World War it was rewritten and published by Macmillan.)
Speech on Robert Burns at the London Burns Club in September (Elgin
Northern Scottish Office).
With C. Sheridan Jones, *Sun Yat Sen and the Awakening of China* (London,
Jarrold).
*The Use of the Tuning Fork in Diagnosing the Outlines of Solid and Hollow
Viscera of the Chest and Abdomen and of Certain Pathological Conditions*
(London, Mayer and Meltzer).

1914   'Some aspects of surgery in the tropics' in *Transactions of the Society of
Tropical Medicine and Hygiene* (priv. reprint.).

1925   D. Masters, *The Conquest of Disease* (London, John Lane), preface.
D. Masters, *New Facts about Cancer* (London, John Lane), preface.
First Aid, illustr. 50 colour diagrams (London, Bale).

2 General Bibliography

B. Abel Smith, *The History of the Nursing Profession* (London, Heinemann, 1960).

A. C. Benson and Viscount Esher (eds), *The Letters of Queen Victoria* (London, Murray, 1907).

G. Cecil, *Life of Robert, Marquis of Salisbury* (4 vols, London, Hodder & Stoughton, 1921–32).

N. Cantlie, *A History of the Army Medical Department* (Edinburgh, Churchill and Livingstone, 1974).

N. Cantlie and G. Seaver, *Sir James Cantlie* (London, Murray, 1939).

N. Corbet Fletcher, *The Annals of the Ambulance Department* (St John Ambulance Association, London, 1949).

H. A. L. Fisher, *History of Europe* (London, Arnold, 1936).

J. Grigg, *The Young Lloyd George* (London, Eyre and Methuen, 1973).

J. Grigg, *Lloyd George: The People's Champion* (London, Eyre and Methuen, 1979).

S. Koss, *Asquith* (London, Allen Lane, 1976).

B. Martin, *Strange Vigour: A Biography of Sun Yat Sen* (London, Heinemann, 1944).

B. Oliver, *The British Red Cross in Action* (London, Faber, 1966).

J. Piggott, *Queen Alexandra's Royal Army Nursing Corps* (London, Lee Cooper, 1975).

R. Taylor, *The Life of Lord Salisbury* (London, Allen Lane, 1975).

Chapter 1

E. Barron, Introduction to 2nd ed. of *Scottish War of Independence* (Inverness, Carruthers, 1934).

I. Brown, *Summer in Scotland* (London, Collins, 1952).

H. M. Knox, *250 Years of Scottish Education* (Edinburgh, Oliver & Boyd, 1953).

I. Simpson, *Education in Aberdeenshire* (University of London Press, 1947).

3rd Statistical Account of Banffshire (Glasgow, Collins, 1961).

3rd Statistical Account of the County of Aberdeen (Glasgow, Collins, 1960).

3rd Statistical Account of Aberdeen (Edinburgh, Oliver & Boyd, 1953).

J. Strong, *A History of Secondary Education in Scotland* (Oxford, Clarendon Press, 1909).

A. Wright, *History of Education and the Old Parish Schools of Scotland* (Edinburgh, Menzies, 1898).

The Parker Committee of Inquiry Report, 1888 [C5336][C5425] P.P.XLI, 603, 641.

Commemorative Brochure on Fochabers', Fochabers Bi-Centenary Committee (Alloa, 1976)

…ʋion (Edinburgh, Lindsay, 1946).

…f Muscles in Latin (Myographia nova sive musculorum …yne, 1684).

…ring Cross Hospital and Medical School (London,

…don, Chapman & Hall, 1934).

Charing Cross (London, Cassell, 1967).

…bles with Explanations in English (London, 1754)

…n, Reports of Chapter for 1876 and 1877.

St John Ambulance Association Committee, Annual Reports for 1878–87. Also Supplementary Report of Central Committee, February 1879.
Police Files, V and K Division Reports, 1876–84.
Charing Cross Hospital Gazette, 1882–7.
Miscellaneous press cuttings in the Order of St John collection, 1878–87, including *Daily Chronicle*, *Morning Post* and *Standard*.

Chapters 3 and 4

J. Cantlie, 'History of raising the V.M.S.C.' in *Charing Cross Gazette*, July 1900– January 1901.
Sir G. Hunter and J. Cantlie, 'Appeal for volunteers for the Medical Staff Corps' (Cantlie Papers).
Communiqué to Sir G. Hunter from the Army Medical Department requesting name most suited for post of officer in command, 3 March 1885 (Cantlie Papers).
Press cuttings on raising the VMSC, 1883–5, from the *British Medical Journal*, *Era, College and Hospital Intelligence, Globe, Standard, Lloyds Weekly, People, Lancet, Belfast Evening News, Scotsman, Times, Court Society Review, Manchester Express, Aberdeen Journal, St Stephen's Review, Morning Advertiser, Observer, Canadian Militia Gazette* and others (Cantlie Papers).
Press cuttings on lecture on 'Degeneracy amongst Londoners', *c*. 31 January 1885, from the *Standard, Observer, Scotsman, Aberdeen Free Press, Illustrated News, Kent Examiner, Daily Chronicle, Globe, Lloyds Weekly, Weekly Despatch, Crieff Journal, Belfast News Letter, Modern Society, Tit Bits, Tyneside Echo* (Cantlie Papers).
Press cuttings on speech on 'Life in London hygienically considered' given at the YMCA, Exeter Hall, Strand, from the *Daily Telegraph*, *Globe, Health* on 28 October 1885; from *Referee* on 1 November and from *Modern Society*, *North East Daily Gazette* and others, n.d.

Chapters 4–7 (Hong Kong)

J. M. Braga, *Hong Kong and Macau* (Macau, 1960).
J. Cantlie and S. Jones, *Sun Yat Sen and the Awakening of China* (London, Jarrold, 1912).
C. H. Choa, 'History of Medicine in Hong Kong' in *The Medical Directory of Hong Kong* (Hong Kong Federation of Medical Societies, 1970).
E. J. Eitel, *Europe in China* (Taipei, Cheng Wen Publishing, 1968).
G. B. Endacott, *A History of Hong Kong* (Oxford, OUP, 1973).
G. B. Endacott and A. Hinton, *Fragrant Harbour: A Short History of Hong Kong* (Oxford, OUP, 1962).
B. Harrison, *The First 50 Years: University of Hong Kong* (Hong Kong University Press, 1962).
V. H. Jarrett, *Old Hong Kong* (South China Morning Post, 1933–35).
P. M. A. Linebarger, *The Political Doctrines of Sun Yat Sen* (Baltimore, Johns Hopkins Press, 1963).
Li Shu Fan, *Hong Kong Surgeon* (Hong Kong, Li Shu Fan Medical Foundation, 1964).
Lo Hsiang Lin, *Hong Kong and Western Cultures* (Honolulu, East West Center Press, 1964).
Lo Hsiang Lin, *Sun Yat Sen and his European and American Friends* (Taipei, Chung Yang Wen Ku, Kung Ying She, 1951).

L. Ride and Jen Yu Wen, *Sun Yat Sen: Two Essays* (Centre of Asian Studies, Hong Kong University, Hong Kong Collection, 1970).

H. Z. Schiffrin, *Sun Yat Sen* (University of California Press, 1968).

Lyon Sharman, *Sun Yat Sen* (New York, Stanford University Press, 1934).

J. Wu, *Sun Yat Sen* (Taipei, Commercial Press, 1971).

P. Manson Bahr and A. Alcock, *Life of Sir Patrick Manson* (London, Cassell, 1927).

B. Shepherd, *An Index of Streets, Houses and Leased Lots of Victoria, Victoria Peak and Kowloon in the colony of Hong Kong* (Hong Kong, Kelly and Walsh, 1894).

H. G. W. Woodhead, *The Truth about the Chinese Republic* (London, Hutchinson, 1920).

China Mail 1887–96, Public Records Office, Hong Kong.

Official Papers – Public Record Office, Kew, London
FO 17/1234, 1239, 1240, 1286.

Official Papers – Hong Kong
Colonial Surgeon's Reports, with particular reference to 1887–96. Hong Kong Sessional Papers.

Report on the Blue Book 1887–1896. British Parliamentary Papers.

Historical and Statistical Abstract of the Colony of Hong Kong, 1841–1870.

O. Chadwick, *Report on the Sanitary Conditions of Hong Kong, 1882*. British Parliamentary Papers.

Hong Kong Government Gazette, 1887–96.

Report for the Governor into Arrangements of Medical Department. Apps B and C on the duties of the Medical Officer of Health, 1895. Hong Kong Sessional Papers.

References to the 'Inquiry into the College of Medicine for the Chinese' (Hong Kong Hansard, July 1896).

Report of the Committee appointed by H.E. the Governor to inquire into and report on the best organisation for a College of Medicine for the Chinese, 1896. Hong Kong Sessional Papers.

Correspondence between H.E. the Governor and Mr Belilios concerning the latter's proposed grant to College (31 July and 4 August 1896, Hong Kong Sessional Papers).

References to police scandal, 13 September 1897, Hong Kong Hansard. Also *Report on Government Corruption, 1897*. Parliamentary Papers.

Plague: Colonial Reports – annual, 1894, 1895, 1896.

Coolies' strike: Colonial Reports, 1895.

Land Register, Land Registry, 1888–1910.

Minutes
Minute Book of Senate. Minute Book of Court for College of Medicine for the Chinese, 1887–96.

Minute Book of Hong Kong Medical Society, 1887–96.

Chapter 8

Sun Yat Sen, *Kidnapped in London* (London, China Society, 1969).

Official Papers – Public Record Office, Kew, London
FO 17/1718, 1286.

Reports on kidnapping in *China Mail* and all leading British newspapers, October 1896.

Chapter 9

R. Heussler, *Yesterday's Rulers: The Making of the British Colonial Service* (New York, Syracuse University Press/London, OUP, 1963).

P. Manson Bahr, *History of the School of Tropical Medicine in London 1899–1949* (London, Lewis, 1956).

J. J. Skertcheley, *The Ethnography of Leprosy in the Far East* (priv. print. from lecture to Royal Society of Queensland, 6 March 1897).

J. E. Stone, *Hospital Organisation and Management* (London, Faber, 1932).

Report on the London School of Tropical Medicine 1899–1903. Cragg's Prize (priv. print. from a speech at the Mansion House, 1912).

A. G. McBride, *The History of the Dreadnought Seamen Hospital at Greenwich* (priv. print. by SHS). SHS Collection.

Minutes of the Seamen's Hospital Society 1897–1903. SHS Collection.

SHS Annual Report 1977. SHS Collection.

Record of Meetings of Lecturers. SHS Collection.

Record of Members of Schools Committee. SHS Collection.

Press reports from the *Lancet*, *British Medical Journal* and *The Times*, December 1896 – September 1899.

Leaflet of Appeal for the Seamen's Hospital Society stating aims of London School of Tropical Medicine. n.d. Cantlie Papers.

Chapter 10

F. J. Wood, *The History of the Maidstone Companies, RAMC (V)* (Maidstone, Kent Messenger, 1907).

'Short history of the Regent St. Polytechnic' in the Annual Prospectus.

Salvation Army Story (London, Salvationist Publishing, 1974).

'Short history of the Working Men's College in Camden, in association with the Frances Martin College for Women', in the Prospectus for 1978–9.

Polytechnic Magazine, 1899–1901.

Journal of Tropical Medicine, August 1896–1901.

First Aid, 1896–1901.

British Medical Journal and *Lancet*, 1896–1901.

Press cuttings from British and Canadian newspapers, Cantlie Papers.

Chapter 11

W. Marshall, *Scottish Airs, Melodies, Strathspeys and Reels for the Pianoforte, Harp, Violin and Cello* in two Vols with Introduction in the 2nd Vol. by J. Mc.G. (Edinburgh, Robertson, 1822). 2nd Vol. pub. posthumously.

J. Scott Skinner, *The Harp and Claymore*, with Introduction by Gavin Greig (Glasgow, Bayley and Ferguson and reprint. Louth, Celtic Music, 1982).

K. C. Wong and L. T. Wu, *History of Chinese Medicine* (Tientsin Press, China, 1932).

M. Bingham, *Henry Irving and the Victorian Theatre* (London, Allen & Unwin, 1978).

Minutes of the Royal Society of Tropical Medicine, 1907–26.

Official Papers, Public Record Office, Kew, London
CO 129/295, CO 129/297, CO 129/298, CO 129/299, CO 129/300, CO 273/257, FO 17/1718.
First Aid, 1901–05.
British Medical Journal and *Lancet*, 1901-07.
Journal of Tropical Medicine, 1901-07.
Transactions of the Society of Tropical Medicine, 1907–26.
Hong Kong College of Medicine Appeal, 1909. Cantlie Papers.
Leaflet giving names of members of Pellagra Commission and stating aims. Cantlie Papers.

Chapter 12

F. Treves, *The Tale of a Field Hospital* (London, Cassell, 1900).
S. Unwin (ed.), *The Work of V.A.D. London 1 during the War* (London, Allen & Unwin, 1920).
'A short history of St. John Ambulance Association'. Centenary leaflet, 1977.
First Aid, 1905–14.
Polytechnic Magazine, 1901–14.
Scheme for the Organisation of Voluntary Aid in England and Wales (HMSO, 1909).
The Red Cross, 1914.
Minutes of BRCS Executive Committee, relevant dates.
Annual Reports for County of London Branch, BRCS, relevant dates.

Chapter 13

Wong and Wu, *History of Chinese Medicine*.

Offical Records, Public Record Office, Kew, London
FO 371/1093, 1094, 1095, 1096, 1097, 1098.
FO 371/1310, 1311, 1312, 1313, 1314, 1315, 1316.
FO 371/1591, 1609, 1623, 1624, 1626.

Chapters 14–18

J. H. Abrahams, *My Work with the London Ambulance Column 1915–1918*. (MS, British Red Cross Society, Barnet Hill, 1915–18).
G. Bowman, *The Lamp and the Book* (London, Queen Anne Press, 1967).
T. Bowser, *The Story of a British V.A.D. in the Great War* (London, Melrose, 1917).
H. Davidson, *The American Red Cross in the Great War* (New York, Macmillan, 1919).
L'Abbé F. Klein, *La Guerre vue d'une Ambulance, Armonier de l'Ambulance Americaine* (Paris, A. Colin, 1915).
L. Melis, *Contribution à l'Histoire du Service de Sauté de l'Armée au Cours de la Guerre 1914–18*. (Bruxelles, Imp. typo de l'Institut Certographique Militaire, 1932).
G. A. Moore (Col. G. A. Moore, Deputy Chairman, Committee St John Ambulance Brigade), *Birth and Early Days of our Ambulance Trains in France* (London, Bale, 1922).
H. S. Souttar, *A Surgeon in Belgium* (London, Arnold, 1915).

J. Terraine, *Mons: The Retreat to Victory* (London, Batsford, 1960).

J. Terraine, *To Win a War: 1918 the Year of Victory* (London, Sidgwick and Jackson, 1978).

S. Unwin (ed.), *The Work of V.A.D. 1.*

'A Report of the Belgian Red Cross', 31 December 1915.

Presence de la Croix Rouge Français (Paris, Édition Larrieu-Bournel, 1974).

'La Croix Rouge Français: Notes et Études, documentaires', 14 March 1973.

American Ambulance Field Service. Diary of Section VII, 1917.

G. Hendrix, *Les Principes Fondamentaux de la Prothèse Orthopédique du Membre Inférieur d'après l'Étude des Membres Artificiels – Types, Confectionnés dans les Ateliers de Prothèse du Service de Santé de l'Armée Belge, à Rouen* (Paris, Maloine, 1917).

'Reports by the Joint War Committee and the Joint War Finance Committee of the BRCS and the Order of St John of Jerusalem in England on Voluntary Aid rendered to the Sick and Wounded at home and abroad and to the Prisoners of War, 1914–18.'

Minutes of the BRCS War Executive Committee, 1914–18.

Report of Order of St John on formation of VAD Joint Committee and War Office directive on General Service Scheme by Sir Richard Temple, Commisioner, St John Ambulance Association, Deputy Controller in Chief, Territorial Branch, 20 September 1915 (St John Papers).

Minutes of the BRCS Joint Women's VAD Committee, 1915. Imperial War Museum.

Minutes and papers concerning various women's corps – Green Cross, Khaki Cross etc., 1914–18. Imperial War Museum.

The Times Red Cross Supplement, 21 October 1915.

Polytechnic Magazine, 1914–18.

The Times, August 1914–December 1918.

Nursing Times, August 1914–December 1918.

British Journal of Nursing, January 1916–December 1916.

The Red Cross, August 1914–December 1923.

First Aid, 1914–18.

Journal of RAMC, July 1914–December 1918.

Lancet, 1914–18.

British Medical Journal, 1914–18.

Journal of Tropical Medicine, 1914–18.

The Queen, 1914–18. Undated cuttings. Cantlie Papers.

The Ladies Field, November and December 1918.

Book of press cuttings on the work of the British Ambulance Committee working for the Croix Rouge. BRCS Papers, Barnet Hill, 1914–18.

Correspondence and cuttings from newspapers of St John Ambulance Association. St John Papers, 1914–18.

Index

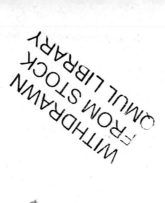